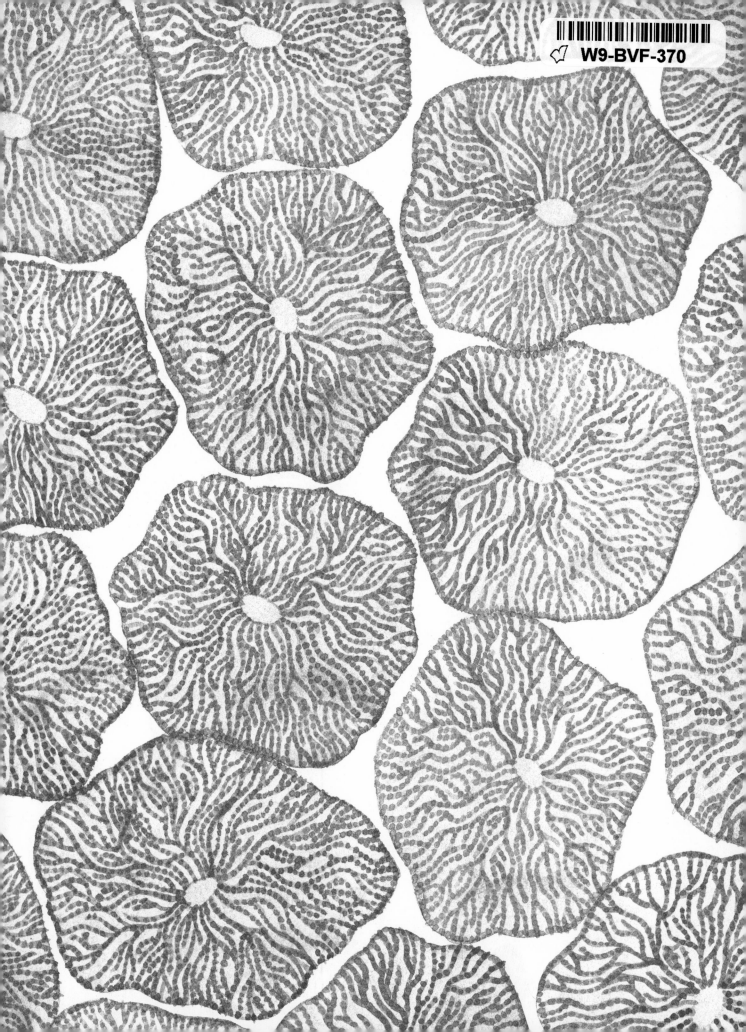

NURSE'S CLINICAL LIBRARY™

# GASTROINTESTINAL DISORDERS

*NURSING85* BOOKS™
SPRINGHOUSE CORPORATION
Springhouse, Pennsylvania

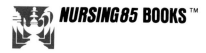

**NURSING85 BOOKS**™

**Nurse's Clinical Library**™
*Other volumes in this series:*
Cardiovascular Disorders
Respiratory Disorders
Endocrine Disorders
Neurologic Disorders
Renal and Urologic Disorders
Neoplastic Disorders
Immune Disorders

**Nurse's Reference Library**®
Diseases
Diagnostics
Drugs
Assessment
Procedures
Definitions
Practices
Emergencies

**New Nursing Skillbook**™ **series**
Giving Emergency Care
  Competently
Monitoring Fluid and
  Electrolytes Precisely
Assessing Vital Functions
  Accurately
Coping with Neurologic
  Problems Proficiently
Reading EKGs Correctly
Combatting Cardiovascular
  Diseases Skillfully
Nursing Critically Ill Patients
  Confidently
Dealing with Death and Dying

**Nursing Photobook**™ **series**
Providing Respiratory Care
Managing I.V. Therapy
Dealing with Emergencies
Giving Medications
Assessing Your Patients
Using Monitors
Providing Early Mobility
Giving Cardiac Care
Performing GI Procedures
Implementing Urologic
  Procedures
Controlling Infection
Ensuring Intensive Care
Coping with Neurologic
  Disorders
Caring for Surgical Patients
Working with Orthopedic
  Patients
Nursing Pediatric Patients
Helping Geriatric Patients
Attending Ob/Gyn Patients
Aiding Ambulatory Patients
Carrying Out Special
  Procedures

**Nursing Now**™ **series**
Shock
Hypertension
Drug Interactions
Cardiac Crises
Respiratory Emergencies
Pain

**Nursing85 Drug Handbook**™

**Nurse's Clinical Library**™

**Editorial Director**
Helen Klusek Hamilton

**Clinical Director**
Minnie Bowen Rose, RN, BSN, MEd

**Art Director**
Sonja E. Douglas

**Clinical staff**
**Clinical Editor**
Joanne Patzek DaCunha, RN

**Drug Information Manager**
Larry Neil Gever, RPh, PharmD

**Contributing Clinical Editors**
Nan Cameron, RN, BSN; Susan M.
Glover, RN, MSN; Sandra L. Nettina,
RN, MSN; Janet Peterka, RN, BSN,
MBA; Nina P. Welsh, RN

**Acquisitions**
Susan Hatch Brunt, Bernadette M.
Glenn

**Editorial staff**
**Editors**
Lisa Z. Cohen, Nancy Holmes,
Patricia Minard Shinehouse, Loralee
Choman Moclock

**Contributing Editors**
Laura Albert, Barbara Hodgson,
Frederick Nohl, Joan Twisdom-Harty

**Copy Supervisor**
David R. Moreau

**Copy Editors**
Dale A. Brueggemann, Diane M.
Labus, Jo Lennon, Doris Weinstock

**Contributing Copy Editors**
Laura Dabundo, Tim Gaul, Linda
Johnson, Rebecca Van Dine

**Production Coordinator**
Sally Johnson

**Editorial Assistants**
Mary Ann Bowes, Maree DeRosa

**Design staff**
**Designers**
Matie Anne Patterson, Mary Wise

**Illustrators**
Michael Adams, Marian Banks,
Dimitrios Bastas, Maryanne
Buschini, David Christiana, John
Cymerman, Design Management,
Marie Garafano, Jean Gardner,
Robert Jackson, Robert Phillips,
George Retseck, Eileen Rudnick,
Dennis Schofield, Lynn Waldo

**Production staff**
**Art Production**
Robert Perry (manager), Diane Fox,
Donald Knauss, Sandy Sanders,
Craig T. Siman, Robert Wieder

**Typography**
David C. Kosten (manager), Ethel
Halle, Diane Paluba, Nancy Wirs

**Manufacturing**
Deborah C. Meiris, Wilbur D.
Davidson (managers), T.A. Landis

Special thanks to Matthew Cahill,
Vonda Heller, Thomas J. Leibrandt,
and Elaine Shelly, who assisted in
preparation of this volume.

The clinical procedures described and
recommended in this publication are based
on research and consultation with medical
and nursing authorities. To the best of our
knowledge, these procedures reflect cur-
rently accepted clinical practice; nevertheless, they can't be considered absolute
and universal recommendations. For individual application, treatment recommendations must be considered in light of the
patient's clinical condition and, before administration of new or infrequently used
drugs, in light of latest package-insert information. The authors and the publisher
disclaim responsibility for any adverse effects resulting directly or indirectly from the
suggested procedures, from any undetected errors, or from the reader's misunder-
standing of the text.

**Library of Congress Cataloging in
Publication Data**
Main entry under title:
Gastrointestinal disorders.
  (Nurse's clinical library)
  "Nursing84 books."
  Includes bibliographies and index.
1. Gastrointestinal system—Diseases.
2. Gastrointestinal system—Diseases—
Nursing.    I. Series. [DNLM:
1. Gastroenterology—nurses'
instruction. WI 100 G2589]
RC802.G375 1984   616.3'3   84-20242
ISBN 0-916730-75-1

*Cover:* Color-enhanced large bowel X-ray.
Photograph by Howard Sochurek.

*Inside front and back covers:* Liver
lobules.

# CONTENTS

# CONTRIBUTORS AND CLINICAL CONSULTANTS

## Contributors

*At the time of publication, the contributors held the following positions:*

**Debra C. Broadwell, RN, PhD, ET**
Associate Professor of Nursing, Nell Hodgson Woodruff School of Nursing, Emory University, Atlanta

**Sally A. Brozenec, RN, MS**
Assistant Professor/Practitioner-Teacher, Rush University College of Nursing, Rush–Presbyterian–St. Luke's Medical Center, Chicago

**DeAnn M. Englert, RN, MSN**
Clinical Nurse Specialist, St. Luke's Episcopal Hospital, Houston

**Barbara S. Henzel, RN, BSN**
Staff Nurse, Gastrointestinal Department, Hospital of the University of Pennsylvania, Philadelphia

**Cynthia Ann LaSala, RN, BSN**
Staff Nurse, Emergency Department, Boston University Medical Center

**Angie Zaharopoulos Patras, RN, MS**
Assistant Professor/Practitioner-Teacher, Operating Room and Surgical Nursing Department, Rush–Presbyterian–St. Luke's Medical Center, Chicago

**Frances W. Quinless, RN, PhD**
Assistant Professor, Rutgers University College of Nursing, Newark, N.J.

**Hazel V. Rice, RN, MS, EdS**
Associate Chairman and Director, Division of Nursing, Southern College of Seventh Day Adventists, Orlando (Fla.) Center

**Starr Shelhorse Sordelett, RN, MSN, CCRN**
Assistant Professor of Nursing, John Tyler Community College, Chester, Va.

**Carol E. Smith, RN, PhD**
Associate Professor, Graduate School of Nursing, University of Kansas College of Health Sciences, Kansas City

**Nancy S. Storz, EdD, RD**
Adjunct Assistant Professor, University of Pennsylvania School of Nursing, Philadelphia

**Marian Walsh, RN, MS**
Practitioner-Teacher, Rush–Presbyterian–St. Luke's Medical Center, Chicago

## Clinical Consultants

*At the time of publication, the clinical consultants held the following positions:*

**Lolita M. Adrien, RN, MS, ET**
Enterostomal Clinical Nurse Specialist, Stanford (Calif.) University Medical Center

**Edmund Martin Barbour, MD**
Assistant Clinical Professor of Medicine, Wayne State University, Detroit; Chief of Gastroenterology, Oakwood Hospital, Dearborn, Mich.

**Roxanne Aubol Batterden, RN, CCRN**
Primary Nurse I, Surgical Intensive Care Unit; Lecturer, Intensive Care, University of Maryland, Baltimore

**Marjorie Davis Beck, RN**
Charge Nurse, GI Procedure Unit, Abington (Pa.) Memorial Hospital

**George J. Brodmerkel, Jr., MD**
Head of Division of Gastroenterology, Allegheny General Hospital, Pittsburgh

**Florence D. Bull, RN, BSEd**
Nurse Clinician, Nutritional Support, East Tennessee Baptist Hospital, Knoxville

**Leonard V. Crowley, MD**
Clinical Assistant Professor, Department of Laboratory Medicine and Pathology and Department of Family Practice, University of Minnesota, Minneapolis; Pathologist, St. Mary's Hospital, Minneapolis

**Tobie Virginia Hittle, RN, BSN, CCRN**
Head Nurse, Intensive Care Unit, The Genesee Hospital, Rochester, N.Y.

**Nancy H. Jacobson, RN, MSN**
Medical-Surgical Nursing Consultant, Philadelphia

**Raymond E. Joseph, MD**
Assistant Professor of Medicine, Jefferson Medical College, Thomas Jefferson University, Philadelphia

**Marsha Evans Orr, RN, MS**
Patient Education Coordinator, St. Joseph's Hospital Health Center, Syracuse, N.Y.

**Harriet E. Pilert, RN, MS, ET**
Enterostomal Therapist, Church Hospital, Baltimore

**Harrison Johnston Shull, Jr., MD**
Assistant Clinical Professor of Medicine, Vanderbilt University Hospital, Nashville

**Karen Wielgosz St. Marie, RN, MSN, CANP**
Adult Nurse Practitioner, Health Care Plan Medical Center, West Seneca, N.Y.

**Mark S. St. Marie, MD**
Consulting Gastroenterologist, Mercy Hospital, Buffalo

**Lawrence L. Tretbar, MD, FACS**
Professor, Clinical Surgery, University of Missouri School of Medicine, Kansas City

**Susan A. VanDeVelde-Coke, RN, MA, MBA**
Project Director, Health Sciences Center, Winnipeg, Manitoba

**Charles Wagner, MD**
Gastroenterologist, Abington (Pa.) Memorial Hospital and Holy Redeemer Hospital, Huntingdon Valley, Pa.; Assistant Clinical Professor of Medicine, University of Pennsylvania School of Medicine, Philadelphia

# FOREWORD

Gastrointestinal (GI) disorders are the leading cause of hospitalization in the United States. Chronic GI disorders affect 20 million Americans. And GI disorders constitute the third largest source of the total economic burden of illness in the United States, surpassed only by cardiovascular diseases and the combined category of accidents, poisonings, and violence.

Despite these statistics, the National Digestive Diseases Educational Program found in a survey that many people do not consider GI disorders a serious health problem. What's more, many people fail to appreciate how diverse and complex they are. GI disorders may involve the digestive tract or its accessory organs—the liver, gallbladder, and pancreas. They range from mild constipation to life-threatening fulminant hepatitis. Some disorders—like Crohn's disease and ulcerative colitis—continue to mystify us; their causes remain obscure and their cures, equally elusive.

As nurses, our role in managing GI disorders varies greatly, reflecting the wide spectrum of associated physical and psychological effects. We need to be aware that assessing and correctly interpreting GI signs and symptoms is often far from simple. Because the GI system offers no convenient normal values—such as pulse rate or respirations—you'll have to combine sharp skills of auscultation, percussion, palpation, and inspection with reliable history taking. And you'll have to recognize that GI signs and symptoms are notoriously nonspecific; what looks like transient indigestion may in fact herald impending cardiac crisis.

GASTROINTESTINAL DISORDERS provides everything you need to know to perform this challenging role confidently. This comprehensive volume opens with a well-illustrated review of GI structure and function. The introductory chapter traces the processes of digestion, absorption, and elimination orchestrated by numerous hormones, enzymes, and other secretions. It also explains the pathologic mechanisms of GI dysfunction. The second chapter describes the systematic, three-part assessment of the GI tract, including the oral, abdominal, and rectal examinations, and outlines the steps to formulate nursing diagnoses—the building blocks of our nursing care plans. The third chapter outlines the diagnostic tests that confirm GI disorders and describes our role before, during, and after such tests. Whether that role is to perform a bowel preparation before a lower GI series or to watch for bleeding after liver biopsy, our kind explanations and expert care can do much to ease the patient's anxiety and discomfort.

The remaining chapters in this volume cover specific GI disorders, including current information on pathophysiology, medical management, and nursing management. Within each chapter, *Pathophysiology* reviews etiology, characteristic signs and symptoms, and effects on other body systems; *Medical management* focuses on current diagnosis and treatment; and *Nursing management* addresses the disorder through the steps of the nursing process—assessment, nursing diagnosis, intervention, and evaluation.

Throughout this volume, numerous color illustrations, photographs, charts, graphs, and patient-teaching aids amplify the text and provide readily accessible, useful information. Two appendices provide supplementary information on mouth disorders and GI drugs.

Today, advances in prevention, diagnosis, and treatment of GI disorders allow many patients to live longer, more productive lives. As a result, your role in patient teaching and nursing care is more important than ever. This volume will help you—and your colleagues at all professional levels—meet this challenge effectively.

DEBRA C. BROADWELL, RN, PhD, ET
Associate Professor of Nursing
Nell Hodgson Woodruff School of Nursing
Emory University
Atlanta

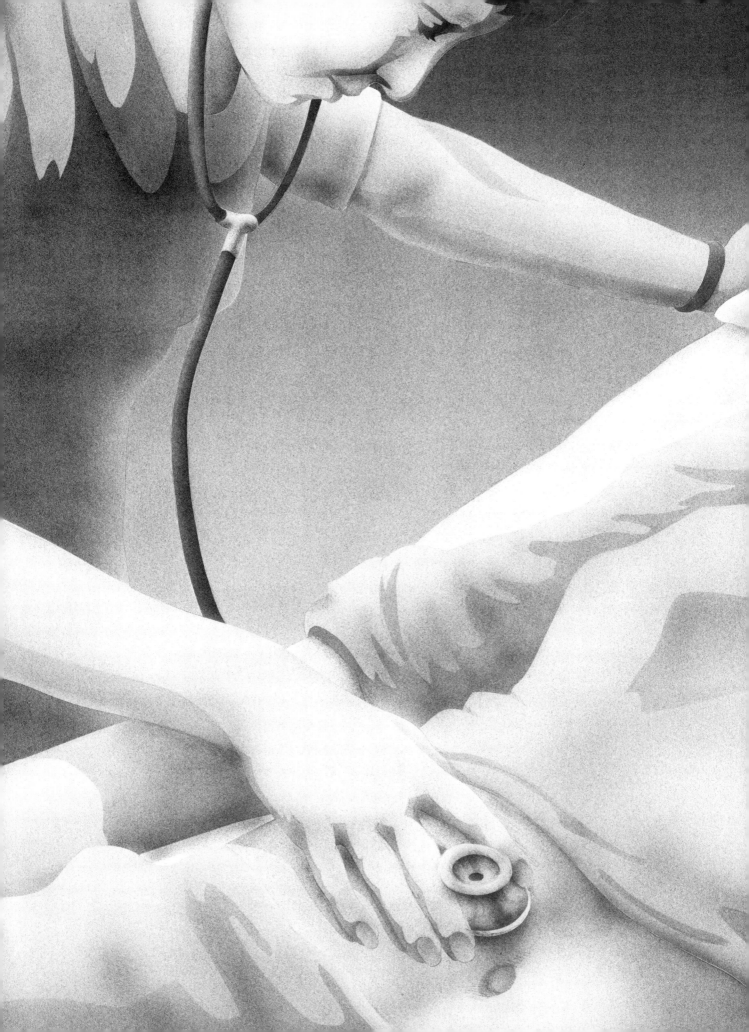

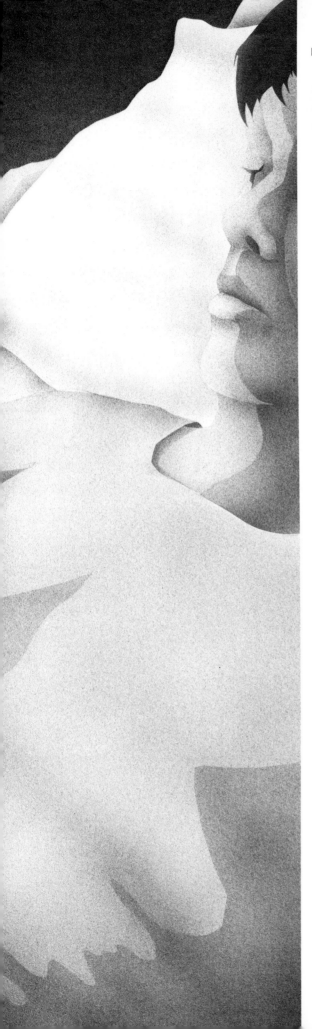

# FUNDAMENTAL FACTS

# 1 REVIEWING G.I. MECHANISMS

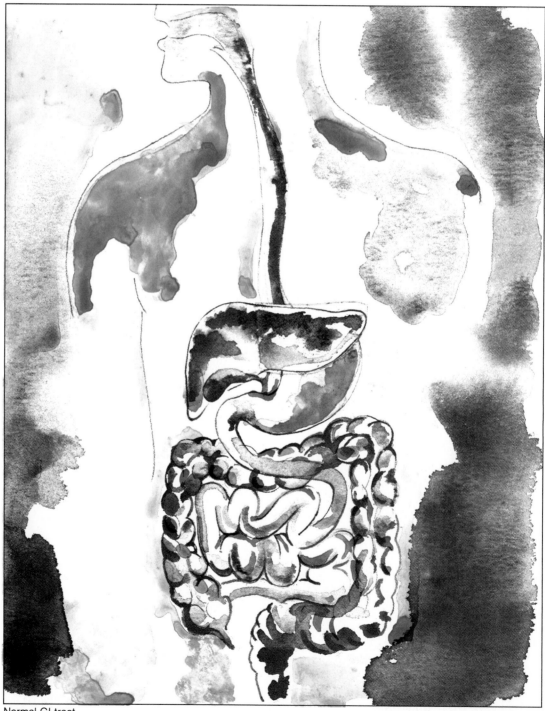

Normal GI tract

The gastrointestinal system profoundly affects every body system. Its pivotal role in digestion supplies essential nutrients to fuel the brain, heart, and lungs, sustaining life. What's more, GI function shapes the quality of life by its impact on overall health.

Because GI disorders affect just about everyone at one time or another, you're sure to deal with them frequently—no matter where you practice nursing. Such disorders range from simple changes in bowel habits, such as constipation, to severe and potentially fatal disorders, such as fulminant hepatitis. You'll be expected to play a prominent role in preventing and controlling these disorders, and in promoting good health through good nutrition. In this chapter, we'll review GI structure, function, and pathology—the knowledge base you'll need to provide effective patient care.

## NORMAL G.I. FUNCTION

The gastrointestinal tract is primarily responsible for digestion and absorption of food and elimination of metabolic wastes. It breaks down food—fats, proteins, and carbohydrates—into molecules that are small enough to permeate cell membranes, thereby providing cells with the necessary fuel to function. The GI tract prepares food for cellular absorption by altering its physical and chemical composition.

The GI tract is also responsible for helping defend the body against pathogens. Its intact mucous membranes, for example, bar the spread of ingested bacteria and indigenous bowel flora. Lymph nodes in the palatine tonsils contain T and B lymphocytes that protect against pathogens. Lymphatic tissue in the small intestine, called Peyer's patches, performs the same function. Intestinal and gastric secretions contain immunoglobulins, primarily immunoglobulin A (IgA), that stimulate the immune response. And gastric acid in the stomach destroys many pathogens because of its low pH.

### The role of saliva

Digestion begins in the mouth through chewing and the chemical action of saliva. First, saliva lubricates foods to stimulate the taste buds and to promote swallowing. Its proteolytic enzymes and antibodies destroy bacteria and wash them away from the teeth. Its nearly neutral pH protects tooth enamel from dissolving in an overly acidic environment.

Saliva promotes the hydrolysis of starch through the actions of the enzyme amylase (also called ptyalin). In the mouth, amylase breaks down 5% to 10% of starches into the simpler sugars dextrin and maltose. In the stomach, amylase continues to break down starches until it's inactivated by hydrochloric acid.

Saliva secretion is controlled by sympathetic and parasympathetic innervation. Sympathetic stimulation inhibits secretion of saliva, whereas parasympathetic stimulation promotes it. During the psychic phase of saliva secretion, efferent nerves leading to the salivary glands are activated by the sight, smell, or thought of appetizing food, and the mouth prepares to receive food. However, if food looks or smells foul, parasympathetic stimulation slows or ceases. During the gustatory phase, parasympathetic stimulation increases secretion of saliva to lubricate food and to promote swallowing. During the gastrointestinal phase, parasympathetic stimulation can evoke continued secretion, especially if irritating or foul-tasting food has been swallowed.

### Two stages of deglutition

Once food has been chewed and mixed with saliva (see *Where digestion begins,* page 12), voluntary tongue movement pushes food toward the back of the mouth to the oropharynx. The oropharynx serves only as a passageway for food and air; no digestion occurs there.

During the first, or pharyngeal, stage of deglutition, food in the oropharynx stimulates swallowing receptor areas and a number of involuntary actions occur: the soft palate rises to prevent food from entering the nasopharynx, the epiglottis closes, the larynx and hyoid bone rise to prevent tracheal aspiration of food, the tongue rises to seal off the mouth, the upper esophageal sphincter relaxes, the esophagus opens, and a peristaltic wave begins in the laryngopharynx to force food into the esophagus. This sequence of events advances food from the mouth to the esophagus in about 1 to 3 seconds.

During the esophageal stage of deglutition, peristalsis propels the food bolus toward the stomach. The circular esophageal musculature constricts above the bolus and relaxes below it. Longitudinal muscles in the esophagus shorten, and neuron receptors in the submucosa transmit messages through the myenteric plexus to the tunica muscularis to initiate peristalsis. The esophageal wall secretes mu- *(continued on page 13)*

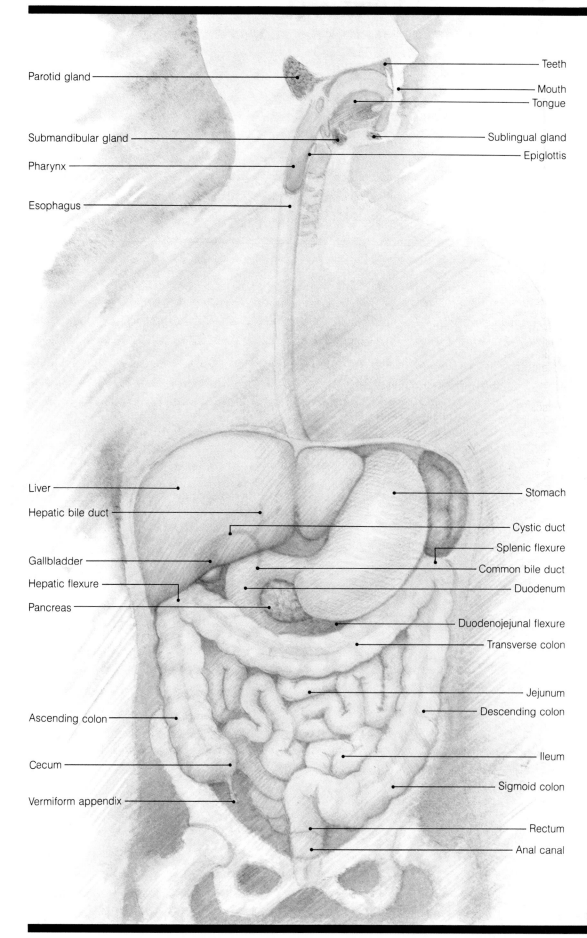

Parotid gland

Submandibular gland

Pharynx

Esophagus

Teeth

Mouth

Tongue

Sublingual gland

Epiglottis

Liver

Hepatic bile duct

Gallbladder

Hepatic flexure

Pancreas

Ascending colon

Cecum

Vermiform appendix

Stomach

Cystic duct

Splenic flexure

Common bile duct

Duodenum

Duodenojejunal flexure

Transverse colon

Jejunum

Descending colon

Ileum

Sigmoid colon

Rectum

Anal canal

# GI structure and innervation

The GI tract is a hollow tube with glands and accessory organs—salivary glands, liver, gallbladder, and pancreas. Its walls alternate muscle tissue with nerve tissue and blood vessels to regulate peristalsis, digestion, and absorption.

## Cellular anatomy
The innermost layer (tunica mucosa, or mucosa) consists of epithelial and surface cells and loose connective tissue. Epithelial cells, convoluted into millions of villi that increase the absorptive surface area, secrete gastric and protective juices and absorb nutrients. The surface cells overlie connective tissue (lamina propria), supported by a thin layer of smooth muscle (muscularis mucosae).

The submucosa (tunica submucosa) encircles the mucosa. It's composed of loose connective tissue, blood and lymphatic vessels, and a nerve network (submucosal, or Meissner's plexus). Around this layer lies the tunica muscularis, composed of skeletal muscle in the mouth, pharynx, and upper esophagus, and of longitudinal and circular smooth muscle fibers elsewhere in the tract. During peristalsis, longitudinal fibers shorten the length of the lumen and circular fibers reduce lumen diameter. At points along the tract, circular fibers thicken to form sphincters. Between the two muscle layers lies another nerve network—myenteric, or Auerbach's, plexus. The stomach wall contains a third, oblique, muscle layer.

The GI tract's outer covering—the tunica adventitia in the esophagus and rectum, the tunica serosa elsewhere—consists of connective tissue protected by epithelium. This visceral peritoneum covers most of the abdominal organs and is contiguous with an identical layer (parietal peritoneum) lining the abdominal cavity. The visceral peritoneum becomes a double-layered fold around the blood vessels, nerves, and lymphatics supplying the small intestine and attaches the jejunum and ileum to the posterior abdominal wall to prevent twisting. A similar mesenteric fold attaches the transverse colon to the posterior abdominal wall.

## GI innervation
Distention of the submucosal or myenteric plexuses stimulates neural transmission to the smooth muscle, initiating peristalsis and mixing contractions. Parasympathetic stimulation—via the vagus nerve for most of the intestines and the sacral spinal nerves for the descending colon and rectum—increases gut and sphincter tone and frequency, strength, and velocity of smooth muscle contractions. Vagal stimulation also increases motor and secretory activities. Sympathetic stimulation, via spinal nerves from levels T6 to L2, reduces peristalsis and inhibits GI activity.

**Structure of GI tract wall**

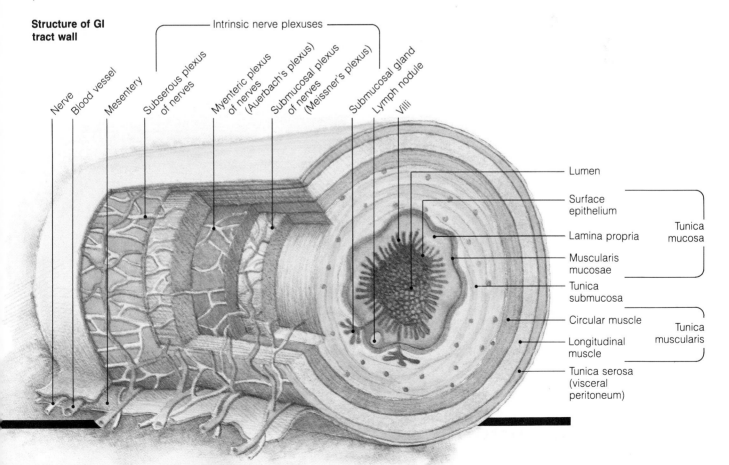

Intrinsic nerve plexuses

Nerve
Blood vessel
Mesentery
Subserous plexus of nerves
Myenteric plexus of nerves (Auerbach's plexus)
Submucosal plexus of nerves (Meissner's plexus)
Submucosal gland
Lymph nodule
Villi

Lumen
Surface epithelium
Lamina propria — Tunica mucosa
Muscularis mucosae
Tunica submucosa
Circular muscle — Tunica muscularis
Longitudinal muscle
Tunica serosa (visceral peritoneum)

# Where digestion begins

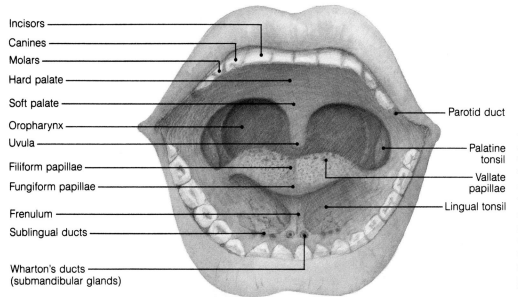

Incisors
Canines
Molars
Hard palate
Soft palate
Oropharynx
Uvula
Filiform papillae
Fungiform papillae
Frenulum
Sublingual ducts
Wharton's ducts
(submandibular glands)

Parotid duct
Palatine tonsil
Vallate papillae
Lingual tonsil

**T**he mouth and its structures assist with taste, mechanical and chemical digestion, and swallowing. These functions often overlap.

### Border structures
The lips, covered externally by skin and internally by mucous membrane, contain blood vessels, skeletal muscle, fat, and sensory receptors to judge food temperature and texture. The cheeks are formed by skin, the buccinator muscle (which aids in chewing), subcutaneous fat, nerves, and mucous membrane. The cheeks confine food to the mouth and lubricate it with secretions from mucous glands that open opposite the last molar teeth.

The hard and soft palates form the roof of the mouth. The hard palate contains two maxillae and two palatine bones covered by mucous membrane that is thick, pale, corrugated, and divided at midline by the palatine raphe. Posteriorly, the soft palate separates the mouth and nasopharynx; its arched opening (fauces), with the uvula suspended at the posterior midpoint, leads to the oropharynx. Besides defining the mouth, these structures and the

tongue also aid in swallowing.

### Taste
The tongue, anchored to the hyoid bone on the floor of the mouth by a fold of mucous membrane (frenulum), is composed mostly of intrinsic skeletal muscle. Beneath the epithelium at the base of the tongue sit large masses of lymphoid tissue, the lingual tonsils. The tongue's apex and base are covered by papillae—rough projections that help mobilize food. Forming an inverted V on the tongue's posterior dorsal surface, the vallate papillae contain taste buds that determine food bitterness. The whitish filiform papillae, covering the anterior two thirds of the dorsum and sides of the tongue, help move food but contain no taste buds. The deep red fungiform papillae, located chiefly at the apex and sides of the tongue, contain taste buds that detect sour, salt, and sweet. Additional taste buds appear on the soft palate and pharynx.

### Mechanical digestion
The teeth (32 in the adult) cut, tear, and grind the food that the cheeks and tongue push into place. The crown, the tooth's visible part, joins the neck,

which is hidden by dense fibrous gum tissue (gingivae). The periodontal ligament locks the root of each tooth into the bony sockets (alveoli) of the alveolar processes projecting from the mandible and maxilla.

The crown contains the body's hardest substance—enamel (97% calcified tissue, 3% organic matter and water), which provides a cutting surface and protects against acid secretions. Dentin, calcified tissue harder than bone, lies directly under the enamel and gives the tooth its shape and rigidity. Below the gum line, dentin is covered by cementum, a bonelike tissue to which the periodontal ligament attaches. The dentin layer encases the pulp cavity, which contains connective tissue permeated by capillaries, nerves, and lymph vessels. This tissue nourishes the dentin and is pain-sensitive; for example, infection increases blood flow and pressure, causing pain. All nerves, blood, and lymph enter the tooth through an opening at its base (apical foramen) and run through the pulp by way of the root canal.

### Chemical digestion and swallowing
Three pairs of salivary glands convey their secretions through ducts to soften, lubricate, and break down ingested food. The submaxillary (submandibular) glands discharge both serous secretions and mucus through Wharton's ducts, located posteriorly on either side of the frenulum. Anteriorly, the sublingual glands secrete thick, stringy mucus onto the mouth floor through many tiny, separate ducts. The largest glands (parotid) secrete serous fluid containing the digestive enzyme salivary amylase (ptyalin) through ducts in the cheeks.

After chewed food mixes with saliva, the tongue, cheeks, and soft palate move it toward the oropharynx, where sensory receptors initiate the swallow reflex.

cus to lubricate the bolus and promote peristalsis.

At the end of the esophagus lies the lower esophageal sphincter (LES), or cardiac sphincter. This circular muscle remains closed, except when receiving food, to prevent reflux of highly acidic gastric juices. When the peristaltic wave propels the food bolus through the esophagus, the LES relaxes just long enough to permit the bolus to enter the stomach. (See *Sites and mechanisms of gastric secretion,* pages 14 and 15.)

## The stomach

Digestion continues in the stomach through the action of gastric secretions, such as hydrochloric acid, gastrin, pepsinogen, mucus, and intrinsic factor. Through a churning motion, the stomach breaks food into tiny particles, and peristalsis mixes it with gastric juices. Although weak peristaltic waves occur continuously in the stomach, their frequency and force increase as stomach volume increases. Normally, peristalsis propels chyme—the watery food bolus mixed with digestive juices—toward the pylorus at a rate of three waves a minute. However, when these waves reach the pylorus, they cause its sphincter to contract so that much of the chyme is propelled back to the stomach body for further processing. Eventually, chyme passes through the pyloric sphincter and empties into the duodenum. The solid portion of food particles remains in the stomach until it liquefies—usually from 1 to 6 hours.

**Gastric emptying.** Neural impulses, chyme, and hormonal effects control the rate of gastric emptying. As the stomach fills and distends, neural impulses increase the rate of peristalsis to propel digested food forward. Excessive distention, though, tends to slow gastric emptying. Vagal stimulation (from anxiety or strong emotion) after a meal also influences the rate of gastric emptying.

The composition of chyme also affects gastric emptying. Carbohydrates pass through the stomach rapidly because salivary amylase has partly broken them down into simpler sugars. Proteins stay in the stomach longer than carbohydrates, since pepsin must break them down into simple compounds called proteoses, polypeptides, and peptones. Fats remain in the stomach the longest time even though the enzyme lipase breaks down only a small percentage of fats to glycerol, fatty acids, and glycerides. But once fats enter the duodenum, they stimulate the enterogastric reflex to inhibit gastric motility and secretion, thereby allowing increased digestion time in the small intestine.

Highly acidic duodenal chyme (pH below *(continued on page 16)*

## How neural impulses trigger swallowing

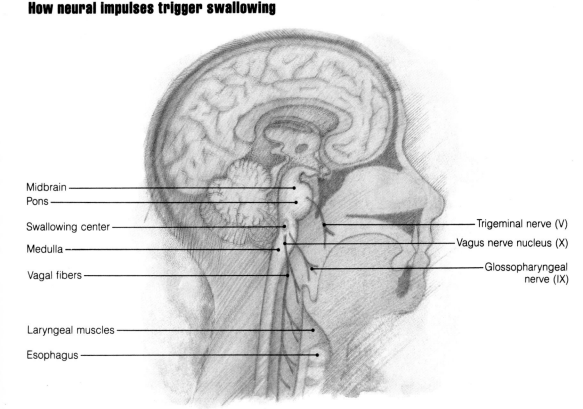

Midbrain
Pons
Swallowing center
Medulla
Vagal fibers
Laryngeal muscles
Esophagus

Trigeminal nerve (V)
Vagus nerve nucleus (X)
Glossopharyngeal nerve (IX)

Before peristalsis can begin, the neural pattern to initiate swallowing illustrated here must occur. First, food pushed to the back of the mouth stimulates swallowing receptor areas that surround the pharyngeal opening. These receptor areas transmit impulses to the brain by way of the sensory portions of the trigeminal (V) and glossopharyngeal (IX) nerves. Then, the brain's swallowing center relays motor impulses to the esophagus by way of the trigeminal (V), glossopharyngeal (IX), vagus (X), and hypoglossal (XII) nerves, causing swallowing to occur.

# Sites and mechanisms of gastric secretion

The stomach lies beneath the diaphragm, its inner curve attached to the liver's underside by a double fold of peritoneum (lesser omentum). Its outer curve attaches to a fold of peritoneum (greater omentum), which extends to the transverse colon and hangs apronlike over the small intestine.

The lower esophageal, or cardiac, sphincter (LES) divides the esophagus and stomach; the pyloric sphincter, the stomach and duodenum. Between these sphincters lie the fundus, body, antrum, and pylorus.

The stomach wall has four layers: the outer serosa; the three-tiered muscularis with circular, longitudinal, and oblique layers of smooth muscle; the submucosa; and the mucosa. Intense wrinkles (rugae) that corrugate the empty stomach's mucosa allow the organ to

quadruple its capacity during digestion.

### Mucosal cell secretions
Three types of glands secrete 2 to 3 liters of gastric juice daily through the stomach's gastric pits. Cardiac glands near the LES and pyloric glands in the pylorus secrete a thin mucus. Gastric glands in the stomach's body and fundus secrete hydrochloric acid (HCl), pepsinogen, intrinsic factor, and mucus.

Specialized cells line the gastric glands, gastric pits, and surface epithelium. Mucous cells in the necks of the gastric glands produce a thin mucus; those in the surface epithelium, a protective alkaline mucus. Both substances lubricate food and protect the stomach from self-digestion by corrosive enzymes and acids.

Argentaffin cells in gastric glands produce the hormone

**Stomach structures**

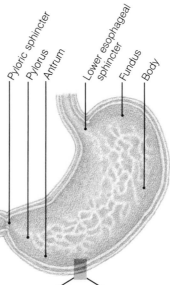

Pyloric sphincter
Pylorus
Antrum
Lower esophageal sphincter
Fundus
Body

**Gastric mucosa**

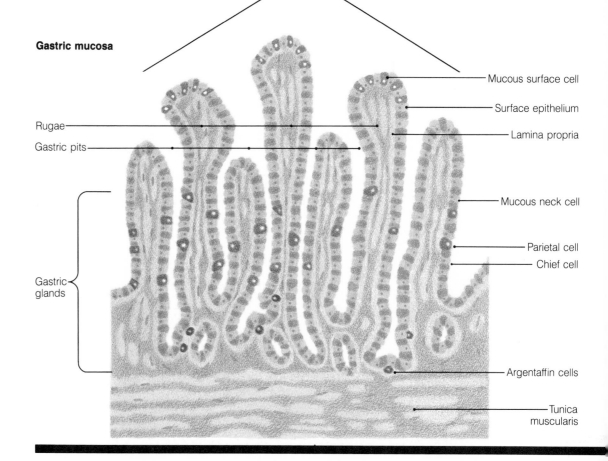

Rugae

Gastric pits

Gastric glands

Mucous surface cell

Surface epithelium

Lamina propria

Mucous neck cell

Parietal cell

Chief cell

Argentaffin cells

Tunica muscularis

gastrin. Chief cells, primarily in the fundus, produce pepsinogen—the inactive precursor of the proteolytic enzyme pepsin, which breaks proteins into polypeptides.

Large parietal cells scattered throughout the fundus secrete HCl and intrinsic factor. HCl enzymatically degrades pepsinogen into pepsin and maintains the acid environment favorable for pepsin activity. It also helps disintegrate nucleoproteins and collagens, hydrolyzes sucrose, and inhibits bacterial proliferation. Intrinsic factor promotes vitamin $B_{12}$ absorption in the small intestine.

### Three stages of gastric secretion
The first (cephalic) stage of gastric secretion occurs at the sight, smell, taste, or thought of food. Parasympathetic stimulation via the vagus nerve causes HCl and pepsinogen to collect in the stomach in anticipation of food.

The second (gastric) phase begins when food enters the stomach. Distention of the stomach wall, parasympathetic impulses, and the chemical makeup of protein, spices, caffeine, or alcohol (called secretagogues) stimulate the antrum to release gastrin into the blood. Gastrin circulates to the stomach mucosa, where it spurs chief and parietal cells to produce more digestive HCl and pepsinogen.

The third (intestinal) phase occurs as food empties into the small intestine and stimulates release of intestinal gastrin, which, in turn, promotes gastric juice secretion.

### Intestinal inhibition of gastric secretion
The hormones secretin, cholecystokinin, enterogastrone, and gastric inhibitory peptide are thought to be secreted into the blood by the intestine when fat and protein are present. These hormones travel back to the stomach mucosa, where they inhibit gastric secretions and gastric motility. Distention and certain characteristics of duodenal chyme, such as its excessive acidity, also inhibit gastric secretion.

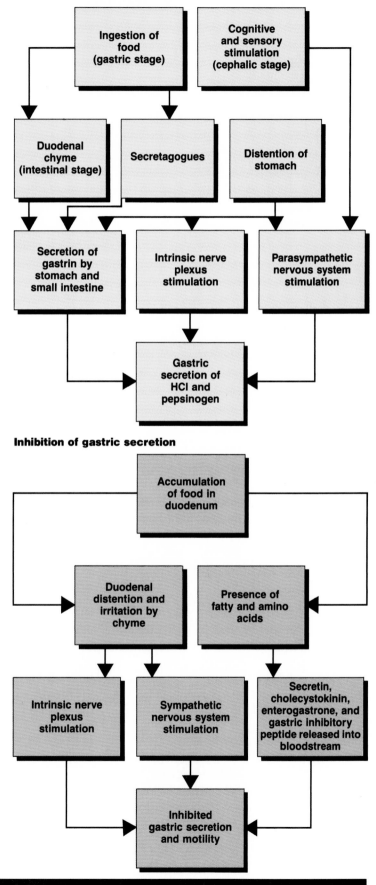

# Small intestine: Its form affects absorption

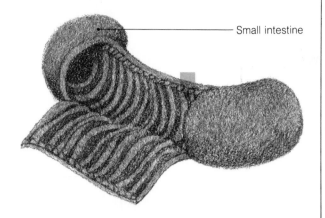

Small intestine

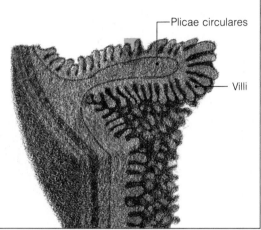

Plicae circulares

Villi

**N**early all digestion and absorption takes place in the 20′ (6.1 m) of small intestine coiled in the abdomen in three major sections: the duodenum, jejunum, and ileum. The duodenum, about 10″ (25 cm) long, extends from the stomach and contains the hepatopancreatic ampulla (ampulla of Vater, or Oddi's sphincter), an opening that drains bile from the common duct and pancreatic enzymes from the main pancreatic

duct. About 40% of people have an accessory duct (duct of Santorini) leading from the head of the pancreas and draining into the duodenum just above Oddi's sphincter.

The jejunum, about 7½′ (2.3 m) long, follows the duodenum and leads to the ileum, about 12′ (3.7 m) long. The small intestine ends in the lower right abdominal quadrant at the ileocecal valve, a sphincter that empties almost nutrient-devoid chyme into the large intestine.

**A specialized mucosa**
Multiple projections of the intestinal mucosa increase the surface area for absorption several hundredfold. Circular projections (plicae circulares) are covered by further projections (villi), each containing a lymphatic vessel (lacteal), a venule, capillaries, an arteriole, nerve fibers, and smooth muscle. Surmounting each villus sit almost 2,000 microvilli resembling a fine brush (hence, brush border). The villi are lined with columnar

---

3.5) also activates the enterogastric reflex, which inhibits gastric motility until highly alkaline pancreatic juices neutralize the chyme. The hormones secretin, cholecystokinin, and gastric inhibitory peptide, secreted by the small-intestine mucosa, inhibit gastric motility by their effects on target organs like the pancreas and gallbladder. (See *Understanding digestive hormones,* page 18, and *Understanding digestive enzymes,* page 19.)

### The small intestine
Although limited amounts of water, salts, and alcohols are absorbed in the stomach, most digestion and absorption take place in the 20′ (6 m) of small intestine, whose four layers are highly specialized for this purpose.

Multiple projections of the innermost *mucosal layer* enhance surface area and increase absorptive efficiency. (See *Small intestine: Its form affects absorption.*) Circular projections (plicae circulares) are covered by threadlike projections (villi), which, in turn, are covered by minute cylindrical projections (microvilli). Peyer's patches also mark the mucosa, espe-

cially in the ileum, and assist in defense against pathogens. The *submucosal layer,* which encircles the mucosa, contains a network of nerves and lymphatic and blood vessels that transport absorbed nutrients. Around this layer lies the *tunica muscularis,* consisting of longitudinal and circular muscle fibers, which is thicker at the proximal end to support frequent peristalsis. The outer *serous layer* is contiguous with the peritoneum, which attaches the small intestine to the abdominal wall to prevent twisting.

Through a churning motion and peristalsis, the small intestine mixes chyme with intestinal secretions and pushes it along the digestive tract. A forward-backward motion known as segmental contraction ensures thorough mixing and enhances blood and lymph circulation. Rhythmic shortening and lengthening of the millions of intestinal villi also aids mixing.

Although chyme typically advances quite slowly in the small intestine, distention triggers the myenteric reflex, which produces more rapid and forceful peristalsis. The com-

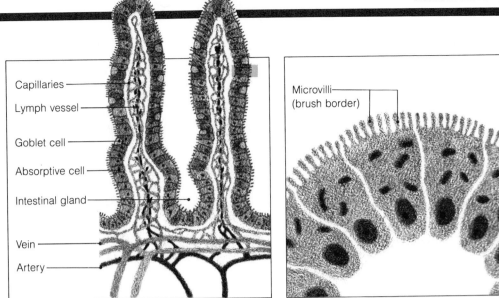

Capillaries
Lymph vessel
Goblet cell
Absorptive cell
Intestinal gland
Vein
Artery

Microvilli
(brush border)

epithelial cells, which dip into the lamina propria between the villi to form intestinal glands (crypts of Lieberkühn).

The type of epithelial cell dictates its function. Mucus-secreting goblet cells are found on and between the villi on the crypt mucosa. In the proximal duodenum, specialized Brunner's glands also secrete large amounts of mucus to lubricate and protect the duodenum from potentially corrosive acidic chyme and gastric juices.

Other important epithelial cells include Paneth's, argentaffin, undifferentiated, and absorptive cells. *Paneth's* cells are thought to regulate intestinal flora. Duodenal *argentaffin* cells produce the hormones secretin and cholecystokinin. *Undifferentiated* cells deep within the intestinal glands replace the epithelium. *Absorptive* cells consist of large numbers of tightly packed microvilli over a plasma membrane containing transport mechanisms for ab-

sorption and producing enzymes for the final step in digestion.

The intestinal glands primarily secrete a watery fluid that bathes the villi with chyme particles. Fluid production results from local neural irritation and possibly from hormonal stimulation by secretin and cholecystokinin. The microvillous brush border secretes a wide variety of hormones and digestive enzymes that catalyze final nutrient breakdown.

position of chyme also influences intestinal transit time, which may require 3 to 10 hours.

The ileocecal valve—a membranous fold dividing the small and large intestines—remains closed to facilitate absorption in the small intestine and to prevent bacterial reflux from the large intestine. It opens to allow passage of chyme in response to gastrin secretion and the gastroileal reflex, triggered by food entering the stomach.

## A close look at absorption

By the time chyme reaches the ileocecal valve, all its nutritional value has been absorbed.

**Water and electrolytes.** Water readily diffuses across the small intestinal wall; in fact, only about 0.5 liter of the 5 to 10 liters of water entering the intestine remains unabsorbed. Sodium is absorbed by active transport in the jejunum, while potassium, magnesium, and phosphate are absorbed throughout the small intestine. Chloride diffuses with sodium, except in the ileum where it's actively transported.

**Vitamins.** Most water-soluble vitamins are absorbed by diffusion, except vitamin $B_{12}$, which combines with intrinsic factor (a glycoprotein secreted by the stomach) and is actively transported in the ileum. Fat-soluble vitamins (A, D, E, K) briefly combine with bile salts to form water-soluble micelles that are absorbed by diffusion.

**Carbohydrates.** Absorbed primarily in the duodenum and upper jejunum, glucose and galactose move by active transport; fructose, by diffusion.

**Proteins.** Amino acids and partially digested dipeptides and tripeptides are absorbed by active transport. Peptides are then broken down to constituent amino acids before release into the bloodstream.

**Fats.** Glycerol and free fatty acids briefly combine with bile salts to form micelles that are absorbed by diffusion. Bile salts are recycled to the liver, while absorbed fats combine with cholesterol, phospholipids, and protein to form chylomicrons. In this form, absorbed fats diffuse into the lacteals of the villi, flow into the lymphatic system, and eventually

## Understanding digestive hormones

| Hormone | Source | Activating substances | Action |
|---|---|---|---|
| Gastrin | Gastric mucosa of pylorus | Partially digested proteins in pylorus | • Stimulates release of gastric juice rich in pepsinogen and hydrochloric acid |
| Gastric inhibitory peptide | Mucosa of small intestine | Fats, sugar, acids, and partially digested proteins in intestine | • Inhibits gastric secretion and motility<br>• Stimulates intestinal secretion and pancreatic insulin production |
| Villikinin | Mucosa of small intestine | Chyme in intestine | • Stimulates intestinal villi movements |
| Secretin | Duodenal mucosa | Partially digested proteins, fats, and acids in duodenum | • Stimulates secretion of low-enzyme, high-bicarbonate pancreatic juice<br>• Stimulates secretion of bile by liver<br>• May enhance cholecystokinin activity in producing pancreatic enzymes and may inhibit gastric motility, acid secretion, and pyloric sphincter contraction |
| Pancreozymin | Duodenal mucosa | Partially digested proteins, fats, and acids in duodenum | • Stimulates pancreatic juice |
| Cholecystokinin | Duodenal mucosa | Partially digested proteins, fats, and acids in duodenum | • Stimulates secretion of high-enzyme pancreatic juice<br>• Inhibits gastric emptying and secretion and intestinal motility<br>• Stimulates gallbladder contractions leading to release of bile |

drain through the thoracic duct into the left subclavian vein.

After absorption, the products of carbohydrate, protein, and fat digestion are taken up by body cells for energy use or storage in response to elevated blood insulin levels. Glucose is stored as glycogen, a polysaccharide, primarily in the liver and skeletal muscle. Protein synthesized from amino acids is also stored in the skeletal muscle. Fats are stored as triglycerides, primarily in the adipose tissue.

### The large intestine
The large intestine serves two major functions: to absorb water and to store feces. (See *Large intestine: Its role in fluid and electrolyte absorption,* page 22.) In the intestine, peristalsis and segmental contractions bring waste material into contact with the colon wall for water absorption and propel it toward the rectum for elimination. Initiated by vagal stimulation or intestinal wall distention, peristaltic waves typically progress from one end of the intestine to the other, moving waste material at the rate of ½″ to 1″ (1.27 to 2.54

cm) per minute. Three or four times a day, more powerful segmental contractions move larger masses of waste material forward.

Rectal distention by waste material, or feces, stimulates the defecation reflex, which initiates peristaltic waves in the descending colon and relaxes the internal sphincter. (Gastric distention may also stimulate this reflex.) Voluntary relaxation of the external sphincter aided by Valsalva's maneuver permits defecation.

Feces normally consist of 75% water and 25% solids (such as cellulose and other indigestible fiber), bacteria, unabsorbed minerals, fat and fat derivatives, desquamated epithelial cells, mucus, and small amounts of digestive enzymes and secretions. Their normal brown color results from metabolism of bile pigments to stercobilin. Fecal odor results from the presence of indole and skatole, end products of protein catabolism by bacterial action in the large intestine.

### Accessory organs assist digestion
Organs that assist in digestion but are not part of the GI tract include the pancreas, liver,

## Understanding digestive enzymes

| Digestive enzyme | Source | What it acts on | What it produces |
|---|---|---|---|
| **Saliva** | | | |
| Amylase (ptyalin) | Salivary gland | Starch | Dextrin, maltose |
| **Gastric juice** | | | |
| Pepsin | Stomach | Proteins | Polypeptides, peptides, proteoses (partially digested proteins) |
| Gastric juice | Stomach | Emulsified fats | Fatty acids, glycerol |
| **Bile** | | | |
| (Contains no enzymes) | Liver (stored in and released from gallbladder) | Unemulsified fats | Emulsified fats |
| **Pancreatic juice** | | | |
| Trypsin | Pancreas | Proteins, polypeptides | Proteoses, peptides, amino acids |
| Chymotrypsin | Pancreas | Proteins, polypeptides | Polypeptides, amino acids |
| Lipase | Pancreas | Bile-emulsified fats | Fatty acids, glycerol |
| Amylase | Pancreas | Starch | Maltose, isomaltose |
| Nucleases | Pancreas | Nucleic acids | Nucleotides |
| Carboxypeptidases | Pancreas | Polypeptides | Smaller polypeptides |
| **Intestinal juice** | | | |
| Enterokinase | Duodenal mucosa | Trypsinogen | Trypsin |
| Aminopeptidases | Duodenal mucosa | Polypeptides | Smaller polypeptides |
| Dipeptidase | Duodenal mucosa | Dipeptides | Amino acids |
| Sucrase | Duodenal mucosa | Sucrose | Glucose, fructose |
| Lactase | Duodenal mucosa | Lactose | Glucose, galactose |
| Maltase | Intestinal villi | Maltose | Glucose |
| Nucleotidase | Intestinal villi | Nucleotides | Nucleosides, phosphoric acid |
| Nucleosidase | Intestinal villi | Nucleosides | Purine, pentose |
| Intestinal lipase | Intestinal villi | Fat | Glycerides, fatty acids, glycerol |

and gallbladder. (See *Accessory organs aid digestion,* pages 20 and 21, and *Understanding secretion of bile and pancreatic juice,* page 24.) Besides its vital exocrine function in digestion, the pancreas also performs endocrine functions. It secretes insulin in response to elevated blood glucose levels after ingestion of food. Insulin stimulates uptake and conversion of glucose to glycogen in the liver, thereby lowering blood glucose levels. However, when intestinal absorption of glucose diminishes and blood glucose levels steadily decrease, the pancreas slows insulin secretion and releases glucagon. This catabolic hormone promotes conversion of glycogen to glucose (glycogenolysis) and of stored protein and fats to glucose (gluconeogenesis). Because glycogenolysis occurs more rapidly and is simpler than gluconeogenesis, it typi- (continued on page 23)

# Accessory organs aid digestion

The liver, gallbladder, and pancreas contribute hormones, enzymes, and bile vital to digestion. These organs deliver their secretions to the duodenum through the hepatopancreatic ampulla, also known as the ampulla of Vater or Oddi's sphincter.

### Pancreas: Hormone and enzyme producer

The pancreas, 6″ to 9″ (15.2 to 22.9 cm) long and somewhat flat, lies behind the stomach with its head and neck extending into the curve of the duodenum and its tail lying against the spleen.

The pancreas performs both exocrine and endocrine functions. Its exocrine function involves scattered cells that daily secrete over 1,000 ml of digestive enzymes. Lobules and lobes of the clusters (acini) of enzyme-producing cells release their secretions into ducts that merge into the pancreatic duct. This duct runs the length of the pancreas and joins the bile duct from the gallbladder before entering the duodenum. Vagal stimulation and release of the hormones secretin and cholecystokinin control the rate and amount of pancreatic secretion.

The endocrine function of the pancreas involves the islets of Langerhans, which are located between the acinar cells. Over 1 million of these islets house two cell types: beta and alpha. Beta cells secrete insulin to promote carbohydrate metabolism; alpha cells secrete glucagon, which stimulates glycogenolysis in the liver. Both hormones flow directly into the blood, their release stimulated by blood glucose levels.

### Gallbladder: Bile warden

The gallbladder, 3″ to 4″ (7.6 to 10.2 cm) long and pear-shaped, attaches to the liver's ventral surface by the cystic duct. It stores and concentrates bile produced by the liver, so that its 30- to 50-ml storage load increases up to tenfold in potency. Secretion of the hormone chole-

**Liver, gallbladder, and pancreas**

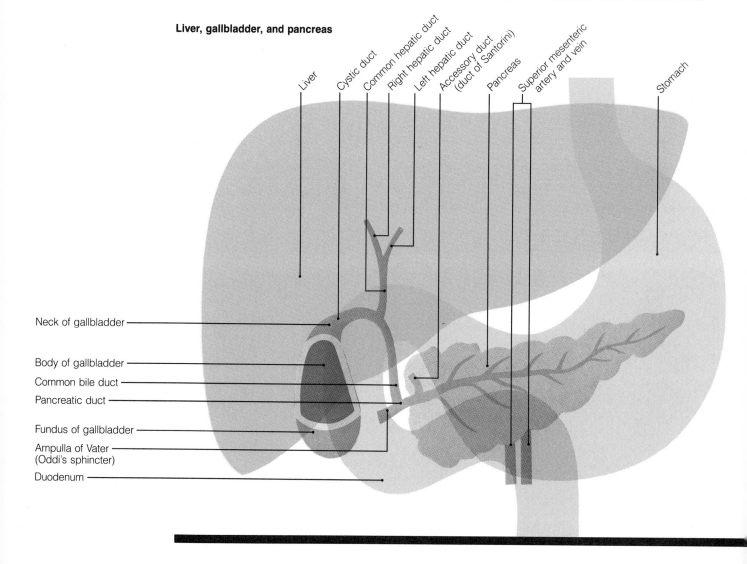

Liver

Cystic duct

Common hepatic duct

Right hepatic duct

Left hepatic duct

Accessory duct (duct of Santorini)

Pancreas

Superior mesenteric artery and vein

Stomach

Neck of gallbladder

Body of gallbladder

Common bile duct

Pancreatic duct

Fundus of gallbladder

Ampulla of Vater (Oddi's sphincter)

Duodenum

**Liver lobule**

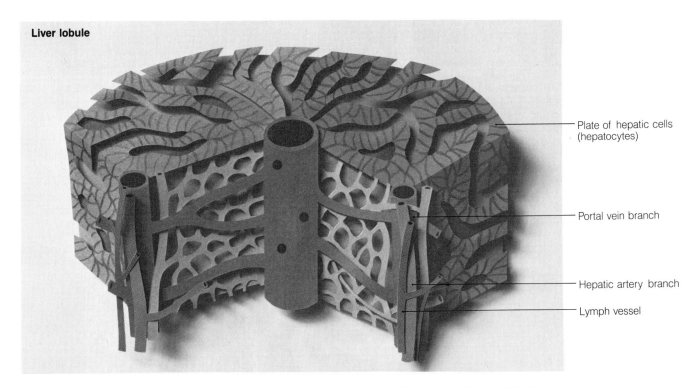

Plate of hepatic cells (hepatocytes)

Portal vein branch

Hepatic artery branch

Lymph vessel

cystokinin causes gallbladder contraction and relaxation of Oddi's sphincter, releasing bile into the common bile duct for delivery to the duodenum. When the sphincter closes, bile shunts to the gallbladder for storage.

### Liver: Bile producer, nutrient storer, blood cleanser

The body's largest gland, the 3-lb (1.4-kg) liver is highly vascular and enclosed in a fibrous capsule in the upper right abdominal quadrant. It's separated by connective tissue into a large right lobe (three fourths of total organ size), a left lobe, and the falciform ligament dividing the two lobes. The right lobe further divides into the right lobe proper and two posterior sections, the caudate and quadrate lobes.

**The liver lobule and bile production.** The liver's functional unit, the lobule, consists of a plate of hepatic cells (hepatocytes) that encircle a central vein and radiate outward. The plates of hepatocytes are separated from each other by sinusoids, the liver's capillary system. Lining the sinusoids are reticuloendothelial macrophages (Kupffer's cells), which remove bacteria and toxins that have entered the blood through the intestinal capillaries.

The sinusoids carry oxygenated blood from the hepatic artery and nutrient-rich blood from the portal vein. Unoxygenated blood leaves through the central vein and flows through hepatic veins to the inferior vena cava. Bile, recycled from bile salts in the blood, leaves through bile ducts (canaliculi) that merge into the right and left hepatic ducts to form the common hepatic duct. This common duct joins the cystic duct from the gallbladder to form the common bile duct to the duodenum.

The liver recycles about 80% of bile salts into bile, combining them with bile pigments (biliverdin and bilirubin—the breakdown products of red blood cells) and cholesterol. The liver produces about 500 ml of this alkaline bile in continuous secretion. Increased bile production can result from vagal stimulation, release of the hormone secretin, increased liver blood flow, and the presence of fat in the intestine.

**Diversified functions.** The liver has several other important functions. It metabolizes digestive end products by regulating blood glucose levels. When glucose is being absorbed through the intestine (anabolic state), the liver stores glucose as glycogen. When glucose isn't being absorbed or when blood glucose levels fall (catabolic state), the liver mobilizes glucose to restore blood levels necessary for brain function. In addition to glucose, the liver maintains stores of nutrients, such as iron, copper, and vitamins A, D, and $B_{12}$.

The liver detoxifies body hormones, ingested drugs, and chemicals, such as alcohol and marijuana. In addition, the liver synthesizes vital plasma proteins, such as albumin, for maintaining plasma oncotic pressure; and prothrombin, fibrinogen, and clotting factors V, VII, IX, and X for aiding blood coagulation.

# Large intestine: Its role in fluid and electrolyte absorption

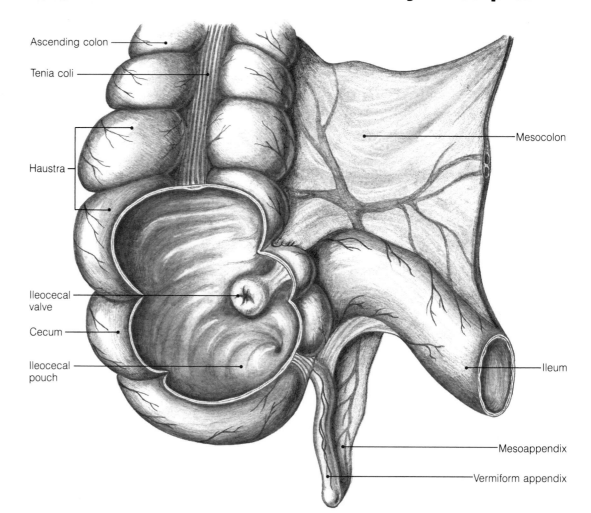

Ascending colon

Tenia coli

Haustra

Ileocecal valve

Cecum

Ileocecal pouch

Mesocolon

Ileum

Mesoappendix

Vermiform appendix

The large intestine, the final section of the GI tract, extends about 5′ (1.5 m). It begins at the juncture of the ileum and cecum with the ileocecal pouch, a blind tube (vermiform appendix) rich in lymph tissue but with no known digestive function. Then it climbs the right abdominal cavity to the liver's lower border (ascending colon), crosses horizontally below the liver and stomach (transverse colon), and descends the left abdominal cavity to the iliac fossa (descending colon).

From there, the sigmoid colon continues to the lower midline of the abdominal cavity, becomes the rectum, and terminates in the anal canal. The anus opens to the exterior through two sphincters. The internal anal sphincter contains thick, circular smooth muscle under autonomic control. The external sphincter contains skeletal muscle under voluntary control.

Circular and longitudinal fibers of the tunica muscularis move and mix intestinal contents, and the longitudinal muscle gives the large intestine its familiar shape. These fibers gather into three narrow bands (teniae coli) down the middle of the colon and pucker the intestine into characteristic pouches (haustra).

The ascending and descending colons attach directly to the posterior abdominal wall for support. The transverse and sigmoid colons attach indirectly through sheets of connective tissue (mesocolon).

**Fluid recycling system**

Although the large intestine produces no hormones or digestive enzymes, it continues the absorptive process. Through blood and lymph vessels in the submucosa, the proximal half of the intestine absorbs all but about 100 ml of the remaining water in the colon plus large amounts of sodium and chloride. The large intestine also harbors the bacteria *Escherichia coli, Enterobacter aerogenes, Clostridium welchii,* and *Lactobacillus bifidus,* which help synthesize vitamin K and break down cellulose into usable carbohydrate. Bacterial action also produces flatus, which helps propel feces toward the rectum. In addition, the mucosa produces alkaline secretions from tubular glands composed of goblet cells. This alkaline mucus lubricates the intestinal walls as food pushes through and protects the mucosa from acidic bacterial action.

cally supports blood glucose levels initially in the catabolic state. For gluconeogenesis, the liver must rely on a supply of amino acids and glycerol from skeletal muscle protein and adipose fat reserves, respectively. Norepinephrine and epinephrine help promote mobilization of these energy reserves. The liver deaminates amino acids to form glucose and converts the by-product ammonia to urea for urinary excretion. Besides using glycerol to form glucose, the liver also converts fatty acids to ketone bodies that can be oxidized as an alternate energy source.

## ABNORMAL G.I. FUNCTION

Although it is one of the most common disorders, GI dysfunction remains poorly understood. Its causes are often obscure; its signs and symptoms, notoriously nonspecific. Moreover, GI dysfunction stems from various pathophysiologic mechanisms that may exist separately or simultaneously. Such mechanisms include tumors, hyperactivity and hypoactivity, malabsorption, infection and inflammation, vascular disorders, intestinal obstruction, and degenerative disease.

### Tumors

Benign or malignant tumors—the result of abnormal cellular growth in the gastrointestinal tract—typically produce vague initial symptoms of backache, weakness, and mild abdominal pain. However, tumor growth eventually causes more dramatic and specific symptoms. For example, dysphagia points to esophageal tumor, while ascites and jaundice point to liver tumor. Anorexia and weight loss are also common with most GI tumors. Early diagnosis offers the best hope for curative treatment; advanced tumors tend to metastasize via the blood or lymph system. For example, colorectal cancer is potentially curable in 80% to 90% of patients if early diagnosis allows resection before nodal involvement occurs.

### Hyperactivity and hypoactivity

Altered GI motility or secretion may cause hyperactivity or hypoactivity. The common peptic ulcer results from hyperactivity; constipation results from hypoactivity.

**Peptic ulcer.** Although its precise cause is unknown, predisposing factors associated with peptic ulcer include smoking; irritants such as caffeine, spices, and certain drugs (for example, ibuprofen, indomethacin, salicylates, and steroids); stress; the O blood type; and heredity. Chronic gastric hyperacidity may result in mucosal erosion due to inadequate mucosal blood flow, decreased mucosal resistance, or defective mucus. Mucosal erosion produces ulceration, which may eventually lead to penetration of surrounding organs, such as the pancreas. Other complications of peptic ulcer include perforation, hemorrhage, and pyloric obstruction.

**Constipation.** A common mechanical obstruction associated with hypoactivity, constipation may result from decreased dietary bulk; inadequate fluid intake; or atonicity due to laxative abuse, seasonal inactivity, bed rest, stress, or hypothyroidism. Untreated constipation may lead to fecal impaction.

Since the autonomic nervous system controls GI function, any factor that influences this system may cause hyperactivity or hypoactivity. Among the most common factors are drugs and stress. Bacterial or chemical toxicity, as in botulism and lead poisoning, is another factor. Spinal cord trauma resulting in quadriplegia may cause permanent hypoactivity.

### Malabsorption

The impaired uptake of essential nutrients, malabsorption boasts a diverse etiology. Its causes include inadequate production of digestive juices (as in pancreatic insufficiency), bacterial proliferation, atrophy or inflammation of the villous lining of the intestine, disturbed lymphatic or vascular flow (as in cardiovascular disorders), loss of absorptive surface area (as in surgical resection), inborn errors of metabolism (as in lactose intolerance), and malnutrition. Mild malabsorption produces little more than transient indigestion; severe malabsorption produces intractable diarrhea, nutrient deficiencies, and clinical starvation.

### Infection and inflammation

Infection and inflammation of the GI tract are both common and diverse.

**Regional ileitis (Crohn's disease) and ulcerative colitis.** Although the exact causes of these inflammatory disorders are unknown, excessive autonomic stimulation, allergy, and autoimmune disorders are among possible causes. Ulcerative colitis typically involves only the mucosa and submucosa of the colon; regional ileitis extends through layers of the intestinal wall and may occur in any part of the GI tract. Patchy or continuous inflammatory lesions, causing hyperemia, fibrosis,

# Understanding secretion of bile and pancreatic juice

The presence of partially digested proteins, fats, and acids in the duodenum stimulates duodenal release of the hormones secretin and cholecystokinin into the blood. Along with vagal stimulation from the brain, secretin triggers the liver to increase bile secretion to the gallbladder, while cholecystokinin contracts the gallbladder to release bile into the duodenum.

These two hormones also promote secretion of pancreatic juices. In response to the same chymous and neural stimuli, secretin triggers exocrine cells in the pancreas to release acid-neutralizing bicarbonates, while cholecystokinin spurs release of digestive enzymes.

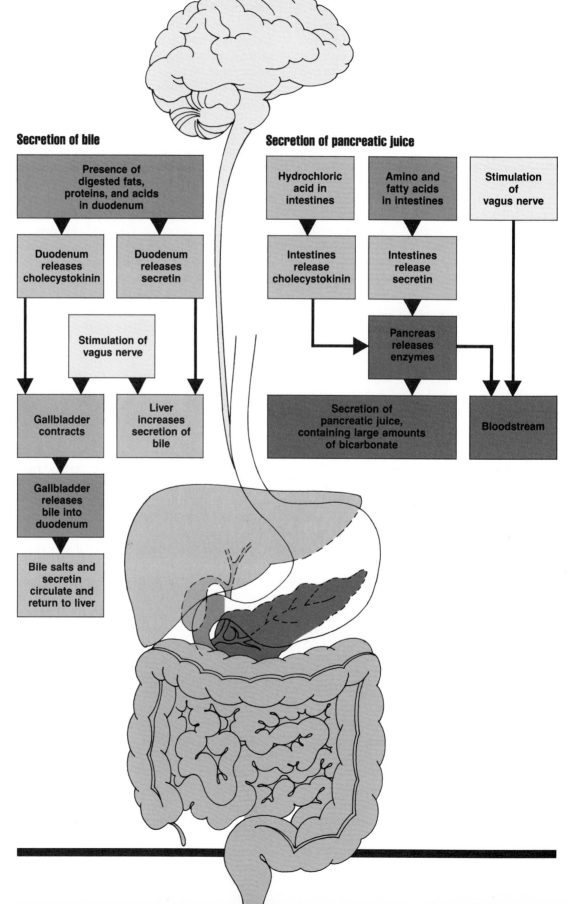

**Secretion of bile**

Presence of digested fats, proteins, and acids in duodenum

Duodenum releases cholecystokinin

Duodenum releases secretin

Stimulation of vagus nerve

Gallbladder contracts

Liver increases secretion of bile

Gallbladder releases bile into duodenum

Bile salts and secretin circulate and return to liver

**Secretion of pancreatic juice**

Hydrochloric acid in intestines

Amino and fatty acids in intestines

Stimulation of vagus nerve

Intestines release cholecystokinin

Intestines release secretin

Pancreas releases enzymes

Secretion of pancreatic juice, containing large amounts of bicarbonate

Bloodstream

and ulceration, are characteristic in both disorders.

**Cholecystitis.** An acute or chronic inflammation of the gallbladder, cholecystitis is usually associated with gallstone disease. Acute cholecystitis develops when gallstones lodge near or within the cystic duct, causing painful distention of the gallbladder. *Escherichia coli,* staphylococci, streptococci, and *Salmonella* commonly cause secondary infection, producing a fibrinopurulent exudate over the gallbladder's surface. Chronic cholecystitis develops insidiously or following repeated attacks of acute disease. In chronic cholecystitis, the gallbladder eventually shrinks, becomes fibrotic, and may adhere to neighboring organs.

**Pancreatitis.** This painful, and at times life-threatening, inflammation of the pancreas occurs in acute and chronic forms. Most commonly associated with alcoholism and biliary tract disease, pancreatitis may also result from trauma, use of certain drugs, and perforated peptic ulcer. It involves autodigestion, in which enzymes normally excreted by the pancreas digest pancreatic tissue. Acute pancreatitis is characterized by extreme pain, persistent vomiting, abdominal rigidity, diminished bowel activity, rales at lung bases, and left pleural effusion. Chronic pancreatitis is characterized by constant dull pain with occasional exacerbations, malabsorption, severe weight loss, and hyperglycemia.

**Hepatitis.** Whether of viral or nonviral origin, hepatitis is marked by liver cell necrosis, leading to anorexia, jaundice, and hepatomegaly. Viral hepatitis occurs in three forms: type A, type B, and type non-A, non-B. Type A hepatitis is transmitted via fecal-oral and parenteral routes. It most often spreads through ingestion of contaminated food or water. Also transmitted parenterally, type B hepatitis spreads through contaminated blood, needles, or medical or dental instruments or through contact with semen or saliva. Type non-A, non-B hepatitis is transmitted parenterally by blood transfusions and hemodialysis. In contrast, nonviral hepatitis follows exposure to hepatotoxins, such as carbon tetrachloride and alcohol. Although most patients recover from hepatitis, a few develop chronic active hepatitis, which may progress to cirrhosis or life-threatening fulminant hepatitis.

## Vascular disorders
Whether it is the result of arterial occlusive disease, arteritis, or shock, decreased or interrupted blood flow to the GI tract may result in tissue ischemia or necrosis. Symptoms vary widely, depending on the organs affected.

In acute and chronic occlusive disease, prognosis depends on the location of the occlusion and the presence or development of collateral circulation to offset reduced blood flow. The duration of occlusion also influences acute disease.

## Intestinal obstruction
Intestinal obstruction—characterized by a buildup of gas, fluid, and chyme—produces distention and increased intraluminal pressure. This increased pressure, in turn, impairs blood flow, inhibiting absorption of nutrients, which triggers fluid shift from the intravascular space to the intestinal lumen. Impaired blood flow may also cause tissue ischemia and necrosis, predisposing to bacterial invasion and peritonitis. Untreated complete obstruction may critically reduce intravascular fluid volume, eventually causing fatal hypovolemic shock and vascular collapse.

## Degenerative disease
A dramatic example of degenerative disease, cirrhosis involves diffuse destruction and fibrotic regeneration of hepatic cells. This fibrosis alters liver structure and normal vasculature, impairs blood and lymph flow, and ultimately causes hepatic insufficiency. Impaired hepatic blood flow triggers portal hypertension, which causes blood to back up into the spleen and flow through collateral channels to the venous system. As a result, portal hypertension produces splenomegaly, dilated collateral veins (esophageal varices, hemorrhoids, or prominent abdominal veins), and ascites. Mortality is high; many patients die within 5 years of onset. Among the diverse causes of cirrhosis are alcoholism, biliary tract disease, hepatitis, hemochromatosis, and right heart failure.

## Combine knowledge and skill
The high incidence of GI disorders guarantees you the opportunity to apply this basic understanding of normal and abnormal GI function. As always, your role also demands sharp nursing skills—from assessment to evaluation. You'll be expected to recognize specific GI disorders, to help prevent them through effective teaching in the hospital and the community, and to identify and solve disease-related problems through insightful nursing diagnoses and appropriate care plans.

**Points to remember**

- The GI tract includes the mouth, pharynx, esophagus, stomach, and small and large intestines. This hollow tube also contains salivary glands and accessory organs—the liver, gallbladder, and pancreas.
- The GI tract breaks down food—proteins, fats, and carbohydrates—into molecules small enough to permeate cell membranes, thereby giving cells the needed nutrients to function properly.
- The GI tract consists of four tissue layers: the tunica mucosa with specialized epithelial cells, the tunica submucosa with Meissner's plexus, the tunica muscularis with muscle layers and Auerbach's plexus, and the tunica adventitia.
- Digestion begins in the mouth through chewing and the action of salivary amylase, an enzyme that breaks down starch. However, most digestion and absorption take place in the small intestine.
- The liver's functional unit, the lobule, produces bile; metabolizes fat, carbohydrate, and protein; detoxifies intrinsic and extrinsic toxins; stores nutrients; and synthesizes factors for blood clotting.
- GI disorders can result from tumors, hypoactivity or hyperactivity, malabsorption, infection and inflammation, vascular disorders, intestinal obstruction, and degenerative disease.

# 2 ASSESSING G.I. FUNCTION

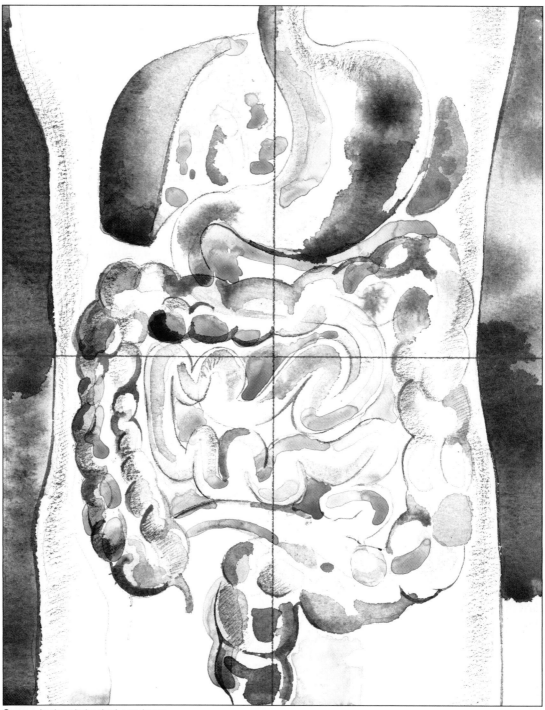

Organs in the abdominal quadrants

The wide-ranging implications of GI symptoms make accurate assessment of the GI tract a difficult but critical nursing task. As you know, GI symptoms can have multiple, markedly dissimilar causes. For example, vomiting may result from pregnancy, cancer, viral infection, or a severe metabolic disorder, such as hyperkalemia. Also, a seemingly innocuous GI symptom may signal a serious disorder in another body system. Indigestion, for example, may signal impending cardiac crisis. With such diverse causes of GI symptoms, how can you meet the formidable challenge of GI assessment?

First, by taking a thorough patient history—an especially important consideration with the GI system—you may discover deep-set psychological problems or stressors that disrupt GI function. By mastering the key assessment techniques of inspection, auscultation, palpation, and percussion, you'll be able to effectively conduct the physical examination. Finally, by keeping your assessment ongoing, you'll be able to prevent development of a secondary GI disorder.

### Prepare the equipment

Begin GI assessment by gathering the necessary equipment. For the oral examination, you'll need a pen light or another light source, gauze pads, a tongue depressor, gloves, and a mouth mirror. For the abdominal examination, you'll need a stethoscope with a diaphragm and bell, a skin-marking pencil, a tape measure, a flexible ruler with centimeter markings, and a percussion hammer. For the rectal examination, you'll need gloves and lubricant. If overhead lighting is insufficient, use a portable lamp. Be sure the room is quiet and free from interruptions so you can correctly auscultate the patient's abdomen.

### Prepare the patient

After introducing yourself to the patient, explain the purpose of the interview. Encourage the patient to ask questions about the assessment, and reassure him in any way possible. Tell him how long the examination should last. Then ask him to void, to put on a hospital gown, and to sit on the examining table.

### NURSING HISTORY AND OBSERVATION

The nursing history will provide a data base you can use to monitor the patient's progress, reactions, and complications throughout hospitalization. If the patient is in great distress or has a poor memory, be sure to obtain information from his family or companions. Note biographical data—particularly the patient's age, sex, and ethnic origin—to help detect predisposition to certain GI disorders. For example, the incidence of esophageal cancer is four times greater in men than in women; ulcerative colitis has a high incidence in Jews.

Be sure to vary your communication techniques during the nursing history. Ask open-ended questions, such as, "What problems have you been experiencing lately?" This tells the patient that you're genuinely interested in what he has to say and allows him to discuss what he feels is important. Also use direct questions, such as "Do you ever have heartburn?" This helps obtain specific clinical information. And remember to practice active listening: try to understand the source of the patient's concern, and allow him time to formulate his responses. Address him by name, and use eye contact appropriately. Also assess the patient's mental status to determine his ability to cooperate. Anxiety, pain, and lethargy can make the history unreliable.

### Discuss the chief complaint

Because GI complaints are often vague, you'll want to elicit as much specific information about the complaint as possible. (See *Checklist for assessing a GI complaint.*) You'll also want to identify factors that aggravate or alleviate the complaint, such as diet or environment. Note the importance the patient attaches to his chief complaint. Does he dismiss it or become anxious when speaking about it? Then, depending on the complaint, ask the following types of questions.

**About pain.** *What does the pain feel like? What symptoms accompany the pain?* Fever, malaise, nausea, vomiting, warmth, redness, and swelling (for example, in the mouth) may indicate viral infection or inflammation of the GI tract. *Do you have heartburn or dyspepsia?* These conditions usually occur after eating spicy foods that produce excess stomach acid; dyspepsia may also occur with hiatal hernia, drug use, or cancer. If the patient has abdominal pain, ask about the relationship of the pain to meals. Peptic ulcer pain usually occurs about 2 hours after meals or whenever the stomach is empty; it may awaken the patient at night. Arterial insufficiency to the bowel usually causes pain 15 to 30 minutes after meals and lasts up to 3 hours. *Do you have rectal pain?* This may indicate local

## Identifying areas of referred pain

Pain may occur relatively near its source or distant from it. These illustrations will help you to identify the areas and causes of referred pain.

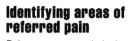

Renal colic

Biliary colic

Cholecystitis, pancreatitis, duodenal ulcer

Small intestine pain

Appendicitis

Colon pain

Ureteral colic

Pancreatitis

Perforated duodenal ulcer, cholecystitis

Penetrating duodenal ulcer

Cholecystitis

Pancreatitis, renal colic

Rectal lesions

problems, such as hemorrhoids. (See *Identifying areas of referred pain.*)

**About dysphagia.** *Where do you feel discomfort during swallowing?* Ask the patient to point to the area of discomfort, because certain disorders affect specific locations during swallowing. *Does solid food, or do both liquids and solids, produce discomfort?* Dysphagia usually results from obstruction or loss of motor coordination. Because cancer is an im-

portant cause of obstruction, ask if the patient has experienced unexplained weight loss. Neurologic disease can cause loss of motor coordination, so ask about additional symptoms, such as dysarthria.

**About nausea and vomiting.** *Do you feel nauseated before vomiting? Is the vomiting projectile?* Projectile vomiting often indicates central nervous system disorders. *Does the vomitus have an unusual odor?* A fecal odor, for example, usually indicates small bowel obstruction. *When do symptoms occur?* Early morning vomiting may result from pregnancy or excessive consumption of alcohol. *Have you vomited blood?* Hematemesis may reflect a GI disorder, such as esophagitis, or non-GI conditions, such as anticoagulant toxicity.

**About diarrhea.** Ask about the frequency of bowel movements. *Do periods of constipation alternate with periods of diarrhea?* This pattern may indicate irritable colon, diverticulitis, or colorectal cancer. *What foods did you eat before the onset of diarrhea?* Food poisoning may cause diarrhea and is usually accompanied by cramping and vomiting. Fever, tenesmus, and cramping associated with diarrhea usually indicate viral infection. *Is the stool bloody?* This may result from inflammation or neoplasm of the bowel. *Is the stool foul-smelling, bulky, or greasy?* This suggests a fat malabsorption disorder. Passage of mucus indicates irritable colon.

**About constipation.** *How would you describe the size, character, and frequency of your bowel movements?* (Many patients mistakenly claim to have constipation.) Inadequate fiber or fluid intake, laxative abuse, and decreased physical activity may lead to constipation. *Do you experience cramping abdominal pain and distention related to constipation?* These symptoms imply obstipation—extreme and persistent constipation caused by intestinal tract obstruction. *Is constipation acute or chronic?* If acute, it's likely to have an organic cause; if chronic, a functional cause. *How would you describe the amount and frequency of flatulence?* Many patients complain of rumbling or growling in their stomach but do not actually expel flatus. If so, determine its associated symptoms (such as bloating) and aggravating factors (such as spicy food).

## Review activities of daily living

Explore the following habits that may influence the patient's chief complaint:

**Diet.** Ask the patient to describe a typical day's menu to help evaluate nutritional status

## Assessing the acute abdomen

| Test | Procedure | Implications of findings |
|------|-----------|--------------------------|
| Hyperesthesia test | Using the point of a pin, gently stroke the abdomen of the supine patient from the upper to the lower areas. | Sharper sensation at any location suggests visceral or parietal peritoneal irritation. |
| Rebound tenderness | With the patient supine, apply deep pressure to the abdomen away from the suspected site of inflammation. Then quickly release pressure. | Pain felt upon release of pressure indicates peritoneal irritation. It may be localized or general. |
| Murphy's sign | As the supine patient takes a deep breath, perform deep palpation in the right upper quadrant, making contact with the gallbladder. | Sharp pain and arrested inspiration suggest cholecystitis. |
| Iliopsoas test | Instruct the supine patient to flex the right hip against moderate resistance over the thigh. Or position the patient on his left side, and have him flex his right leg at the hip. | Pain in the right lower quadrant during psoas muscle contraction suggests an inflamed or perforated appendix. |
| Obturator test | Ask the supine patient to flex his right hip and knee to 90°. Rotate his ankle internally and externally. | Pain in the hypogastric area with obturator muscle involvement suggests a perforated appendix or pelvic abscess. |

and to pinpoint the cause of GI symptoms. Spicy foods, for example, may produce excess stomach acid. Inadequate fiber or fluid intake may cause constipation. Recent weight loss may signal anorexia or cancer.

**Smoking.** Obtain a history of tobacco use. If the patient smokes cigarettes, note the duration in pack years. Cigarette smoking can cause various cancers, esophagitis, and ulcers; pipe smoking, stomatitis or lip cancer.

**Alcohol and caffeine consumption.** Ask the patient about consumption of alcohol or caffeine-containing beverages, and record the type and amount. Excessive alcohol consumption contributes to cancer, esophageal tears, liver disease, and, along with large amounts of caffeine, gastric ulcers.

**Travel.** Ask the patient if he has traveled recently. Ingestion of foreign or contaminated food and water can cause GI distress.

### Review psychosocial history

Begin reviewing the psychosocial history by determining how the patient's chief complaint affects his life-style. Has it impaired his expectations, family life, or social contacts? Then ask about the patient's job. A sedentary job can contribute to constipation; a highly stressful job can lead to ulcers. Occupational exposure to toxins, such as lead, can also cause GI disorders.

Ask the patient about recent emotional distress. Such distress can lead to dyspepsia, nausea, anorexia, gluttony, mouth sores, or idiosyncratic tendencies such as cheek-biting. Fear of treatment may exacerbate the patient's symptoms. And financial difficulties may contribute to poor nutritional habits, stress-related GI symptoms, and inadequate dental and medical treatment.

### Review physical history

Begin the physical history by collecting information on GI disorders, previous hospitalizations, and drug use that may affect GI function. Chronic ulcerative colitis or GI polyposis, for example, may predispose the patient to colorectal cancer. Cesarean section, for example, may cause adhesions and lead to bowel obstruction. Aspirin may irritate the gastric lining, and narcotics can cause constipation. Chemotherapy and steroids may cause stress ulcers, nausea, and vomiting; antibiotics often cause nausea and vomiting. Drug therapy for chronic obstructive pulmonary disease (COPD) may precipitate ulcers. Laxatives, including mineral oil and stool softeners, affect intestinal motility. Habitual use of laxatives may cause constipation (from diminished defecation reflexes).

You'll also need to obtain the family medical history. Inquire about the health of the patient's parents, grandparents, and siblings. Note the cause of death or any known

## Identifying abdominal quadrants and their underlying structures

To help you perform an abdominal assessment and record your findings accurately, divide the patient's abdomen into quadrants. Then learn to recognize the size, shape, and location of abdominal structures within each quadrant.

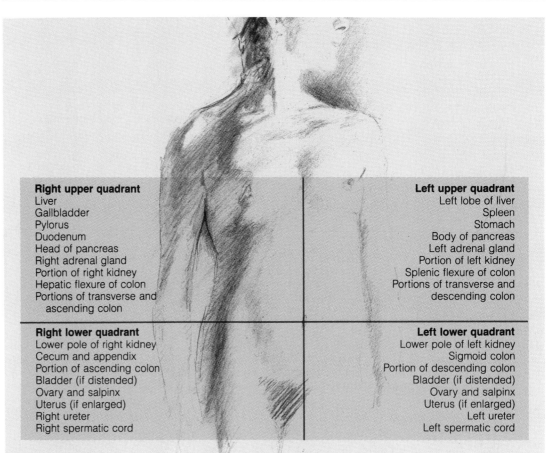

**Right upper quadrant**
Liver
Gallbladder
Pylorus
Duodenum
Head of pancreas
Right adrenal gland
Portion of right kidney
Hepatic flexure of colon
Portions of transverse and
   ascending colon

**Left upper quadrant**
Left lobe of liver
Spleen
Stomach
Body of pancreas
Left adrenal gland
Portion of left kidney
Splenic flexure of colon
Portions of transverse and
descending colon

**Right lower quadrant**
Lower pole of right kidney
Cecum and appendix
Portion of ascending colon
Bladder (if distended)
Ovary and salpinx
Uterus (if enlarged)
Right ureter
Right spermatic cord

**Left lower quadrant**
Lower pole of left kidney
Sigmoid colon
Portion of descending colon
Bladder (if distended)
Ovary and salpinx
Uterus (if enlarged)
Left ureter
Left spermatic cord

illnesses of family members. Be sure to inquire about GI disorders having familial tendencies, such as tumors, gastric ulcers, liver disease, and malabsorption syndromes.

Next, assess the patient's general health by asking about recent fever, weakness, and fatigue. Record the patient's allergies to drugs, food, and environmental elements, and note any previous trauma. Then review the following body systems for symptoms related to GI disorders:

• *Integumentary system.* Generalized jaundice and pruritus may result from hepatocellular damage or biliary obstruction. Pruritus may indicate a problem with bile breakdown and elimination. Telangiectases and a tendency to bruise easily may reflect liver dysfunction.

• *Neurologic and ophthalmologic systems.* Many neurologic disorders, such as cerebrovascular accidents and myasthenia gravis, interfere with nutrition because of difficulty in chewing and swallowing. Uveitis may accompany ulcerative colitis or Crohn's disease.

• *Cardiopulmonary system.* Dyspnea may result from limited respiratory excursion caused by ascites. Signs of congestive heart failure, such as jugular vein distention and tachycardia, often result from liver failure. COPD may

cause constipation due to diaphragmatic weakness and decreased strength to defecate.

• *Lymphatic system.* Swelling of cervical, supraclavicular, or inguinal lymphatics may signal GI cancer.

• *Endocrine system.* Diabetes mellitus may cause diarrhea or constipation. Hypothyroidism can also cause constipation.

• *Urinary system.* Uremia can cause GI bleeding, and various urinary tract disorders can produce abdominal pain.

• *Musculoskeletal system.* Arthritis may occur with ulcerative colitis or Crohn's disease.

### PHYSICAL EXAMINATION

After recording the patient's history, begin the physical by taking his vital signs; then explain the examination procedures that you'll use to examine his mouth, abdomen, and rectum. Tell him that he'll feel some pressure during abdominal palpation. If he is experiencing abdominal pain, tell him that you'll assess the painful area last or not at all.

### Examine the mouth

Unless the patient has an urgent abdominal complaint, begin by examining the mouth. Have the patient remove lipstick, dental appliances, and chewing gum.

Inspect for asymmetry or swelling around the jaws and lips. While the patient opens and closes his mouth, observe carefully for limited motility and for tenderness and crepitus of the temporomandibular joint. Inspect the lips for abnormal color and for lesions. Next, put on a rubber glove or finger cot to palpate the outer lips. Invert the lips and, using your light source, inspect and palpate the inner lips with the patient's jaw closed. Note any lesions, nodules, or fissures, especially at the junction of the upper and lower lips. Note any malocclusion of the patient's bite by retracting his lips while he clenches his teeth. Check for obvious dental caries and for teeth that are missing, broken, stained, displaced, or loose. Then, inspect and palpate the patient's gums (gingivae). They should be pink, moist, and smooth. Note any redness, pallor, hypertrophy, ulcers, bleeding, or tenderness on palpation.

Ask the patient to stick out his tongue so you can check its lateral surfaces. They should be pink and moist and should appear rough because of papillae. Note any paralysis or abnormal movement, such as deviation to one side. Also note swelling, lesions, or coating. Grasping the tongue with a 2″ × 2″ gauze pad, palpate its superior surface and sides. Note any nodules or ulcerations. Ask the patient to touch the roof of his mouth with his tongue while you inspect and palpate the tongue's superior surface and the floor of the mouth. Inspect carefully for ulcers, which are common in this area and may be an early sign of oral cancer. Check the mouth's floor and the oral mucosa for leukoplakia which may be precancerous. Next, inspect and palpate the buccal mucosa. Record abnormalities, such as pallor, redness, excessive salivation or dryness, bleeding, swelling, ulcers or sores, and white patches or plaques. Inspect and palpate the hard and soft palates. Normally, the hard palate is dome-shaped, pale, firm, and transversed irregularly by rugae; the soft palate, pink, cushiony, and without rugae. Note any redness, lesions, patches, petechiae, or pallor.

To examine the patient's pharynx, tilt his head back and hold down his tongue with a tongue depressor. Ask the patient to say "Ah." His uvula and soft palate should rise and remain in the midline. Inspect the anterior and posterior pillars, the tonsils, and the posterior pharynx, which is normally pink and may be slightly vascular. Note abnormali-

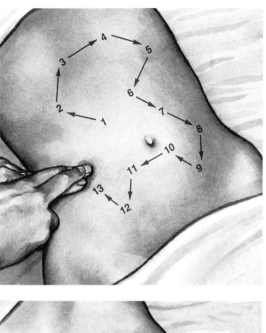

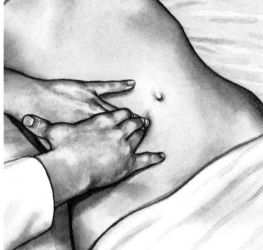

ties, such as uvular deviation; the absence, hypertrophy, or induration of the tonsils; and swelling of the tonsils or the posterior pharynx. Inspect for lesions, plaques, exudate, or a gray membrane. Finally, describe unusual mouth odor in your notes—for example, *sweet and fruity* or *fetid and musty.*

### Examine the abdomen

After completing the oral examination, begin abdominal assessment—but check first for contraindications. Never palpate the abdomen of a patient with suspected appendicitis or a dissecting abdominal aortic aneurysm because of the possibility of rupture. Don't perform palpation on a patient with polycystic kidneys—you may dislodge a cyst. Avoid percussion or palpation on a patient with transplanted kidneys or other organs. And remember that abdominal pain contraindi-

## Performing percussion and deep palpation

Unless your patient is in pain, begin percussion in the right upper quadrant. Otherwise, identify the quadrant in which the patient is experiencing pain. Moving clockwise, percuss each quadrant in a *systematic* pattern, concluding with the painful quadrant. To perform percussion, place the distal phalanx of one middle finger against the body surface, keeping the palm and other fingers raised above the skin. Using the tip of the other hand's middle finger, quickly tap the distal joint of the resting finger. When tapping, remember to remove your upper finger quickly so you don't dampen vibrations.

To perform deep palpation, place the distal portions of the fingers of one hand lightly over the abdominal surface. Superimpose the other hand and apply firm pressure, depressing the lower hand about 3″ (7.6 cm). With the lower hand you should be able to feel abdominal contents.

cates repeated abdominal assessment. (See *Assessing the acute abdomen,* page 29.)

For assessment purposes, the abdomen is divided into four sections: the left upper quadrant, right upper quadrant, left lower quadrant, and right lower quadrant. (See *Identifying abdominal quadrants and their underlying structures,* page 30.) The patient's history should tell you in which quadrant his symptoms are located. Examine all four quadrants, concluding with the symptomatic one. Otherwise, you may elicit pain in the symptomatic quadrant, causing the muscles in the other quadrants to tighten and making examination difficult.

Inspection tells you where to listen closely when you auscultate for bowel and circulatory sounds. Percussion outlines major organs or masses. Palpation helps assess the tenderness, size, mobility, consistency, and location of organs or enlarged masses. Use all four of these techniques in each of the abdomen's quadrants while concentrating on the organ system underlying that section. And remember to perform them in modified sequence—auscultation before palpation and percussion—to avoid stimulating intestinal activity that may produce misleading bowel sounds.

Position the patient on his back, with his knees bent and his arms at his sides, to prevent tensing of the abdominal muscles. Warm your hands and your stethoscope's diaphragm before beginning the examination.

**Inspection: Identifies surface irregularities.** Standing at the supine patient's side, stoop to check abdominal contour. (See *Observing abdominal contour.*) Then, inspect the umbilicus for such abnormalities as blue tinge, which may indicate intraabdominal bleeding or acute pancreatitis (Cullen's sign). Standing at the foot of the examining table, observe the abdomen again for symmetry of contour and for masses. An asymmetrical abdomen may result from previous abdominal trauma or surgery, an abnormal organ, or weak abdominal muscles.

Then, move to the patient's right side, and inspect the abdomen for movement from respiration, peristalsis, and arterial pulsations. Exaggerated abdominal movement during breathing may indicate respiratory distress or severe anxiety. Normal peristaltic movement is rarely visible, even through a thin abdominal wall. If you see strong contractions (peristaltic waves) crossing the patient's abdomen, suspect impending bowel or pyloric obstruction. Report this finding to the doctor. You may see pulsations of the abdominal aorta in the epigastric area. In a thin patient, you may see femoral arterial pulsations.

Inspect the abdominal skin thoroughly. Tense, glistening skin may indicate ascites (effusion and accumulation of serous fluid in the abdominal cavity) or abdominal wall edema. Note any scars, lesions, ecchymoses, striae, rashes, or dilated veins. Also inspect for abdominal hernia, which may become apparent when you ask the patient to cough. Record the location, size, and color of such abnormalities. Many skin and vascular find-

## Observing abdominal contour

Viewing the supine patient's abdomen can help you to identify underlying GI abnormalities. Use the illustrations at right to guide you in identifying abdominal contour and any associated GI conditions.

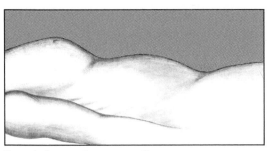

**Rounded:** normal convex profile

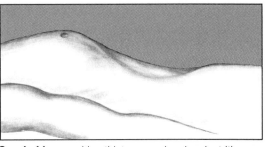

**Scaphoid:** normal in athlete; may signal malnutrition

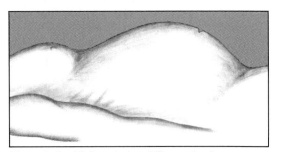

**Distended, with inverted umbilicus:** obesity or gas distention

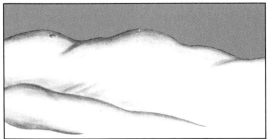

**Upper half distention:** carcinomatosis, pancreatic cyst, or gastric dilation

ings relate to pressure caused by obstruction of the vena cava or portal vein. Jaundice may result from liver disease or splenic hemolysis. Chronic uremia may cause abdominal pallor. Although vascular lesions in the skin may result from various causes, always consider the possibility that the patient has a gastrointestinal disorder.

**Auscultation: Identifies abnormal sounds.** After inspecting the patient's abdomen, use the diaphragm of the stethoscope to exert light pressure, and listen for bowel sounds in all quadrants. Normally, air and fluid movement through the bowel creates irregular bubbling or soft, gurgling noises every 5 to 15 seconds. If you don't hear bowel sounds immediately, listen for at least 5 minutes to confirm their absence—a finding that may indicate paralytic ileus or peritonitis. Report this finding. Conversely, rapid, high-pitched, tinkling bowel sounds or loud, gurgling noises with visible peristaltic waves commonly accompany diarrhea or gastroenteritis and indicate a hyperactive bowel. These findings may also signal an early intestinal obstruction.

Next, use the bell of the stethoscope to listen to vascular sounds and to check for bruits (blowing sounds that seem to elongate the pulsation normally heard over a vessel). Place the bell lightly over the midline to check for bruits of the abdominal aorta resulting from a narrowing of the vessel by arteriosclerosis or a dissecting aortic aneurysm. Also check for bruits over the renal vessel, a result of dilation or constriction.

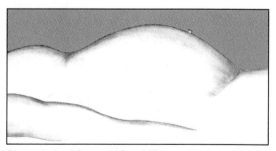

**Distended, with everted umbilicus:** chronic ascites, tumor, or umbilical hernia

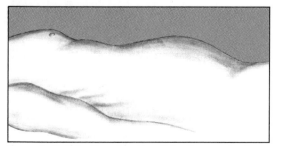

**Lower half distention:** bladder distention, ovarian tumor, pregnancy, or uterine fibroids

Now listen for other abnormal abdominal sounds. A hum—a medium-tone sound created by blood flow in a large, engorged vascular organ, such as the liver or spleen—may signal fluid overload. A friction rub, which sounds like two pieces of sandpaper being rubbed together and which coincides with respiratory movement, may originate in an inflamed spleen or a neoplastic liver.

*Test for edema.* While auscultating the abdomen, watch the imprint left by the bell of the stethoscope. If the circular imprint of a lightly placed stethoscope remains visible on the skin, fluid has probably accumulated within the abdominal wall. This often results from a nutritional deficiency, such as low protein levels.

**Percussion: Detects structural abnormalities.** Percussion is used mainly to check the size of abdominal organs and to detect excessive amounts of fluid or air in the abdomen. Keep the positions of underlying organs in mind, and follow a pattern when you percuss. (See *Performing percussion and deep palpation,* page 31.) Abdominal percussion normally elicits tones ranging from dull or flat (over solids) to tympanic (over air). A sigmoid colon filled with stool produces dullness in the left lower quadrant. You'll usually hear high-pitched, tympanic notes over a section of bowel filled with air (the degree of tympany reflects gaseous bowel distention). If ascites is present, you'll detect dullness when you percuss the patient's flanks. You can also use percussion to assess the liver. (See *Estimating liver size.*) Hepatomegaly is often present with liver or cardiac disease.

**Palpation: Determines size, shape, and position of structures.** When palpating the abdomen, you'll use light and deep palpation and ballottement. To perform light palpation, use your fingertips to depress the abdominal wall a little more than ½" (1.3 cm). Using light palpation, you can determine skin temperature, detect large masses and tender areas, elicit guarding, and assess abdominal vasculature. You can usually palpate the femoral pulse in the groin area, and you can palpate the aortic pulse by pressing the patient's upper abdomen slightly to the left of midline. (Deeper palpation may be necessary to locate this pulse.)

Light palpation may not allow you to feel normal-sized abdominal organs, especially in an obese patient. But if you place your index finger parallel to, and slightly beneath, the right costal margin and ask the patient to take

## Estimating liver size

You can estimate the size and position of the patient's liver through percussion.

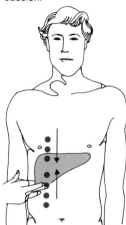

Beginning at the right iliac crest, percuss upward on the midclavicular line (MCL). The percussion note will become dull when you find the lower border of the liver, usually at the costal margin (although it may be lower with liver disease or on deep inspiration). Mark this point. Then, starting under the clavicle, percuss downward along the right MCL. But place your percussion finger between the patient's ribs as you tap to avoid confusing the dull note of the liver's superior border (generally in the fifth to seventh intercostal spaces) with the dull note that comes from percussing bone. Mark the liver's upper border. The distance between the two points you've marked represents the approximate size of the liver's right lobe, normally from 2⅜" to 4¾" (6 to 12 cm).

## Recognizing signs of ascites

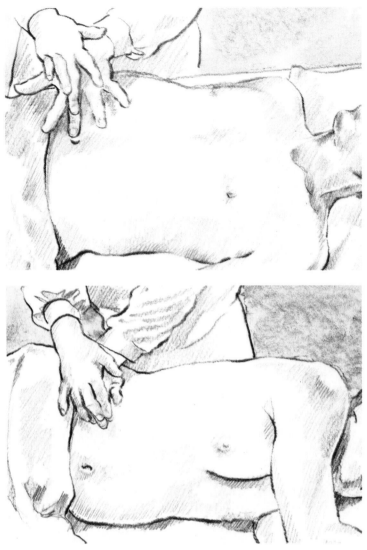

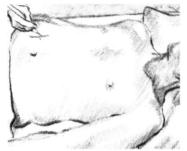

You can detect ascites by testing for shifting dullness and a fluid wave. To test for shifting dullness, have the patient lie on his back. Percuss from the umbilicus outward to the flank. Draw a line to mark the change from tympanic to dull sounds.

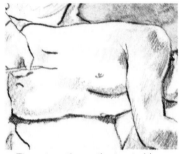

Then, turn the patient onto his side, which causes ascitic fluid to shift. Percuss again and mark the change from tympany to dullness. Any difference between these lines can signify ascites.

Remember, though, that shifting dullness can also result from movement of an engorged loop of bowel, causing dull percussion tones, or from surgical adhesions that prevent fluid from shifting freely.

To test for a fluid wave, have the patient or a staff member press deeply into the midline of the patient's abdomen to prevent vibration from traveling along the abdominal wall. Place one of your palms on one of the patient's flanks. Strike the opposite flank with your other hand. If you feel the blow in the opposite palm, ascitic fluid is present.

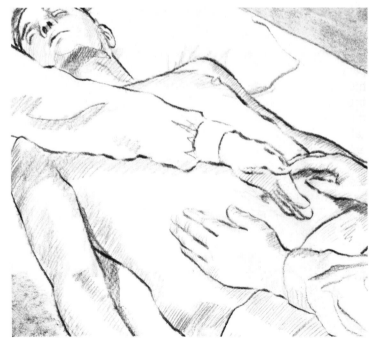

a deep breath, you may be able to feel the liver's lower edge. Normally, this edge stops just below the margin. It feels like a firm, sharp, even ridge with a smooth surface. If the patient grimaces or reports pain during this maneuver, notify the doctor immediately.

Assist the patient to the right lateral position. Then use light palpation under the left costal margin to assess splenic tenderness. If you suspect an enlarged spleen, use very light pressure and observe for signs of discomfort.

Use deep palpation to determine the position of organs and to detect abdominal masses. (See *Performing percussion and deep palpation,* page 31.) Never use deep palpation on a patient who's just had a kidney transplant or on one who has polycystic kidneys. Avoid this technique on a patient with known appendicitis, a tender spleen or another tender organ, or suspected abdominal aneurysm. Also avoid deep palpation of a known abdominal mass because manipulation may cause tumor cells to spread. To assess the inferior liver border, stand at the right of the recumbent patient and face his feet. Hook the fingers of both your hands over the costal margin, and ask the patient to take a deep breath. You should be able to feel the border of the liver's right lobe. Assess it for contour, mobility, consistency, and tenderness.

Use ballottement to detect early rigidity of abdominal muscles caused by inflammation. To perform abdominal ballottement, bounce your fingers upward along the midinguinal line to detect resistance. Also test for a fluid wave and shifting dullness to detect ascites. (See *Recognizing signs of ascites,* page 34.)

**Examine the rectum**
Begin the rectal examination by turning the patient on his left side, with his knees up and his buttocks close to the edge of the examining table. (If the patient is ambulatory, ask him to stand and bend over the examining table.) Spread the buttocks to expose the anus. Rectal skin is normally darker than the surrounding area. Inspect for inflammation, lesions, scars, outpouchings, fissures, and external hemorrhoids. Check for hemorrhoids while the patient strains as though to defecate.

Use a disposable glove and lubricant to palpate the rectum. While the patient strains as though to defecate, use your index finger to palpate any weak anal outpouchings, nodules, or tenderness on movement. Then, explain to the patient that you'll insert your gloved finger a short distance into his rectum

and that this pressure may make him feel as though he needs to defecate. Wait for the anal sphincter to relax, then insert your finger gently and rotate it to palpate as much of the rectal wall as possible. Palpate for any nodules, irregularities, or tenderness and for fecal impaction. Then, obtain a stool sample and test for occult blood.

**Perform ongoing assessment**
Even after completing a thorough GI assessment, you'll need to reassess the patient each time he reports a GI complaint. Don't assume, for example, that previously diagnosed gallstones are causing his current abdominal pain. The nature and location of his pain may have changed, signaling more extensive involvement or perhaps a new disorder. So, to ensure effective care, you'll need to perform ongoing assessment. Keep in mind, though, that some patients may assume that ongoing assessment means that they have a significant health problem. Therefore, you'll need to reassure them that repeated evaluations aid diagnosis and treatment.

**NURSING DIAGNOSES**
With information gathered during GI assessment, you're ready to formulate accurate nursing diagnoses. The nursing diagnosis is a statement identifying the patient's actual or potential health-care problem and the problem's etiology. To formulate a nursing diagnosis, follow these simple steps:
• Establish a baseline assessment using the objective and subjective data you've accumulated. Be sure to identify problems that a nurse can treat.
• Identify the patient's problems related to etiology. Use clear and concise phrasing that suggests interventions or a care plan.
• Write the diagnostic statement using the formula "problem related to etiology;" for example, "fluid volume deficit related to dysphagia" or "alterations in comfort related to nausea and vomiting."

**Assessment: Key to an effective care plan**
Comprehensive GI assessment will help you to interpret the often subtle and misleading signs and symptoms of GI disorders. Mastering this critical first step allows you to construct well-organized and effective care plans. And maintaining continuing assessment will help you to detect significant changes in the patient's condition, to prevent complications, and to improve the prognosis.

**Points to remember**

• Comprehensive GI assessment includes physical and psychosocial histories, as well as oral, abdominal, and rectal examinations.
• Pain, dysphagia, nausea, vomiting, diarrhea, and constipation are the common chief complaints associated with GI disorders.
• Unless the patient has an urgent abdominal complaint, begin GI assessment with the mouth, and then examine the abdomen and the rectum.
• When assessing the abdomen, always perform auscultation before percussion and palpation to prevent spurious bowel sounds.
• Consider all of your assessment data before writing the nursing diagnosis.

# 3 IMPLEMENTING THE DIAGNOSTIC WORKUP

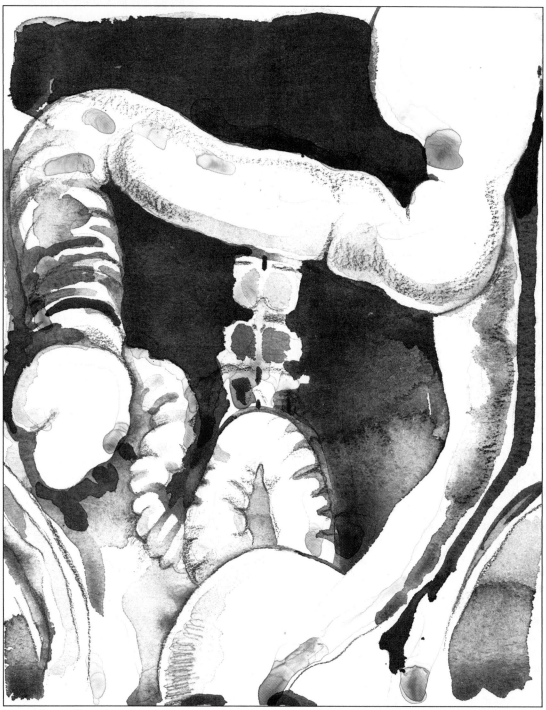

Normal X-ray of large bowel

I f you care for patients with GI disorders, you know how elusive diagnosis can be. These patients often have vague and widespread symptoms that involve other body systems. Usually, tests to assess these symptoms are uncomfortable, emotionally draining, and time-consuming.

Preparing patients for GI tests can also be time-consuming. Your responsibilities include helping patients stay calm, making sure they know about (and adhere to) dietary restrictions, and scheduling tests so they don't conflict with and invalidate each other.

For some tests, like percutaneous liver biopsy, you'll probably assist the doctor. For others, like the basal gastric secretion test, you're likely to collect specimens. And still others, such as the acid perfusion test, you're likely to perform yourself.

Although the doctor will report the results to your patient, you'll probably have to provide supplementary information. Above all, you'll have to help your patient keep his test results in perspective.

In short, you're the patient's guide—telling him what to expect, helping him through, and making sure he understands results. So, obviously, the more you know about GI tests (see *Sites evaluated by GI diagnostic tests,* page 38), the better you can do your job.

## BLOOD AND URINE TESTS
Blood tests are particularly helpful indicators of dysfunctions involving liver and pancreatic disease, biliary disorders, and intestinal malabsorption. Urine tests for bilirubin, urobilinogen, glucose, and galactose also evaluate liver function; D-xylose and vitamin $B_{12}$ tests evaluate ileal function. (See *Blood and urine tests for GI disorders,* pages 40 and 41.)

## GASTRIC ANALYSIS
Two tests measure the stomach's secretion of gastric acid: the basal gastric secretion test and the gastric acid stimulation test. Together, these tests detect abnormal secretion and suggest various gastric and duodenal disorders, but require radiographic studies and endoscopy to pinpoint the cause.

### Basal gastric secretion test
This test measures basal secretion, the secretion of acid between meals. Remember to tell the patient to avoid food and fluids before this test.

To perform the test, a nasogastric tube is inserted into the stomach and attached to continuous suction. Fluoroscopy may be used to determine proper positioning. Gastric contents are withdrawn for 15 minutes and pH is obtained. Then the specimen is discarded. Gastric contents are then collected every 15 minutes for 1 hour. Basal acid output is obtained by adding the results of the four collections together.

Normal values for basal secretion are 0.2 to 3.8 mEq/hour for women and 1 to 5 mEq/hour for men. High values suggest gastric or duodenal ulcers; very high values, Zollinger-Ellison syndrome. Depressed values suggest gastric carcinoma or benign gastric ulcer; no secretion (achlorhydria), pernicious anemia. This test also evaluates the effects of antisecretory drugs, such as cimetidine.

Findings should be correlated with those of the gastric acid stimulation test, which can be performed immediately afterward.

### Gastric acid stimulation test
This hour-long test evaluates integrity of the stomach's parietal cells through testing their ability to secrete acid.

After subcutaneous administration of a drug that stimulates gastric acid output, usually pentagastrin, wait 15 minutes. Then collect four specimens through a nasogastric tube at 15-minute intervals. Label the specimens "Stimulated Contents" and number them.

Normal values for acid secretion following stimulation are 11 to 21 mEq/hour for women and 18 to 28 mEq/hour for men. High levels suggest duodenal ulcers; very high levels, Zollinger-Ellison syndrome. Depressed values can mean gastric carcinoma; achlorhydria, pernicious anemia.

## PERITONEAL FLUID ANALYSIS
In this test, peritoneal fluid samples are extracted by abdominal paracentesis. Sample analysis includes inspection of gross appearance; determination of red and white blood cells, protein, glucose, amylase, ammonia, and alkaline phosphatase levels; and a check for the presence or absence of malignant cells, bacteria, and fungi.

Fluid accumulation in the peritoneal space (ascites) can result from inflammation, infection, tumor, or abdominal trauma or from liver, kidney, or cardiovascular disorders. Cloudy fluid with a high white blood cell count can mean bacterial peritonitis. Fluid containing blood suggests abdominal trauma or a tumor, especially hepatoma. A high amylase content usually indicates pancreatic dis-

## Sites evaluated by GI diagnostic tests

**Liver**
Endoscopic retrograde
  cholangiopancreatography
Percutaneous transhepatic
  cholangiography
Ultrasonography

**Duodenum**
Duodenoscopy
Small bowel enema
Small bowel series

**Gallbladder**
Biliary drainage test
Oral cholecystography
Ultrasonography

**Jejunum and ileum**
Small bowel enema
Small bowel series

**Pharynx**
Barium swallow

**Esophagus**
Acid perfusion test
Barium swallow
Esophageal manometry
Esophagoscopy
pH reflux studies

**Pancreas**
Computerized tomography
Endoscopic retrograde
cholangiopancreatography
Secretin test
Ultrasonography

**Stomach**
Gastric analysis
Gastric emptying studies
Gastroscopy
Upper GI series

**Colon and rectum**
Anorectal manometry
Barium enema
Colonoscopy
Proctoscopy
Sigmoidoscopy

ease. Bile-stained, green fluid can mean acute pancreatitis, ruptured gallbladder, or perforated intestine or duodenal ulcer. An elevated red blood cell count can mean tumor or tuberculosis; excessive elevation, intraabdominal trauma. Protein levels over 3 g/dl can mean malignancy; over 4 g/dl, tuberculosis. High ammonia levels indicate ruptured or strangulated intestine, ruptured ulcer, or ruptured appendix.

## FECAL ANALYSIS

Stool specimen analysis includes examination for occult blood, lipids, bacteria, fecal urobilinogen, and parasites. It's usually indicated with changed bowel habits, diarrhea, constipation, bleeding, or persistent abdominal pain.

Ask the patient to tell you when he feels the urge to defecate. Have clean equipment ready: bedpan, specimen container, and tongue blades. Advise the patient to avoid contaminating stool specimens with urine or toilet tissue.

To collect a random specimen, have the patient defecate into the bedpan. Transfer the stool to a container, using a tongue blade. Secure the lid, label the container, and send it to the laboratory or keep it refrigerated. To collect a timed specimen, begin the collection period with the first stool passed, then collect all stools for the prescribed time.

### Occult blood

Microscopic analysis or chemical testing detects occult blood in feces. Although small amounts of blood (2 to 2.5 ml/day) normally appear in feces, large amounts may indicate GI bleeding. Black, tarry stools (melena) suggest upper GI bleeding; dark maroon stools, lower intestinal bleeding.

Collect a random or timed specimen, as ordered, and test it on a premixed guaiac-impregnated paper such as Hemoccult. Check stool color immediately and again in 5 minutes. A dark blue reaction indicates a positive result; a light blue reaction, a weak positive result; a green reaction, normal.

GI bleeding can be a result of varices, peptic ulcer, carcinoma, ulcerative colitis, dysentery, or hemorrhagic disease. In approximately 80% of patients with colorectal cancer, fecal occult blood tests are positive. A positive test requires additional testing to evaluate the site and extent of bleeding. Common follow-up tests include barium swallow and colonoscopy.

## Lipids

The examination of feces for increased fat (steatorrhea) helps detect malabsorption. Two tests exist, one qualitative and the other quantitative. The Sudan stain, the qualitative test, is generally performed in two steps— first, screening for neutral fat (triglyceride) and then for split fat. The presence of excessive amounts of neutral fat may imply maldigestion; the presence of split fat, malabsorption. Stool samples from patients with pancreatic disease show a marked increase in neutral fat. In most patients with steatorrhea from other causes, there is no increase in neutral fat.

## Bacteria and parasites

Diarrhea can result from bacteria, such as *Escherichia coli, Vibrio cholerae, Shigella,* and *Salmonella;* or from parasites, such as *Giardia lamblia* and *Entamoeba histolytica.*

To allow examination of stools for bacteria, collect a specimen on each of 3 consecutive days. The presence of parasites in feces is difficult to confirm. The specimens should be sent immediately to the laboratory. The presence of *G. lamblia* in one stool is diagnostic.

## MOTILITY STUDIES

GI motility studies commonly evaluate abnormalities in esophageal and rectal peristalsis. Motility studies of the colon and small bowel are still investigational.

All studies use manometric catheters equipped to measure sphincter pressures. When asked to assist with a manometric test, make sure that you can tell your patient what to expect, and that you know how to help insert the catheter either orally or anally.

## Esophageal manometry

This test measures intraluminal pressures of the esophagus and its lower and upper sphincters; it also evaluates the quality of esophageal peristaltic contractions. The test is indicated for patients with dysphagia, odynophagia, heartburn, noncardiac chest pain, regurgitation, and inability to initiate swallows.

During the test, the patient swallows a manometric catheter containing a transducer along its length. Baseline pressures are measured at various esophageal levels, and sphincter pressures are measured before and after swallowing. The duration and sequence of peristaltic contractions are charted as a series of high-pressure peaks. An intraluminal pH electrode can also be attached alongside the catheter to measure intraesophageal pH and to assess gastroesophageal reflux. (Normal esophageal pH is between 6 and 7; a drop to less than 4 indicates reflux.)

Normal lower esophageal sphincter (LES) pressures range from 15 to 25 mm Hg. LES pressures of 0 to 5 mm Hg indicate an incompetent sphincter and are more likely to occur with gastroesophageal reflux. Low pressures may also indicate ascites, pernicious anemia, esophagitis, hiatal hernia, or scleroderma.

High LES pressures (up to 50 mm Hg) indicate a hypertensive sphincter. Causes may include achalasia, diffuse esophageal spasm, and esophageal diverticula or carcinoma.

Upper esophageal sphincter abnormalities occur in most patients with oropharyngeal dysphagia. They may also result from neuromuscular diseases, Zenker's diverticulum, and local and structural lesions, such as oropharyngeal carcinoma, pharyngeal abscess, and proximal esophageal webs.

Peristaltic abnormalities take various forms. Some patients may show changes in the amplitude of peristaltic contractions. Others may show multiple contractions following a swallow, simultaneous contractions without peristalsis following a swallow, spontaneous contractions without a swallow, or no response to a swallow.

In patients with achalasia, peristalsis is weak and absent throughout the esophagus. Patients with diffuse esophageal spasm may retain some peristalsis in the distal esophagus, but they experience simultaneous, repetitive, or spontaneous contractions elsewhere. Patients with esophageal scleroderma have little or no peristalsis in the lower two thirds of the esophagus.

Peristaltic abnormalities may also signal central nervous system disorders, such as multiple sclerosis, myasthenia gravis, and diabetic or alcoholic neuropathies.

## Anorectal manometry

Anorectal manometry, a relatively new test, measures internal and external anal sphincter pressures. It's indicated for patients with unexplained severe constipation, colonic dilation, or alternating constipation and diarrhea.

In this test, a catheter with a deflated balloon is inserted about 3⅞" (10 cm) into the rectum. Then the balloon is inflated and manometric measurements are made as the catheter is pulled back through the sphincters.

When the balloon is distended, the internal *(continued on page 42)*

# Blood and urine tests for GI disorders

| Test | Comments | Normal results | Implications of abnormal results |
|---|---|---|---|
| **Blood and serum** | | | |
| **Alkaline phosphatase** Measures for enzyme activity in bone, intestine, and in liver and biliary systems | | Men: 87 to 222 IU/liter Women: 60 to 197 IU/liter | *Increased* with cholestasis; biliary obstruction; liver metasis; viral, drug-induced, or chronic hepatitis; space-occupying hepatic lesions |
| **Gamma glutamyl transpeptidase (GGT)** Measures the enzyme activity in kidney tubules, liver, biliary tract epithelium, and pancreas; active in amino acid transport | Requires 24-hr alcohol abstention | Women over age 45 and men: 6 to 37 units/liter Women under age 45: 5 to 27 units/liter | *Increased* with acute liver disease (especially from chronic alcohol abuse), obstructive jaundice, liver metastasis, acute pancreatitis |
| **Bilirubin** Measures liver conjugation and excretion of this pigmentary product of erythrocyte breakdown   Indirect (unconjugated, or prehepatic form) | | 1.1 mg/dl or less | *Increased* with hemolytic disorders (from increased erythrocyte destruction), hepatocellular jaundice, viral hepatitis |
|   Direct (conjugated, or posthepatic form) | | Less than 0.5 mg/dl | *Increased* with biliary obstruction, hepatocellular jaundice, viral hepatitis |
| **Cholesterol** Measures liver metabolism and synthesis of this bile acid precursor | Requires overnight fast | 120 to 330 mg/dl | *Increased* with incipient hepatitis, lipid disorders, pancreatitis, or cholestasis resulting from biliary or alcohol disease *Decreased* with cirrhosis or malnutrition (except for biliary or alcoholic cirrhosis with cholestasis) |
| **Transaminases** Measures cytoplasmic enzymes that leak into plasma after cell damage   Serum glutamic-oxaloacetic transaminase (SGOT)   Serum glutamic-pyruvic transaminase (SGPT) |  More specific to liver cells and liver disease than SGOT | 8 to 20 units/liter  Men: 10 to 32 units/liter Women: 9 to 24 units/liter | *Increased SGOT or SGPT* with acute viral or drug-induced hepatitis, biliary obstruction or cirrhosis, pancreatitis, liver metastasis |
| **Lactic dehydrogenase (LDH)** Measures total enzyme level and levels of five isozymes released by damaged liver, heart, blood, and skeletal muscle cells | Isoenzyme LDH$_5$ specific to liver disease | LDH$_5$: 5.3% to 13.4% of total LDH Total LDH: 48 to 115 IU/liter | *Increased LDH$_5$* with hepatitis, cirrhosis, hepatic congestion |
| **Protein electrophoresis** Measures major blood proteins active in transporting bilirubin, fatty acids, and hormones (albumin); and lipids and hormones (globulins)   Albumin   Gamma globulin   Alpha globulin | | Total: 6.6 to 7.9 g/dl    Albumin: 3.3 to 4.5 g/dl Gamma: 0.5 to 1.6 g/dl Alpha$_1$: 0.1 to 0.4 g/dl Alpha$_2$: 0.5 to 1 g/dl | *Decreased albumin and increased gamma globulin* with cirrhosis *Increased alpha globulin* with carcinoma, primary biliary cirrhosis, infection |
| **Prothrombin time** Measures clotting time to determine activity of prothrombin and fibrinogen | | Men: 9.6 to 11.8 seconds Women: 9.5 to 11.3 seconds | *Increased* with vitamin K deficiency or liver disease; value over 2½ times normal probably indicates abnormal bleeding |
| **Ammonia** Measures ability of liver to detoxify ammonia | Arterial value preferred | Less than 50 mcg/dl | *Increased* with acute hepatic necrosis, hepatic encephalopathy, cirrhosis |

## Blood and serum (continued)

| Test | Comments | Normal results | Implications of abnormal results |
|------|----------|----------------|----------------------------------|
| **Hepatitis B surface antigen** Screens for latent or active hepatitis B virus | | Negative | *Present* with acute hepatitis B, chronic active hepatitis, carrier status, hepatoma (in 30% to 40% of patients) |
| **Alpha-fetoprotein** Diagnoses hepatoma (by immunologic assay) | | Nonpregnant patients: less than 30 ng/ml | *Increased* with hepatoma, pancreatic stomach, or biliary cancer |
| **Carotene** Screens for malabsorption of vitamin A precursor, normally absorbed with fats and transported by bile salts | | 48 to 200 mcg/dl | *Decreased* with intestinal fat malabsorption or biliary obstruction |
| **Amylase** Measures pancreatic enzyme active in digestion of starch and glycogen and released with pancreatic damage | | 60 to 180 Somogyi units/dl | *Increased* with acute pancreatitis, cholecystitis, common bile duct obstruction, intestinal obstruction *Normal or decreased* with chronic pancreatitis, cirrhosis, hepatitis |
| **Lipase** Measures pancreatic enzyme active in digestion of fats and released with pancreatic damage | | 32 to 80 units/liter | *Increased* with acute pancreatitis, pancreatic duct obstruction, pancreatic tumor, intestinal obstruction, biliary duct obstruction |
| **Oral glucose tolerance** (See urine test) | | | |
| **D-xylose** (See urine test) | | | |

## Urine

| Test | Comments | Normal results | Implications of abnormal results |
|------|----------|----------------|----------------------------------|
| **Bilirubin (direct)** Measures water-soluble direct form (fat-soluble indirect form never appears in urine) | Can be measured with dipstrip or 1 ictotest at bedside or in laboratory | 0.02 mg/dl | *Increased* with liver disease or biliary obstruction *Absent* with hemolytic anemia |
| **Urobilinogen** Measures ability of liver to process bilirubin reduction products | Can be measured at bedside with dipstrip or sent to laboratory in dark container (to prevent oxidation) | Men: 0.3 to 2.1 Ehrlich units/2 hr Women: 0.1 to 1.1 Ehrlich units/2 hr | *Increased* with hemolytic anemia, hepatitis, cirrhosis *Decreased* with congenital enzymatic jaundice or hemolytic anemia *Absent* with complete obstructive jaundice, and hepatic or extrahepatic biliary obstruction |
| **Oral glucose tolerance** Measures metabolic response to carbohydrate (glucose) | Oral glucose (Glucola) is given to the fasting patient | Serum: 160 to 180 mg/100 ml in 30 to 60 min; fasting levels in 2 to 3 hr   Urine: negative | *Decreased tolerance* (sharp peak, slow fall) with diabetes mellitus *Increased tolerance* (below normal peak) with malabsorption syndrome *Present* with diabetes mellitus |
| **Galactose tolerance** Measures ability of liver to convert galactose to glycogen | | Negative | *Present* with genetic disorders of galactose metabolism *Absent* with extrahepatic obstructive jaundice |
| **D-xylose** Evaluates intestinal absorption of this pentose sugar, normally passed through the liver and excreted intact | Requires overnight fast and ingestion of 25 g of D-xylose | Adults under age 65: Serum: 25 to 40 mg/dl in 2 hr Urine: more than 4 g in 5 hr Adults 65 and older: Serum: 25 to 40 mg/dl in 2 hr Urine: more than 3.5 g in 5 hr and more than 5 g in 24 hr | *Decreased* with cirrhosis, sprue, regional ileitis (jejunum), Whipple's disease, multiple jejunal diverticula |
| **Schilling test** Evaluates intestinal absorption of vitamin $B_{12}$ | | 8% to 40% of original dose of radioactive vitamin $B_{12}$/24 hr | *Decreased* with ileal dysfunction, pernicious anemia, pancreatic insufficiency, bacterial proliferation |

sphincter should relax and the external sphincter should contract. If the external sphincter relaxes, the cause may be loss of muscle tone from aging, cerebrovascular disease, paraplegia, or rectoperineal surgery.

## CONTRAST RADIOGRAPHY

In the tests discussed here, the patient is given a contrast medium (see *Selecting a contrast medium*), and the radiologist observes the medium's action by fluoroscopy. Still photographs (spot films) can be taken during radiography to record areas for later study. Cineradiography, a recent development, allows for filming GI motion—a useful tool for detecting esophageal motility disorders.

The radiologist chooses either a single- or double-contrast study. In single-contrast studies, dilute barium sulfate is used to distend the lumen, and lesions are seen by compression or profile. This method is preferred for patients with suspected diverticulitis or obstruction or for patients who are immobile or unable to cooperate.

In double-contrast (air-contrast) studies, a thin layer of dense barium sulfate is used to line the lumen, which is then distended with air. This method is preferred for viewing mucosal detail, locating polyps, and finding erosive gastritis, inflammatory bowel disease, or early carcinoma.

### Barium swallow

A barium swallow test allows examination of both the pharynx and the esophagus.

An overnight fast precedes the test. Then, as the patient swallows a thick mixture of barium sulfate, cineradiography is used to record pharyngeal action. Next, as the patient swallows the mixture, fluoroscopy is used to examine passage of the liquid through the esophagus. Spot films of the esophageal region may also be taken, usually from lateral angles and from right and left posteroanterior angles.

This test is often done for patients with histories of dysphagia, odynophagia, heartburn, or regurgitation. It can detect strictures, ulcers, tumors, polyps, diverticula, hiatal hernias, esophageal webs, motility disorders, and sometimes achalasia. To detect gastroesophageal reflux and sliding hiatal hernia, the patient may be placed in Trendelenburg's position during the test. Barium swallow results may need confirmation by other tests, such as manometry and endoscopic biopsy.

If a patient scheduled for a barium swallow is also scheduled for cholangiography or a barium enema, be sure barium enema or cholangiography precedes barium swallow, because ingested barium can cloud details on X-ray films.

### Upper GI series

An upper GI series extends the barium swallow by fluoroscopically tracking ingested barium sulfate from the esophagus through the stomach. It's usually combined with a small bowel series, which follows the contrast agent on through the small intestine. Both single- and double-contrast techniques may be used.

When the barium enters the esophagus, its progress is monitored, and spot films may be taken from lateral and right and left posteroanterior angles. When the barium enters the stomach, the patient is turned to coat the stomach lining. If a double-contrast examination is needed, the patient is given tablets, powders, or granules that release carbon dioxide. Glucagon may be given to delay gastric emptying, but not if gastric motility disorders are suspected.

The upper GI series is used to evaluate patients who have trouble swallowing, who regurgitate food, or who report burning or gnawing epigastric pain. It's also used for patients whose nausea, vomiting, and weight loss suggest small bowel disease or for those who show signs of GI bleeding, such as hematemesis and melena. The series helps diagnose gastritis, carcinoma, nervous disorders, hiatal hernias, diverticula, strictures, and (most commonly) gastric and duodenal ulcers.

If the patient has an ulcer, it will fill with barium during a single-contrast study and appear the same on all films. Compression films must be taken or the ulcer may be missed. If a double-contrast study is done, the ulcer will appear empty and outlined with barium.

Radiographic studies revealing tumors or ulcers may suggest, but not confirm, malignancy. For example, malignant tumors appear on X-rays as filling defects that disrupt peristalsis; benign tumors, as nondisruptive outpouchings in the gastric mucosa. Malignant ulcers generally have folds radiating beyond the ulcer crater; benign ulcers, folds radiating only to the crater. Suspected malignancy requires confirmation by biopsy.

An upper GI series can also suggest motility disorders. If a patient's distal esophagus has the appearance of a beak, he may have achalasia. If barium backs up from his stomach into his esophagus, he may have gastroesophageal reflux. But, diagnosis of most motility disorders requires manometry studies.

Oral cholecystography, barium enema, and routine radiography, when ordered, should precede the upper GI series, because ingested barium can cloud subsequent X-rays.

## Small bowel series and enema
The small bowel series and enema require the same fasting preparation as the upper GI series. The patient ingests barium sulfate, and fluoroscopy follows its path through the small intestine. Spot films are taken at specified intervals until the barium reaches the ileocecal valve, usually 45 to 90 minutes after ingestion. For patients with diseases that inhibit small bowel motility (for example, diabetes, sprue, and scleroderma), this time will be longer. A continuous barium column must be maintained, or lesions may be missed.

The small bowel enema is more time-consuming and uncomfortable than the small bowel series, but it distends the bowel better, making lesions easier to identify. The test involves inserting a nasogastric tube, positioning it through the pylorus, and advancing it to the ligament of Treitz. Barium is then quickly infused, followed by water or methylcellulose if a double-contrast study has been ordered.

The small bowel series and enema are indicated with persistent diarrhea or weight loss. Test results may demonstrate small ulcerations and edematous changes, indicating regional ileitis; flecking or fragmenting of the barium, indicating malabsorption syndrome; or filling defects, indicating Hodgkin's disease or lymphosarcoma. Test results may also demonstrate bowel dilation, indicating obstruction, motility disorders, or sprue; thick, distorted fold patterns, indicating amyloidosis, giardiasis, or lymphoma; or thick, regular patterns, indicating ischemia, bleeding, or inflammation. Thickened bowel wall sections interspersed with nodular, narrow sections may indicate regional ileitis.

Small bowel disorders are highly diverse, and generally need further tests to confirm diagnosis. Remember, though, that oral cholecystography, barium enema, and routine radiography, when ordered, should precede tests involving barium ingestion.

## Barium enema
Barium enema, the most common test for suspected lower intestinal disorders, allows radiographic study of the large intestine after barium sulfate is given rectally. Indications include altered bowel habits; lower abdominal pain; and blood, mucus, or pus in the stool. The test helps diagnose inflammatory disorders, colorectal cancer, polyps, diverticula, and large-intestine structural changes such as intussusception.

Either single- or double-contrast studies can be done. Although deep ulcers will show up on a single-contrast study, inflammatory bowel disease may not. Polyps, small mucosal lesions, and subtle, ulcer-caused intestinal bleeding show up better on double-contrast studies. Because proctosigmoidoscopy provides a better view of the rectosigmoid region, it often precedes barium enema.

Before a barium enema, the patient's colon must be free of stool. The prescribed pre-test regimen usually includes restriction to clear liquids and use of laxatives and cleansing enemas. During the test, the patient must "hold onto" the barium; if he can't, insert an enema catheter with an inflatable balloon to retain it. As the barium fills the intestine, spot and compression films are taken. If the double-contrast technique is used, air is injected into the intestine after the barium.

Inflammatory lesions usually appear diffuse, whereas malignant lesions are more sharply defined and filled. A definitive diagnosis of cancer usually requires a biopsy.

## Angiography
Angiography, the radiographic contrast study of the vascular system, can be used to determine the site of GI bleeding and to detect ischemia or angiodysplasia.

In celiac and mesenteric arteriography, a contrast medium is injected into the celiac, superior mesenteric, or inferior mesenteric artery after an 8-hour fast and administration of a cathartic. As the medium flows through the abdominal vasculature, serial radiographs outline the vessels in the arterial, capillary, and venous phases of perfusion.

If angiography reveals the site of GI bleeding, vasopressin may be infused to stem the bleeding. If this doesn't work, the offending artery may be embolized with embolic material, such as aminocaproic acid (Amicar), or an absorbable gelatin sponge (Gelfoam).

## Oral cholecystography
Oral cholecystography allows study of the gallbladder to detect gallstones or to diagnose inflammatory disease or tumors.

## Selecting a contrast medium
Most GI radiographic tests use either barium sulfate or diatrizoate meglumine (Gastrografin) as a contrast medium.

Barium sulfate is better for visualizing mucosal detail, so it's usually preferred. It's also preferred if aspiration is suspected, because Gastrografin is hyperosmolar and could cause pulmonary edema if aspirated into the lungs. The specific barium sulfate preparation used depends on the area to be studied and whether a single- or double-contrast test is to be done.

Gastrografin is preferred when perforation is suspected, especially peritoneal perforation. Because it's water soluble and rapidly reabsorbed, it can leak into the peritoneal cavity without causing problems. Often, Gastrografin is used first to check for perforation, and, if none exists, it's followed with barium sulfate.

# ERCP: Radiography and endoscopy

Endoscopic retrograde cholangiopancreatography (ERCP) uses both radiography and endoscopy to examine the pancreatic ducts and the hepatobiliary tree.

A small, side-viewing endoscope is advanced through the patient's mouth, esophagus, stomach, and duodenum until the ampulla of Vater can be seen. A contrast medium is injected by passing a cannula through the endoscope. Both pancreatic and biliary systems may be visualized.

ERCP is done for patients with suspected pancreatic disease and jaundice of unknown origin and to diagnose duct stones, pancreatic cancer, and cancer of the duodenal papillae or biliary ducts. It's also used to locate cysts, calculi, and stenosis in the pancreatic ducts and hepatobiliary tree, particularly when other radiographic studies, such as ultrasonography, computerized tomography, liver scans, and biliary tract X-rays, are inconclusive.

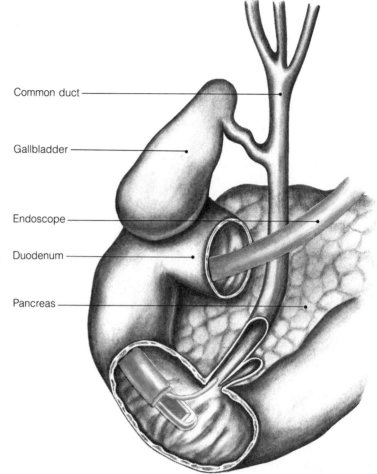

Common duct

Gallbladder

Endoscope

Duodenum

Pancreas

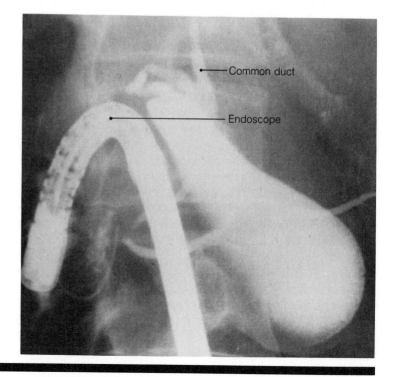

Common duct

Endoscope

Before the test the patient ingests a contrast medium, usually iopanoic acid (Telepaque) tablets. (Be sure the patient isn't allergic to iodine.) When the contrast medium reaches the small intestine, it's filtered by the liver, excreted in the bile, and stored in the gallbladder. The gallbladder is then examined fluoroscopically, and spot films are taken.

If the gallbladder fails to opacify, the patient may have gallstones that stop the contrast material from entering the gallbladder. Or he may have an inflammatory disease, such as cholecystitis or cholelithiasis, that impairs the gallbladder's concentrating ability. He may also have GI symptoms that stop the contrast material from reaching the gallbladder, such as vomiting, diarrhea, gastric or esophageal strictures, malabsorption disorders, liver disease, or elevated (over 2%) bilirubin levels. Because about 25% of healthy patients show little or no gallbladder visualization after a single dose of Telepaque, the test should be repeated to confirm a GI disorder.

After the gallbladder's filling capacity has been examined, the patient may be given a fat stimulus. This will cause the contrast medium to empty into the common bile duct and small intestine, allowing fluoroscopic study of common bile duct patency.

### Percutaneous transhepatic cholangiography
This test allows fluoroscopic examination of the biliary ducts after a fast and injection of a contrast medium into a biliary radicle. The test opacifies the biliary ducts independently of function.

Percutaneous transhepatic cholangiography helps assess biliary duct obstruction and helps differentiate extrahepatic from intrahepatic obstructive jaundice. But with suspected obstructive jaundice, noninvasive procedures are usually performed first.

## ULTRASONOGRAPHY AND COMPUTERIZED TOMOGRAPHY
Cheaper than CT scan and posing no risk of radiation, ultrasonography is preferred in cases where either test produces equally accurate results (for example, in diagnosing biliary tract and liver disease). But CT scan is preferred for examining the pancreas and for examining obese patients.

### Ultrasonography
Besides differentiating between obstructive and nonobstructive jaundice, ultrasonic examination of the gallbladder and biliary system helps diagnose cholelithiasis and cholecystitis when results of cholecystography are inconclusive. Although ultrasonography can detect gallstones, polyps, and carcinoma in the gallbladder and is highly accurate in assessing biliary duct size, it can't always identify the cause of biliary obstruction.

Liver ultrasonography can detect metastases and hematomas and can be used with liver-spleen scanning to identify cold spots—areas that don't pick up the radionuclide—as tumors, abscesses, or cysts.

Pancreatic ultrasonography aids diagnosis of pancreatitis, pseudocysts, and pancreatic carcinoma. Splenic ultrasonography identifies splenomegaly and, when used after liver-spleen scanning, identifies cold spots as cystic or solid lesions.

### CT scan
CT scan, computer-assisted cross-sectional X-ray, detects mainly biliary tract, liver, and pancreatic disorders. The test can be done with or without a contrast medium, but using a medium accentuates tissue density differences and helps detect biliary dilation.

CT views of the biliary tract and liver can detect disease; distinguish between obstructive and nonobstructive jaundice; and identify abscesses, cysts, hematomas, and tumors. Views of the pancreas can detect carcinoma, abscesses, pseudocysts, and acute and chronic pancreatitis. If tumors are found, biopsy may be necessary to determine malignancy.

Barium studies, when ordered, should be performed at least 4 days before CT scan.

## NUCLEAR IMAGING
Nuclear imaging examines concentrations of ingested or injected radiopaque substances in the body. Because the substances contain only traces of radioactivity, they pose little or no danger to patients. However, radioactive uptake in one test can cloud the results of other tests, so no more than one radionuclide study can be scheduled on the same day.

### Gastric emptying studies
These radionuclide studies assess ability to empty solid or liquid material. They're commonly done for patients with emptying disorders resulting from peptic ulcer, ulcer surgery, diabetes, or gastric neoplasia.

In a solid emptying study, the patient eats a cooked egg white containing the sulfur colloid 99m technetium ($^{99m}$Tc). He's then placed in a supine position under a gamma camera, and images are recorded every 2 minutes for 60 minutes. In a liquid emptying study, the patient drinks 150 ml of orange juice and 150 ml of normal saline solution containing $^{99m}$Tc.

### Liver-spleen scanning

Nuclear imaging of the liver and spleen is usually the best way to find hepatocellular disease, hepatic metastases, and focal disease. It also helps diagnose hepatomegaly, splenomegaly, and hematoma after abdominal trauma. But, it is nonspecific for focal disease, and it may not find tumors, cysts, and abscesses smaller than ¾″ (2 cm) in diameter.

The test begins with an I.V. injection of a colloid such as $^{99m}$Tc. Next, the patient is positioned under a rectilinear scanner or a gamma camera to record the distribution of radioactivity in the liver and spleen.

In a healthy patient, the liver and spleen images appear equally bright. Any difference in intensity indicates a difference in colloidal uptake. If the spleen shows greater uptake than the liver, the patient could have cirrhosis, chronic active hepatitis, or portal hypertension from extrahepatic causes.

Patchy colloid distribution with an enlarged liver and spleen may mean cirrhosis; even distribution with liver enlargement, hepatitis. Focal defects—tumors, cysts, and abscesses—appear as cold spots, areas of no uptake. Metastases need biopsy to confirm diagnosis, cysts need ultrasonography, and abscesses need gallium scanning or ultrasonography.

Nuclear imaging can also locate sites of GI bleeding, especially in patients who don't require immediate attention. The patient is given an I.V. injection of $^{99m}$Tc, then studied under a scintillation camera. Normally, the bleeding site must be detected within 10 to 15 minutes following injection. After this interval, the liver, spleen, and kidneys take up too much of the colloid, making detection difficult.

### HIDA scan

The HIDA scan (technetium-labeled iminodiacetic acid [$^{99m}$Tc HIDA]), a recent procedure, evaluates hepatobiliary function. It's useful in diagnosing acute cholecystitis, and, because it requires less patient preparation, it provides quicker results than oral cholecystography.

After a fast, the patient receives an I.V. injection of $^{99m}$Tc HIDA. A gamma camera is used to record the colloid's progress through the liver, bile ducts, gallbladder, and duodenum. Too little radioactivity in the liver

suggests hepatocellular disease; none at all in the gallbladder and duodenum, biliary obstruction.

### ENDOSCOPY

In GI endoscopy, a fiberoptic endoscope is passed through the patient's mouth and into his esophagus, stomach, and duodenum; or it is passed through his anus and into his large intestine. Because endoscopy is an invasive procedure, it usually follows radiographic studies in a diagnostic GI workup.

Endoscopy is becoming more popular. Technology has made fiberoptic instruments more flexible and their use more tolerable. Also, endoscopy allows specimens to be taken under direct vision, using biopsy, lavage, cytology brush, or culture swab; and it permits removal of polyps and other foreign bodies.

Endoscopy can be used to confirm X-ray findings and, when combined with biopsy, to differentiate between benign and malignant lesions. Because endoscopy allows close internal examination of tissue, it sometimes identifies small or surface lesions undetected by X-ray. Finally, endoscopy uses no radiation.

### Esophagogastroduodenoscopy

Esophagogastroduodenoscopy allows visualization of the esophageal, stomach, and upper duodenal lining via an endoscope passed through the patient's mouth into his esophagus, then down into his stomach and duodenum.

The procedure detects inflammation, ulcers, varices, strictures, hiatal hernias, mucosal lesions, periampullar carcinoma, regional ileitis, and Mallory-Weiss syndrome. It can be used to detect small or surface lesions that don't show up on X-rays, to differentiate between gastric and duodenal ulcers, and (when used with a barium swallow) to differentiate between benign and malignant ulcers.

Esophagogastroduodenoscopy is often indicated for patients with acute or chronic GI bleeding, pernicious anemia, esophageal injury, dysphagia, odynophagia, substernal pain, and persistent epigastric discomfort unexplained by X-ray findings.

### Proctosigmoidoscopy

Proctosigmoidoscopy provides visualization of the distal sigmoid colon, the rectum, and the anal canal. First, the anal sphincters are examined digitally. Then a rigid sigmoidoscope is inserted into the anus to examine the rectum and distal sigmoid colon. (If a flexible

# Assisting during colonoscopy

To guide your patient through a colonoscopy, first review your understanding of the procedure. In this test, a colonoscope is inserted into the anus, after which a small amount of air is insufflated to locate the bowel lumen. The scope is then advanced through the rectum into the sigmoid colon. After the scope has passed the splenic flexure, it's advanced through the transverse colon and the hepatic flexure into the ascending colon and cecum.

Abdominal palpation or fluoroscopy may guide the colonoscope through the large intestine. If the scope's tip gets lodged in the colon, fluoroscopy can help locate it and adjust the entry angle. During the examination, suction may be used to remove blood or secretions that obscure vision.

Biopsy forceps or a cytology brush may be passed via a channel in the colonoscope to get specimens for histologic and cytologic examination, respectively; an electrocautery snare may be used to remove polyps.

### Prepare the patient
• Explain to the patient that this test permits examination of the large intestine's lining. Tell him that a flexible instrument will be passed through his anus and that the procedure takes approximately 30 to 60 minutes. Assure him that the colonoscope is well lubricated to ease its insertion, that it will feel cool at first, and that he may feel the urge to defecate when it's inserted and advanced. Tell him who will perform the test and where.
• Advise the patient that his large intestine must be thoroughly clean in order to be clearly visible. Instruct him to maintain a clear liquid diet for 48 hours before the test and a complete fast for 8 hours before the test.
• On the evening before the test, give him 3 tbsp (45 ml) castor oil or 10 oz (296 ml) magnesium citrate. Give warm tap water or sodium biphosphate enemas 3 to 4 hours before the test, as ordered, until the return is clear. (Preps may vary depending on the institution). Don't administer a soapsuds enema, because this irritates the mucosa and stimulates mucous secretions, hindering the examination.
• Tell the patient that he may receive a sedative such as diazepam (Valium) during the procedure to help him relax.

### Assist during the procedure
• Place the patient on his left side with his knees flexed, and drape him. (Patient's position may need to be changed if there is difficulty advancing the scope.) Tell him to breathe deeply and slowly through his mouth as the doctor inserts his gloved, lubricated index finger into the anus and rectum and palpates the mucosa. After a water-soluble lubricant has been applied to the patient's anus and to the colonoscope tip, tell the patient that the colonoscope is about to be inserted.
• When the scope reaches the descending sigmoid junction, if necessary, help the patient to a supine position. This will smooth the scope's advance and may also help it negotiate the splenic flexure.
• If the examiner removes a tissue specimen, immediately place it in a specimen bottle containing 10% formalin; immediately place cytology smears in a Copeland jar containing 95% ethyl alcohol.
• During the test, watch vital signs and be supportive.
• Afterwards, encourage the patient to rest and to expel the air in his bowel. Also, watch for complications (intestinal perforation, excessive bleeding, and retroperitoneal emphysema).

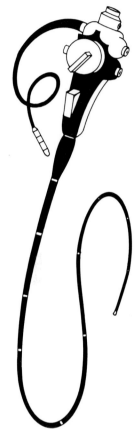

sigmoidoscope is used, the descending colon can also be seen; if a rigid sigmoidoscope is used, the procedure can be done at bedside because the sigmoidoscope is portable.) Finally, a proctoscope, a rigid instrument that is shorter than a sigmoidoscope, is inserted into the anus to further examine the lower rectum and anal canal.

Proctosigmoidoscopy is done for patients with diarrhea, constipation, rectal bleeding, and abdominal pain—usually to supplement other inconclusive tests or to confirm radiographic findings. It helps detect hemorrhoids, hypertrophic anal papillae, polyps, fissures, fistulas, abscesses, and inflammatory, infectious, and ulcerative bowel disease.

Proctosigmoidoscopy identifies colon cancer in about 50% of patients with the disease. With biopsy, it helps distinguish malignant from benign tumors. Proctoscopy is routine before a barium enema, because a barium enema doesn't adequately visualize the colon's lower 6″ to 10″ (15 to 25 cm).

### Colonoscopy
When proctosigmoidoscopy and a barium enema yield negative or inconclusive results, colonoscopy can be performed. This procedure examines the lining of the large intestine, using a flexible endoscope inserted anally. Abdominal palpation may help advance the endoscope through the intestine, and fluoroscopy can be performed as it moves. (See *Assisting during colonoscopy.*)

# Inserting GI tubes

**Nasogastric tube**

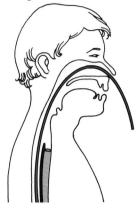

**Orogastric tube**

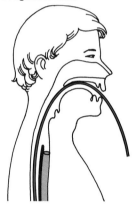

You may be asked to insert, or to assist during insertion of, a gastric or duodenal tube during testing for gastrointestinal disorders. The test's success—and the patient's safety—may depend on how well you prepare the patient and how skillfully you handle the tube.

Some tubes are passed nasally; others, orally. For example, a gastric analysis test requires a Levin or other nasogastric (NG) tube. A biliary drainage test requires an oral duodenal tube, such as a Rehfuss. When a patient has a deviated septum or has had nasal surgery, you may have to pass an NG tube orally, though this route is less comfortable for the patient.

### Prepare the patient
• First, give the patient written material explaining the test purpose and how it will be conducted. Also, supply pre-test instructions, such as fasting times.
• If the patient wears dentures or glasses, have him remove them when you insert the tube. With most tests, he'll be able to wear them after the tube's in place. If the test requires a long waiting period, tell the patient beforehand, so he can bring something to read or otherwise occupy himself.
• Show the patient relaxation techniques he can use during the procedure, and offer him emotional support.

### Insert the tube
• If the test calls for a Levin tube, use a #16 or 18 French. To measure the proper length, place the tube's distal end at the tip of the patient's nose, and run the tube to his earlobe and from there to the tip of his xiphoid process.

The average adult's pylorus is at the 55- to 60-cm level, so any tube inserted beyond that mark will likely begin to kink. (If a patient has had a gastric resection, position the tube at the 50-cm level and confirm by fluoroscopy.)
• Smear a water-soluble lubricant over the tube's distal end, but don't plug the openings. Make sure the tube has no sharp edges or burrs.
• *Nasal tube passage.* Place the patient in a sitting position, and insert the tube into the nostril through which he breathes more easily, usually the larger one. Rotate the tube inward as you advance it. Continue with a slight downward deflection until the patient feels the tube in the back of his throat.
• *Oral tube passage.* Position the tube's distal end far back on the patient's tongue. Then ask him to flex his head and to swallow with his teeth apart.
• With either insertion, ask the patient to swallow as you advance the tube. If the test allows him to have water, ask him to sip some through a straw, and advance the tube a few inches with each swallow.
• When you've inserted the tube, confirm placement of the distal end in the patient's stomach by aspirating stomach contents, by injecting a little air into the tube and auscultating gurgling in the epigastric region, or by fluoroscopy. Note: If the patient coughs frequently during insertion, the tube may be in his trachea or coiled in his pharynx. If so, remove it immediately, let him rest, and begin again.

Colonoscopy is indicated with a history of undiagnosed constipation and diarrhea, anorexia, persistent rectal bleeding, or lower abdominal pain or to confirm conditions diagnosed by other means, such as radiographic studies. It's used to diagnose inflammatory and ulcerative bowel disease and colonic strictures and lesions, to locate the origin of lower GI bleeding, and to check for recurring polyps or malignant lesions. It's also helpful as a follow-up test in inflammatory bowel disease.

## OTHER STUDIES
Various other tests help diagnose GI disorders. Of those described below, the first five are invasive tests; the sixth, noninvasive.

### Small bowel biopsy
In small bowel biopsy, a mucosal specimen is evaluated for malabsorption disorders.

The procedure requires the patient to swallow a tube and capsule, which is fluoroscopically guided through the stomach and into the small bowel to the ligament of Treitz, the preferred biopsy site.

Small bowel biopsy can confirm diagnoses of small bowel disorders and differentiate malabsorption syndromes. A dilated lacteal system indicates lymphangiectasis; villous atrophy with plasma-cell infiltration in the lamina propria indicates nontropical (celiac) sprue. Clubbed villi with normal epithelial cells indicate Whipple's disease.

This test can be performed as an inpatient or outpatient procedure.

### Percutaneous liver biopsy
Percutaneous liver biopsy involves needle aspiration of a segment of core tissue for histologic analysis.

Be sure the patient has fasted for 6 hours

before the test, which is usually done at the patient's bedside using a local anesthetic. During insertion of the needle, tell the patient to exhale and hold his breath on expiration for 5 to 10 seconds to prevent accidental puncture of the pleural cavity or diaphragm. (See *Performing a liver biopsy,* page 50.)

This procedure helps confirm diffuse hepatocellular diseases, such as cirrhosis and hepatitis, and multifocal lesions, such as tumors and granulomas. Liver biopsy is contraindicated in patients with clotting defects.

## Secretin test
This 3-hour test most accurately measures pancreatic exocrine function, the secretion of enzymes, water, and electrolytes into the duodenum.

Begin the test by inserting a double-lumen nasogastric tube into the stomach. Once the double lumen is passed into the stomach, continuous aspiration of the stomach begins. The proximal lumen end is attached to continuous suction so there is no further contamination of duodenal contents. Collect three 20-minute basal collections. Then, have the doctor inject the secretin I.V. Collect four more 20-minute collections. Make sure to collect all specimens under oil and keep them refrigerated until you can send them to the laboratory for analysis.

If the collected fluid is voluminous or if it shows abnormally high bicarbonate or enzyme levels, the patient may have pancreatic carcinoma, pancreatic ductal obstruction, chronic pancreatitis, or advanced pancreatic insufficiency.

## Acid perfusion test
The acid perfusion (Bernstein) test helps differentiate epigastric or retrosternal pain caused by angina pectoris from pain caused by esophagitis. This test is best performed during the esophageal manometric study to detect motility changes and pain.

If you're asked to perform this test, first be sure your patient abstains from antacids for 24 hours, food for 12 hours, and fluids and smoking for 8 hours. Then insert a nasogastric tube, marked 30 cm (11¾″) from the tip, into the patient's stomach and aspirate the contents. Then withdraw the tube to the 30-cm mark, which places its end in the esophagus.

Alternately instill 0.9% normal saline solution and 0.1-*normal* HCl solution through the tube, without telling the patient when you change solutions. If he has pain or burning during perfusion of the acidic solution, he may have esophagitis. Immediately return to the saline solution until his pain subsides. Confirm the results, if ordered, by repeating perfusion of both solutions. If the patient experiences no discomfort after 30 minutes of acidic perfusion, the results are negative.

Occasionally, a patient with esophagitis has pain during perfusion of both solutions. Also, a patient with asymptomatic esophagitis may have no pain during the test.

## Biliary drainage test
This test aids diagnosis of cholelithiasis when cholecystogram results are inconclusive or incompatible with clinical signs and symptoms. It evaluates bile for white blood cells, cholesterol crystals, mucus, bacteria, and parasites such as *G. lamblia.*

Be sure the patient fasts for 8 hours before the test. Then, insert a single-lumen tube, such as a Rehfuss tube, into the stomach and aspirate contents. Slowly advance the tube until aspirated secretions become clear, golden, and alkaline, indicating correct duodenal placement. Collect "A" bile (clear, golden bile in the duodenum).

Next, to increase the flow of bile into the duodenum, instill 30 to 45 ml of warmed magnesium sulfate (33% solution), or give an I.V. injection of .02 mcg/kg body weight of sincalide (Kinevac). You should obtain 30 to 60 ml of "B" bile (concentrated bile from gallbladder), which can be centrifuged and analyzed microscopically.

Cholesterol crystals and calcium bilirubinate pigment usually indicate cholelithiasis.

## NURSING ROLE IN DIAGNOSTIC STUDIES
GI tests are often tedious, frightening, uncomfortable, and even painful for the patient. So you have an important role in helping patients through such tests.

## Prepare patients physically
When more than one test is ordered, make sure scheduling is proper. For example, a barium enema should be scheduled several days before a small bowel or upper GI series, because barium takes that long to pass through the GI tract.

A test's success may depend on adequate pre-test preparation. Check the patient's history for hypersensitivity to iodine (ask about seafood allergies) or contrast media and obtain signed consent forms for invasive tests.

Know which tests require fasting and for

## Performing a liver biopsy

To perform percutaneous liver biopsy using a Menghini needle, the doctor follows these steps:

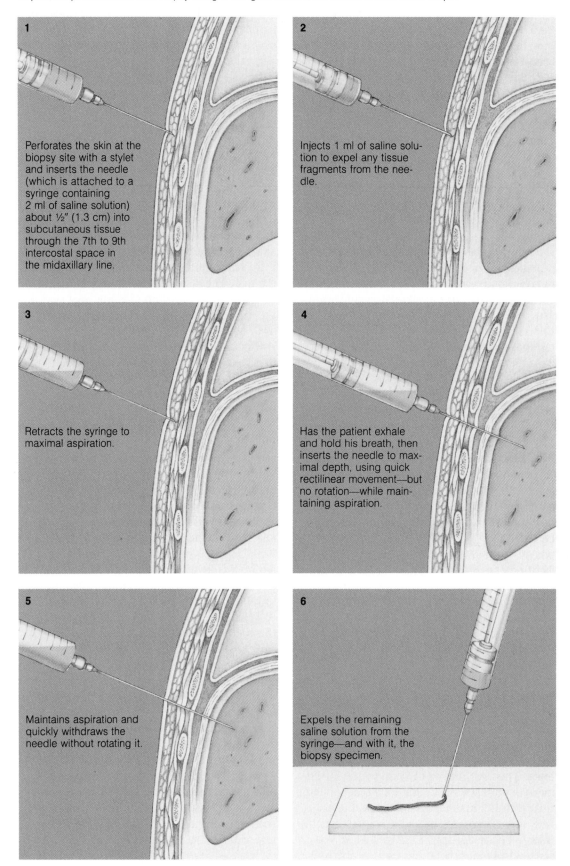

**1**
Perforates the skin at the biopsy site with a stylet and inserts the needle (which is attached to a syringe containing 2 ml of saline solution) about ½" (1.3 cm) into subcutaneous tissue through the 7th to 9th intercostal space in the midaxillary line.

**2**
Injects 1 ml of saline solution to expel any tissue fragments from the needle.

**3**
Retracts the syringe to maximal aspiration.

**4**
Has the patient exhale and hold his breath, then inserts the needle to maximal depth, using quick rectilinear movement—but no rotation—while maintaining aspiration.

**5**
Maintains aspiration and quickly withdraws the needle without rotating it.

**6**
Expels the remaining saline solution from the syringe—and with it, the biopsy specimen.

how long and which require advance medication. For example, endoscopy requires fasting for at least 6 hours before administration. Oral cholecystography requires Telepaque tablets the night before, and I.V. cholangiography may require injections of Cholografin 6 to 24 hours before.

If your patient's scheduled for lower intestinal studies, such as colonoscopy, remember to have him ingest clear liquids for at least 2 days. Give oral laxatives and enemas to clear the colon of residual feces that could obscure results.

Don't give enemas the last 2 to 4 hours before a barium enema; doing so can cause irritation, increased mucus secretion, and motility changes. When giving enemas to the elderly and those with abdominal distention, watch for perforation: abdominal pain, fever, weakness, a drop in blood pressure, a rise in pulse rate, and bleeding from the rectum. And after repeated enemas, watch for potassium depletion and sodium retention.

Be sure you understand how medications and diet influence test results. For example, don't give nitrates to patients scheduled for esophageal manometry for diagnosis of diffuse esophageal spasm, because nitrates would mask results. And see that patients scheduled for contrast studies observe diet restrictions.

### Prepare patients emotionally
Give emotional support before, during, and after tests. Before, tell the patient and his family what the test is, why it's being done, how long it will last, any medications that will be given, and what the patient will feel. Emphasize any pre-test instructions, such as fasting periods, and explain the reason for them. Also explain the post-test care you'll give and what complications are possible.

### Put patients at ease
Most GI studies cause some anxiety. Anxiety can cause palpitations, hyperventilation, increased gastric acid secretion, and intestinal spasm, thereby increasing discomfort and altering the results of some tests. It can also result in pylorospasm, delayed gastric emptying, and colonic spasm that prevents barium retention during radiography. Anxiety may even make some tests inadvisable—endoscopy, for example, which requires patient cooperation to minimize the risk of perforation.

Reducing the patient's stress relieves his discomfort, lowers the risks, and helps ensure accurate test results.

### Be ready to assist in testing
You should be ready to help with most GI tests. Have sedatives, such as diazepam, on hand—after checking for patient allergies to medications. When appropriate, have atropine or glucagon ready to decrease saliva, gastric secretions, and motility. Remember, medications given during testing can alter level of consciousness. So take precautions, such as removing a patient's dentures.

Have suction available to remove oral secretions and to prevent aspiration. In procedures where secretions drain from the patient's mouth, position the patient on his left side with his chin tilted downward. Monitor vital signs and ensure a patent airway.

You'll be asked to help collect most stool, urine, and blood specimens. Have the needed equipment ready, oversee specimen collection, and deliver labeled specimens to the laboratory. Also know how to help during such procedures as percutaneous liver biopsy.

### Monitor patients after testing
After diagnostic tests, especially invasive ones, monitor vital signs. Watch for bleeding, pain, and dyspnea. If a topical anesthetic was used to anesthetize the patient's throat, check for the gag reflex before allowing oral food and fluid intake.

After liver biopsy, tell the patient to lie on his right side for 1 to 2 hours. Check for bleeding, bile peritonitis, and pneumothorax. Signs of bleeding into the liver include shock, tenderness, and rigidity around the puncture site. Maintain bed rest for 24 hours. Expect the patient to feel localized pain and referred shoulder pain, but report prolonged pain.

Monitor elimination of barium after tests that use it. Give a mild laxative, if needed.

Remember, most diagnostic tests tire patients both physically and mentally. Provide a peaceful environment for rest afterward and, if appropriate, limit visitors.

### Interpret diagnostic tests
When tests are completed, you'll be using results to interpret signs and symptoms, to determine the patient's needs, to establish a nursing diagnosis, and to evaluate progress.

You'll be called on to explain the medical and nursing diagnoses to the patient and to identify needed therapies, preventive measures, and life-style changes. Offering emotional support and allowing time for discussion will help him accept his diagnosis and make therapy successful.

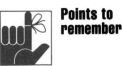

**Points to remember**

• Diagnostic tests for GI disorders can be extensive and complicated. Commonly, patients have many vague symptoms that necessitate multiple testing.
• You need to understand GI tests because they can involve you at every stage: preparation, procedure, and follow-up care.
• Most GI tests involve some patient discomfort, so your role in preparing your patients physically and emotionally is crucial.
• A patient's diet or medications can influence test results, so for some tests you'll have to set restrictions.
• After testing, regularly assess the patient's physical and mental needs to ensure optimal care and to help establish an accurate diagnosis.

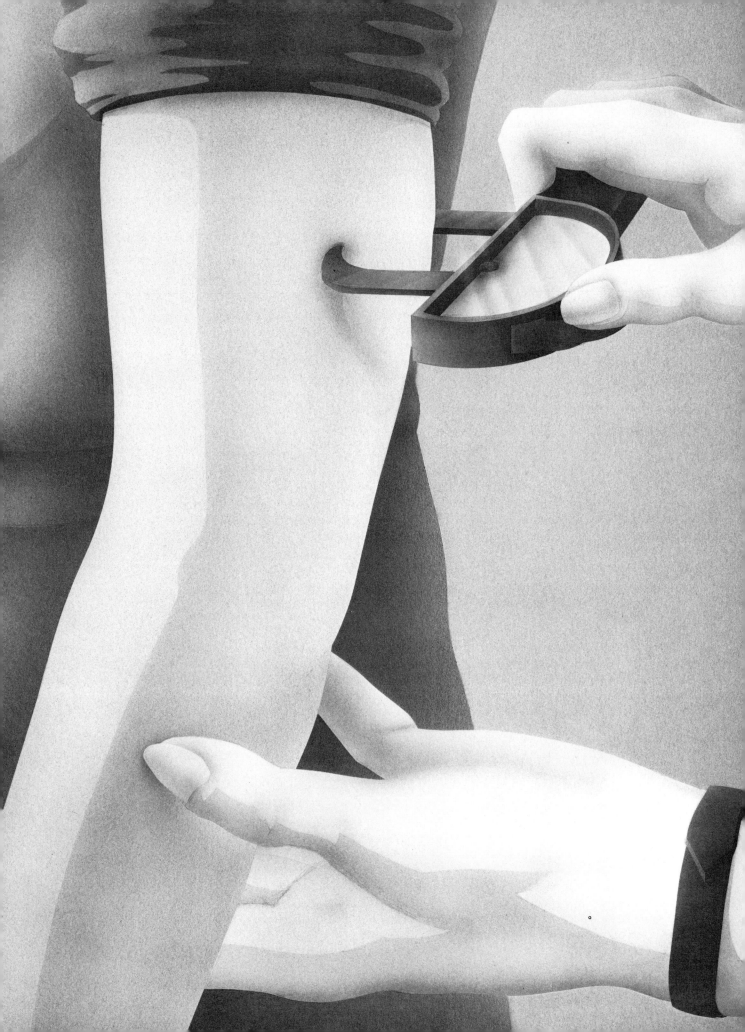

# NUTRITIONAL DISORDERS

# 4 CORRECTING NUTRITIONAL PATTERNS

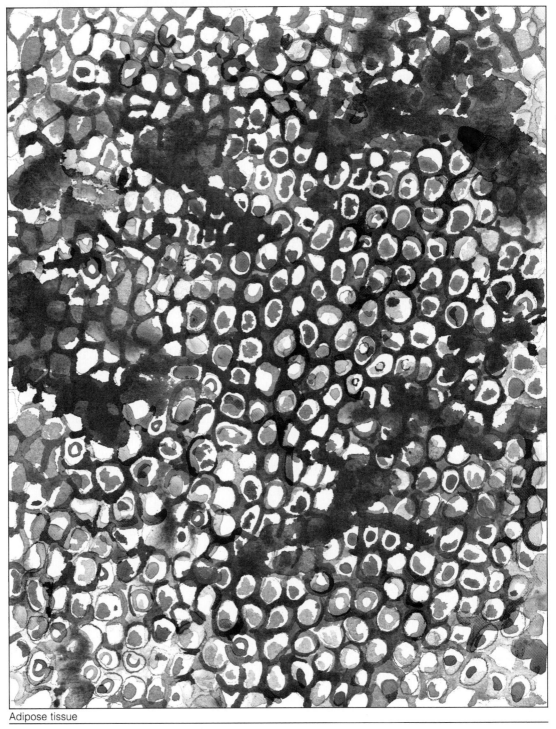

Adipose tissue

Although an emaciated teenage girl and a morbidly obese middle-aged man may seem like striking opposites, they share a common disorder: malnutrition. Broadly defined as faulty or poor nutrition, malnutrition results from a *deficiency or excess* of nutrients. Typically, it develops gradually and may stem from physiologic, psychological, or environmental factors.

Why is malnutrition so significant? First of all, it increases vulnerability to disease in almost every body system. Second, it multiplies surgical risks. And, when malnutrition causes gross changes in body weight, as in anorexia nervosa and obesity, it often colors self-image and impairs social interaction. Obviously, then, nutritional assessment is one of your key tasks. To perform it effectively, you'll need to collect a thorough diet history; conduct a complete physical examination, including anthropometric measurements; and evaluate laboratory test results. Understanding the pathophysiology and current treatment for malnutrition will help you collect and correctly interpret your assessment data.

## PATHOPHYSIOLOGY OF UNDERNUTRITION

Undernutrition results from food intake that's inadequate to meet the body's energy demands (primary undernutrition) or from conditions that impair digestion, absorption, or use of food or that increase energy demands (secondary undernutrition).

**Primary undernutrition.** *Protein-calorie malnutrition,* the most common type of severe primary undernutrition, appears in two forms: kwashiorkor and marasmus. Kwashiorkor—a disorder involving acute protein depletion—produces generalized edema, skin lesions, hair changes, and fatty infiltration of the liver. Marasmus—the severe depletion of both protein and calories—causes growth retardation in children and wasting of subcutaneous fat and muscle. Often these two disorders exist concurrently, a condition called *marasmic kwashiorkor* or *protein-energy malnutrition.* Although severe primary undernutrition is relatively rare in the United States, mild and subclinical primary undernutrition—often seen in marginal vitamin and mineral deficiencies—certainly isn't. In fact, iron deficiency anemia is common in the United States, as are deficiencies of vitamins A, $B_6$, and C. Undernutrition primarily affects children, adolescents, pregnant and lactating

women, and the elderly. Why is it so widespread? Economic, social, and educational factors may all be part of the answer. Community programs for feeding the poor simply can't eradicate all cases of undernutrition. Lack of social interaction, especially common in the elderly, may cause loneliness, apathy, and depression and may encourage a monotonous diet of toast, tea, and canned soups. Lack of education may contribute to poor food choices of refined sweets and empty-calorie foods instead of widely available enriched flour, cereals, and other healthful food products. Indiscriminately following fad diets may foster undernutrition by eliminating one or more foods or by restricting intake to only one food, such as grapefruit. Even the commonly followed vegetarian diet may cause undernutrition if it doesn't include adequate vegetable proteins.

Excessive dieting—common practice among female adolescents who strive to emulate gaunt fashion models—may lead to *anorexia nervosa*. This psychological disorder is characterized by loss of 25% or more of body weight due to self-inflicted starvation. It sometimes coexists with bulimia—a disorder involving episodes of binge-eating followed by self-induced vomiting and use of cathartics and diuretics. Typically, anorexia nervosa affects an adolescent or young adult female from a middle- or upper-middle-class family. What's most baffling, she's usually intelligent and charming, as well as attractive at her normal weight. Fortunately, the anorectic victim now has a brighter prognosis. Years ago, only 25% of these patients were cured, compared to 75% today. In addition, mortality has decreased to about 5%.

**Secondary undernutrition.** Metabolic or endocrine disorders, such as juvenile diabetes, may impair digestion, absorption, or use of food, causing secondary undernutrition. Extensive burns, prolonged low-grade fever, and wasting diseases, such as cancer, increase the basal metabolic rate, thereby increasing energy demands. For example, a 1° F. increase in body temperature raises energy demands at least 5%, and extensive burns can increase them three or four times. If caloric intake fails to keep pace with increased energy demands, undernutrition inevitably results.

## Effects of starvation

Prolonged or severe undernutrition—starvation—has devastating, and potentially fatal, effects. (See *Starvation: Depleting the body's*

## Preventing iatrogenic malnutrition

Hospitalization may aggravate or even trigger malnutrition, increasing the cost and duration of medical care. Fortunately, you're in an ideal position to prevent iatrogenic malnutrition by identifying patients at risk. Begin by asking yourself questions like these:
• Is the patient frequently scheduled for tests at mealtimes?
• Is emotional stress reducing his appetite?
• Has he been receiving low-calorie infusions or a nutritionally inadequate diet for a prolonged period?

Next, review the patient's drug regimen since many drugs interfere with digestion, absorption, or use of nutrients. Many chemotherapeutic drugs, for example, damage normal cells, like those of the intestinal epithelium, resulting in diarrhea. The anticonvulsants phenytoin, phenobarbital, and primidone can cause folate deficiency. Isoniazid (INH) and penicillamine act as vitamin $B_6$ antagonists. Neomycin and the tetracyclines can interfere with calcium absorption. Chronic use of cathartics depletes electrolytes and fluid, and many diuretics cause significant potassium loss.

Finally, ask about alcohol intake. Chronic alcohol abuse causes many vitamin and mineral deficiencies.

## Starvation: Depleting the body's energy reserves

Typically, a healthy diet supplies adequate carbohydrate, fat, and protein to satisfy energy demands and to maintain *nitrogen balance*—the equal rate of protein synthesis and protein breakdown. However, starvation forces the body to draw on its reserves of glycogen, protein, and fat to meet energy demands. Glycogen, found in both the liver and muscle, is mobilized first and converted to glucose. However, the available glycogen can support blood glucose levels only for about 6 to 12 hours.

In *acute starvation,* muscle protein is deaminated and converted to glucose in the liver, with the remaining nitrogen (urea) excreted in the urine. Lipolysis also increases in response to depressed blood insulin levels, releasing free fatty acids for energy.

*Prolonged starvation* triggers several adaptive changes that increase use of fat, thereby sparing protein reserves. Basal metabolism slows, and blood insulin levels decrease further, stimulating glucagon secretion and increased lipolysis. Ketone bodies replace glucose as the brain's major energy source, inhibiting release of muscle protein.

Starvation ultimately depletes fat and muscle protein reserves, forcing the body to break down visceral protein for energy—a potentially fatal last resort. Of course, significant weight loss alone may cause death beforehand.

In *starvation with stress,* markedly increased basal metabolism boosts energy demands. The resulting rise in serum catecholamine, glucocorticoid, and glucagon levels inhibits release of insulin and free fatty acids, causing hyperglycemia. Depletion of muscle protein occurs rapidly, and visceral protein may be sacrificed earlier to satisfy energy demands.

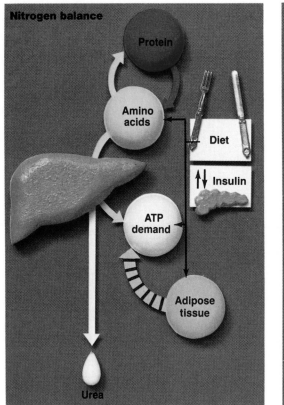

Nitrogen balance

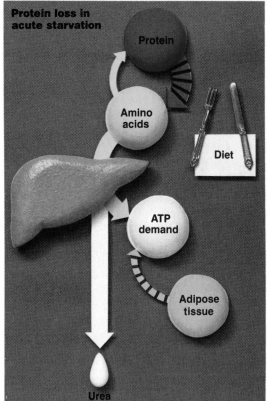

Protein loss in acute starvation

*energy reserves,* pages 56 and 57.) These effects include protein loss, reduced renal perfusion, fluid and electrolyte imbalance, and vitamin deficiencies.

**Protein loss.** Both somatic (muscle) and visceral (organ) protein, the body's major protein reserves, serve specific functions. *Somatic protein* forms the lean mass of skeletal muscle, accounting for about 45% of body weight. It participates in redistribution of amino acids to support visceral protein synthesis and contributes to muscle's tensile property. Depletion of somatic protein results in generalized muscle weakness, which can involve the diaphragm and intercostal muscles and can impair ventilation.

*Visceral protein* includes liver secretory proteins (albumin and transferrin) and immune proteins (lymphocytes and antibodies). Depletion of visceral protein increases susceptibility to infection, delays wound healing, diminishes oxygenation, and encourages third-space fluid shifts, among other deleterious effects.

**Renal perfusion.** Starvation reduces renal perfusion, slowing glomerular filtration. As the body increases lipolysis to protect its protein reserves, urea nitrogen levels fall (as a result of decreased gluconeogenesis) while ammonium nitrogen levels rise (stimulated by aci-

dosis), causing excretion of large amounts of dilute urine.

**Fluid and electrolyte imbalance.** Initial weight loss primarily depletes water and salt, which reduces blood volume and may cause dehydration. Moderate potassium loss produces no adverse effects, but gradual depletion of calcium and phosphorus leads to osteoporosis.

**Vitamin deficiencies.** Starvation quickly depletes ascorbic acid and most B complex vitamins. Loss of thiamine, riboflavin, and niacin interferes with metabolism. Niacin also plays a role in fat synthesis and glycolysis, and vitamin $B_6$ plays a role in protein metabolism. Vitamin $B_{12}$ and folic acid participate in the formation of red blood cells (RBCs). Since vitamins A, D, and $B_{12}$ are normally stored in the liver in excess, they're not as quickly depleted as the other vitamins.

## PATHOPHYSIOLOGY OF OVERNUTRITION

In the United States, overnutrition and its effect—obesity—are widespread and rank among the most pervasive public health problems. In fact, the 1983 height and weight tables released by the Metropolitan Life Insurance Company reflect a trend toward heavier body weight. During a 30-year period, the average weight for men rose 11 lb; for

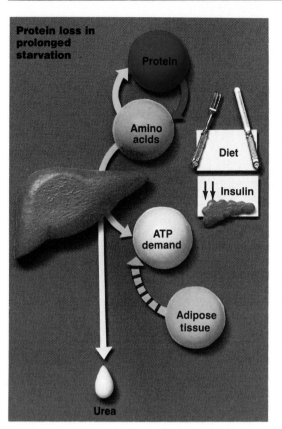

Protein loss in prolonged starvation

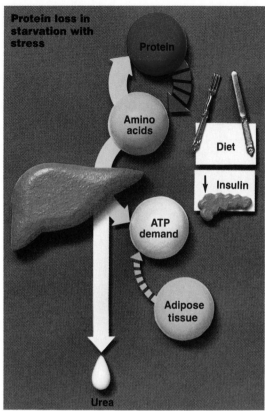

Protein loss in starvation with stress

women, 5 lb. Selective Service data over the past 50 years also confirm this trend. The United States Ten-State Nutritional Survey and the Health and Nutrition Examination Survey indicate that 1 in 4 adults and more than 1 in 10 children are overweight or obese. Also, obesity is more common in women than men, especially black women and those of lower socioeconomic status.

### What causes obesity?

Obesity, the accumulation of fat exceeding 20% of total body mass, results from caloric intake that surpasses energy demands (see *How lipid transport operates,* page 58). Infrequently, it results from overt metabolic disorders such as Cushing's syndrome, hypothyroidism, and Prader-Willi syndrome. Usually, though, its causes are not so obvious and much more complex, probably reflecting the interaction of many factors, including heredity; capacity for thermogenesis; hypothalamic control mechanisms; and structural differences within the GI system, including the structure and prevalence of fat cells and intestinal length.

**Heredity.** Although diet and activity level are important factors in obesity, heredity also plays a prominent role. Research shows that identical twins are more similar in weight

than are fraternal twins or other siblings and that the weight of adopted children more closely resembles that of their biologic parents than that of their adoptive parents. Also, children with two obese parents have a 75% chance of becoming obese. When neither parent is obese, the risk falls to less than 10%.

**Fat cells.** How the body stores fat may also influence obesity. Recent research has improved our understanding of how fat cells develop. Fat accumulates by an increase in either the number or size of fat cells. During two developmental stages, the first years of life and adolescence, a relatively fixed number of fat cells become established in subcutaneous tissue. Overeating during these stages increases the size and number of fat cells, producing a hyperplastic obesity that is especially resistant to treatment. Obesity that begins in adulthood, the hypertrophic form, is characterized by an increase in the size but not the number of fat cells.

**Deficient thermogenesis.** The body's ability to activate thermogenesis—the increased production of heat and dissipation of energy—may be an adaptive response to overeating that maintains stable weight. Thermogenesis occurs in brown adipose tissue distributed in the scapular, axillary, and nape regions; along the large blood vessels in the thorax and abdomen; and between the rib bases. Animal studies show that the obese have limited ability to activate thermogenesis or to increase brown tissue reserves in response to overeating.

**Intestinal length.** The obese tend to have overly long intestines, thereby promoting increased caloric intake owing to a greater absorptive surface. Decreased intestinal motility resulting from poor diet or sedentary life-style also enhances caloric intake.

**Hypothalamic control mechanisms.** The hypothalamus plays a pivotal role in regulating food intake. However, the exact mechanism for short- and long-term regulation—and how

this may contribute to obesity—remains unclear.

*The glucostatic theory* proposes that a satiety center in the ventromedial section of the hypothalamus inhibits eating in response to elevated blood glucose or fatty acid levels, while a feeding center in the lateral hypothalamus stimulates eating in response to decreased glucose and fatty acid levels. This explanation for short-term regulation of food intake is still unconfirmed.

*Current theory* states that inhibition of nerve fibers in the posterior hypothalamus by serotonin produces a sensation of satiety while stimulation of fibers in the hypothalamus by

## How lipid transport operates

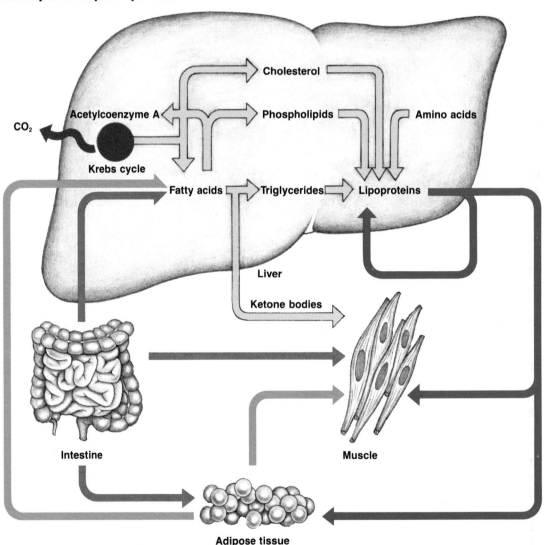

**Key:**

Fatty-acid breakdown in liver

Lipoproteins

Albumin-bound fatty acids

Chylomicrons

Reviewing lipid transport will help you understand how excessive caloric intake gradually builds fat reserves. After absorption from the small intestine as chylomicrons, lipids are transported to the liver, adipose tissue, and muscle. In the liver, they're broken down to fatty acids, which are then used to satisfy energy demands, or are converted to phospholipids and triglycerides.

Triglycerides are transported as lipoproteins to muscle and adipose tissue for storage. If caloric intake is insufficient, adipose tissue releases free fatty acids or albumin-bound molecules to satisfy energy demands. However, if intake is sufficient or excessive, adipose tissue simply stores accumulating triglycerides, resulting in obesity.

dopamine encourages eating. Total adipose tissue mass governs long-term regulation of food intake. Apparently, a feedback mechanism operates whereby the desire for food on one day reflects the intake on previous days. Inadequate food intake gradually depletes fat reserves, stimulating hunger.

*The set-point weight theory* attempts to explain why most people tend to maintain a fairly stable weight despite daily variations in food intake. This specific weight, or set-point of fat reserves, influences the body's intake and basal metabolic rate and acts as a physiologic barrier to dieting. Instead of reducing fat reserves in response to decreased food intake, the body lowers its metabolic rate and expends calories more efficiently.

**Psychosocial factors.** Of course, obesity doesn't result from physiologic factors alone. Some individuals eat simply because food is in front of them or in response to environmental cues. Reminders of food and eating abound in the United States. Some individuals can't pass a bakery or a delicatessen without sampling its foods. Television and radio advertising often inspire a trip to the refrigerator or to a local grocery store. Any celebration or minor occasion becomes an opportunity for snacking. Emotional upset may trigger defensive or protective eating. The ability to identify valid hunger signals, such as internal gastric contractions, is often lost, and food no longer serves its purpose of simple nourishment. Food may be used as a reward or a bribe, as a substitute for love or security, or for some other vicarious purpose. A sedentary life-style, due to numerous labor-saving devices and the tendency to drive rather than walk and to watch rather than participate in sports, also contributes to weight gain.

### Effects of obesity
Obesity increases the risk of disease and impairs overall body function. The risks of diabetes, hypertension, and atherosclerosis are greater among the obese. Gallbladder disease, gout, degenerative arthritis, and renal disease are also more common.

Obesity taxes the heart and circulatory system, particularly during exercise, and may eventually precipitate heart failure. It can cause breathing difficulty and, in some patients, the pickwickian syndrome—characterized by increased RBCs, facial flushing, and hypoventilation. In addition, obesity increases the risk of complications during pregnancy and delivery.

Excessive intake of specific nutrients by the obese or normal weight individual also can be damaging. For example, fat-soluble vitamins A and D aren't readily excreted when taken in excess. Instead, relatively large amounts are stored in the liver. Hypervitaminosis A causes deep bone pain, anorexia, hair loss, scaly dermatitis, irritability, and liver enlargement, among other symptoms. Hypervitaminosis D can cause metastatic calcification of soft tissues, kidney stones, headache, nausea, and weakness.

### MEDICAL MANAGEMENT
Although diagnosis of severe undernutrition or morbid obesity is simply a matter of observation, a thorough patient history, physical examination, and laboratory tests are needed to determine the cause of malnutrition (see *Laboratory tests: Key to nutritional assessment,* page 60). This evaluation can also pinpoint patients with mild or subclinical nutritional disorders, thereby allowing prompt treatment.

### Energy demands guide treatment
Because energy demands directly influence nutritional status, they must be considered for effective treatment. Typically, energy demands fluctuate during an individual's life span. They rise during periods of rapid growth (infancy through adolescence) and periods of stress (trauma, disease, pregnancy, and lactation). And they fall gradually after age 25, with the natural slowing of basal metabolic rate and reduced physical activity associated with aging. In fact, the basal metabolic rate and the activity level are the two major factors that influence energy demands. Basal metabolism expends roughly 1 kcal/kg of body weight per hour for men and slightly less for women. Activity levels are typically described as light, moderate, or strenuous, although lists matching specific activities with caloric expenditure per hour are available. Digestion, or the specific dynamic action of food, usually accounts for about 10% of total energy demands.

Calorimetry, or measurement of released body heat during activity, also helps assess energy demands. Direct calorimetry requires a closed, carefully controlled environment and is more difficult and expensive to perform than indirect calorimetry. Indirect calorimetry involves fitting the patient with a respirometer so that oxygen is inhaled from one container and carbon dioxide exhaled into another. It determines the ratio of expired carbon dioxide to oxygen consumed, or the respiratory quo-

# Laboratory tests: Key to nutritional assessment

Blood and urine tests provide the most precise data about nutritional status. In fact, they often reveal nutritional problems before they're clinically apparent. Typically, these tests evaluate three basic substances: nutrients absorbed from the GI tract or products for cellular use; waste products en route to the kidneys, lungs, or liver; and blood components.

## Serum vitamins and minerals
Vitamins commonly screened for deficiency include A, B, $B_{12}$, folic acid, ascorbic acid, beta carotene, and riboflavin. Zinc, calcium, magnesium, and other minerals may also be measured.

## Serum nutrients
Glucose levels help assess suspected diabetes or hypoglycemia. Cholesterol and triglyceride levels help differentiate the type of hyperlipoproteinemia.

## Nitrogen balance
This test reveals the difference between nitrogen intake and output. A negative nitrogen balance indicates inadequate intake of protein or calories.

## Hemoglobin and hematocrit
Decreased levels can occur in protein-calorie malnutrition, but they can also reflect overhydration, hemorrhage, and hemolytic disease. Normal or elevated values may occur in underhydration.

## Serum iron
Reduced serum iron levels—combined with elevated total iron-binding capacity; decreased hemoglobin and hematocrit levels; and the presence of hypochromatic, microcytic cells—may indicate iron deficiency.

## Serum transferrin (ST)/Total iron-binding capacity (TIBC)
Decreased transferrin levels may indicate visceral protein depletion and, together with reduced TIBC, diverse protein-losing conditions, such as nephrotic syndrome and iron overload.

## Serum albumin
Reduced levels may indicate visceral protein depletion due to GI disease, liver disease, or nephrotic syndrome. However, reduced levels also occur in overhydrated states. Normal or elevated levels occur in underhydration.

## Total lymphocyte count (TLC)
The TLC falls in protein-calorie malnutrition, reflecting impaired cell-mediated immunity.

## Delayed hypersensitivity skin testing
This test also assesses cell-mediated immunity. One or more positive responses, in 24 to 48 hours, to intradermally injected common recall antigens (mumps virus, *Candida*, streptokinase-streptodornase) indicate intact cell-mediated immunity. A negative response, a delayed response, or no response may indicate protein-calorie malnutrition. Trauma, sepsis, and chemotherapy may also suppress immunity.

## Creatinine height index (CHI)
This calculated value, based on creatinine clearance and the patient's height, reflects muscle mass and estimates muscle protein depletion. Reduced CHI may indicate protein-calorie malnutrition; however, it may also indicate impaired renal function.

---

tient (RQ). One liter of oxygen consumed represents 4.82 kcal of released energy. The procedure can be performed with the patient at rest or active. Use of dietary substrates, such as carbohydrate and fat, can also be measured by indirect calorimetry. Carbohydrate, the most efficient fuel, has an RQ of 1. Protein and fat have RQs of approximately 0.8 and 0.7, respectively.

Continuous electronic monitoring of the heart rate helps assess energy expenditure. This procedure doesn't interfere with the patient's normal activity; however, the relationship between heart rate and oxygen consumption varies among individuals and must be determined beforehand for a baseline.

### Treatment for overnutrition
No group in the United States is more susceptible to fads, quackery, and other dubious (diet-related) practices than the overweight. Typically, legitimate treatment for overnutrition involves one or more techniques—most commonly, dieting, exercise, drugs, surgery, or behavior modification.

### Dieting
Recommended diets may be based on restricted carbohydrate or fat intake, intake of one or two foods alone, or no food intake whatsoever. Typically, these diets are monotonous and inadequate in at least some essential nutrients. Almost all have restricted caloric intake, which ultimately accounts for weight loss if the diet is followed. Initial weight loss typically draws on glycogen and protein stores and reflects loss of water and sodium. When carbohydrate and caloric intake are grossly inadequate, accelerated breakdown of fat and protein can result in ketosis, a partic-

ular hazard to those predisposed to diabetes. Pure protein diets may also be harmful if the diet lacks vitamins and minerals and the protein is of low biologic value. Any inadequate diet should be closely monitored and not prescribed or encouraged for more than a short period of time.

Although a balanced calorie-restricted diet isn't easy to follow, it's the optimal method for achieving weight loss. This diet, based on the four basic food groups, includes two servings from the milk product group, two from the meat or protein group, four from the cereal or grain group, and four from the fruit and vegetable group. Caloric intake is restricted so that the body uses fat reserves to satisfy energy demands. When few high-calorie extras like butter, sugar, sour cream, and salad dressing are added to a balanced diet, the total caloric intake is between 1,000 and 1,200. Also, the recommended dietary allowances (RDAs) for essential vitamins and minerals are typically satisfied by such a diet. Because the patient has some choice in food selection, he exercises control and is more likely to follow the diet. Ultimately, the patient must monitor his own intake for effective dietary changes.

### Exercise
An important part of any weight-reduction program, exercise improves cardiovascular function and muscle tone and enhances caloric expenditure. It also curbs stress and overeating; increases stamina; and improves sleep, rest, and self-image. Of course, exercise must be tailored to the patient's age, ability, and interest.

### Drugs
Unfortunately, there's no magical pill to cure or treat obesity. Amphetamines act on the central nervous system to suppress appetite. However, they can cause physiologic dependence and may lose their appetite-suppressant effect after 10 days. Bulking agents suppress appetite by creating a feeling of fullness or satiety, which helps reduce further food intake. Diuretics remove excess fluids, but chronic use fosters dehydration and electrolyte imbalance. Hormonal therapy with thyroid extract increases basal metabolic rate, producing a transient rise in energy expenditure. Research shows that human growth hormone may help treat obesity by depleting fat reserves yet sparing protein. However, supplies of this hormone are limited.

### Jaw-wiring
A drastic method for reducing food intake, jaw-wiring permits ingestion of liquid food alone, which normally results in weight loss. However, ingestion of high-calorie liquids or pureed solid food may defeat this goal. And, unfortunately, since jaw-wiring fails to reform the patient's eating habits, permanent weight loss is unlikely. Meticulous oral hygiene and frequent dental check-ups are a must with jaw-wiring.

### Four types of surgery
Lipectomy, jejunoileal bypass, gastric bypass, and gastroplasty (gastric stapling) are four surgical procedures to treat obesity that have been used with varying success. Lipectomy, or the excision of subcutaneous fat, is largely ineffective since fat stores return. Jejunoileal bypass, which diverts food past most of the small intestine, has serious potential side effects, namely, chronic diarrhea resulting in severe fluid and electrolyte imbalance and liver failure.

Most frequently recommended, gastric bypass and gastroplasty close off part of the gastric reservoir, limiting food intake (see *Gastric bypass and gastroplasty for morbid obesity,* page 62). Typically, candidates for these procedures must:
• have been at least 40 kg overweight for several years
• have no serious concomitant disease (liver, myocardial, or inflammatory bowel disease or renal failure)
• have a high-risk condition that weight loss would ameliorate
• fail to respond to dietary control and conservative medical management
• show emotional stability and a willingness to comply with extended follow-up care
• be under age 65.

### Behavior modification
Probably the most promising technique for achieving permanent weight loss, behavior modification involves heightening the patient's awareness of his eating habits. First, the patient meticulously records the time and place of eating, his degree of hunger just before eating, his mood and physical position during eating, the presence of others, any activities associated with eating, and the type and amount of food eaten. Behavior modification then strives to improve eating habits by reducing stimuli that trigger high-calorie, rapid, or frequent food intake. The patient is

## Gastric bypass and gastroplasty for morbid obesity

Two surgical procedures limit the size of the gastric reservoir and slow gastric emptying, thereby restricting food intake and encouraging weight loss.

*Gastric bypass surgery* involves separating the fundus from the remainder of the stomach by rows of sutures. A loop of the jejunum is then attached to the fundus, leaving a 12-mm stoma. Because 85% of the stomach is bypassed, the patient feels satisfied after consuming about 4 oz of food or fluids. Additional intake causes discomfort or nausea and vomiting.

*Gastroplasty* involves dividing the stomach by a double row of staples below the fundus. A 12-mm channel in the staple line allows passage of food. This channel is reinforced with sutures to prevent stretching and overly rapid emptying of the fundus. Additional staples also reinforce the lesser curvature of the stomach.

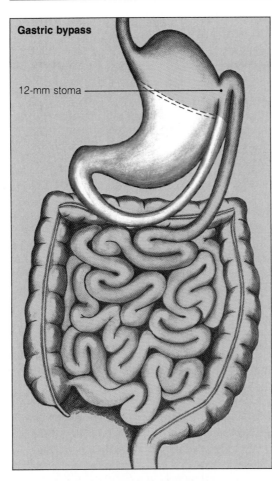

**Gastric bypass**

12-mm stoma

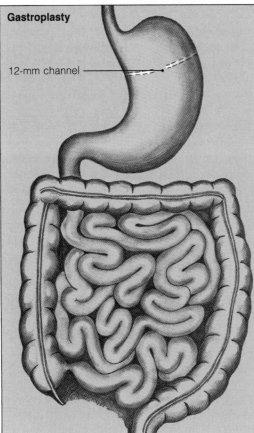

**Gastroplasty**

12-mm channel

instructed to eat slowly in only one location, to chew food more thoroughly, to eat smaller portions on smaller plates, and, generally, to concentrate on what and how much he eats as well as when and why.

Like behavior modification, hypnosis aims to change the patient's eating habits. It involves planting appropriate suggestions or cues for behavior in the patient's subconscious when he's in a passive, trancelike state.

### Treatment for undernutrition

Restoring healthy nutritional status in the underweight is no less challenging than caring for the obese. Ultimately, increased food intake is the only effective treatment for undernutrition, although appetite stimulants or antinauseants may help. By using the patient's caloric needs at his present weight as a baseline, food intake is gradually increased to avoid taxing the digestive system. Protein digestion may be particularly difficult when GI edema complicates prolonged malnutrition. Edema may trigger diarrhea or vomiting until the body adjusts to increased intake.

### Tube feedings

Typically, the ideal candidate for tube feeding is a patient with a functional GI system who can't ingest sufficient food and nutrients for energy. Conditions that warrant tube feeding include anorexia, coma, head and neck surgery, physical impairment (such as fractured jaw or stroke), and hypermetabolic states such as burns. The patient's condition, the type and amount of formula, and the expected duration of therapy determine the type of tube feeding—nasogastric, nasoduodenal, nasojejunal, esophagostomic, gastrostomic, or jejunostomic. The latter three feeding methods require surgical insertion of the feeding tube.

Tube feedings are safer and less expensive than intravenous hyperalimentation (IVH). They also maintain food contact with the gut, preventing atrophy of the intestinal villi.

The volume and concentration of enteral formula delivered by tube feeding are individually tailored to the patient. Protein can be delivered whole or intact, as in milk-based formulas; isolates of protein, such as albumin or casein; or free amino acids, the most elemental form. The choice varies with the ability of the gut to digest and absorb nutrients. Formulas may be lactose-free and low-residue. Although fats, proteins, and carbohydrates vary in type and amount, standard amounts of vitamins and minerals are typically included on the basis of RDA guidelines.

## Intravenous hyperalimentation
In IVH, or total parenteral nutrition, the patient's complete nutrient requirements—all necessary proteins, carbohydrates, water, electrolytes, vitamins, trace elements, and fats—are supplied exclusively by vein. Typically, the IVH solution is delivered to the superior vena cava through an indwelling subclavian vein catheter inserted by the infraclavicular approach or, less commonly, by the supraclavicular, internal jugular, or antecubital fossa approach. The IVH solution itself usually contains 500 ml of dextrose 50% mixed with 500 ml of 8.5% crystalline amino acid solution, or 350 ml of dextrose 50% mixed with 750 ml of 5% to 10% protein hydrolysate solution. Specially prepared solutions have been devised for patients with renal and hepatic failure. Electrolytes, vitamins, and trace elements must be added to the base solution to satisfy daily requirements.

## Nutritional support at home
Recent advances in long-term nutritional support have enabled patients to be discharged from the hospital while receiving IVH or enteral nutrition therapy. Intermittent or bolus feeding allows the patient mobility and a more normal life-style. Even continuous feedings are possible wth proper facilities and patient teaching. However, the patient should be encouraged to return to a normal, oral diet as soon as possible to stimulate the enzyme production and musculature of the gut.

## Psychotherapy
In anorexia nervosa and bulimia, physical intervention alone isn't enough. Psychotherapy is necessary to resolve the underlying emotional conflicts that typically trigger the disorders. The patient must develop better coping skills and change her attitude toward food to gain weight. Depending on the severity of weight loss, tube feeding or IVH may initially be necessary to prevent death.

Because the anorectic patient tends to be manipulative, recovery is typically slow and painstaking. Using inventive and secretive ways, the patient will resist eating and cling to a distorted body image. Despite her emaciated appearance, she will continually insist she's too fat. That's why restoring a healthy body image is a major treatment goal. Often, family therapy plays a role in successful recovery.

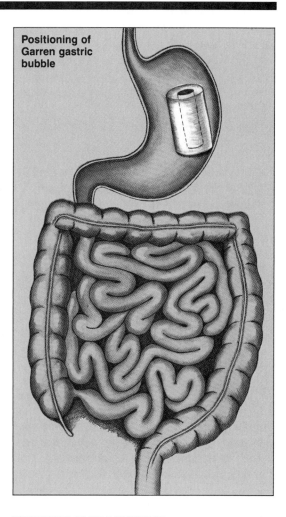

**Positioning of Garren gastric bubble**

## NURSING MANAGEMENT
Assessing nutritional status is surely among your most challenging nursing tasks. Adequate nutrition is vital for optimal health, yet nutritional needs change with age, activity level, and physical condition. Effective assessment requires correlating data from the diet history, the physical examination, and laboratory tests.

During history taking and the physical examination, try to determine the patient's perception of himself. A patient with anorexia nervosa or psychogenic obesity typically has a distorted body image which, until corrected, will thwart all treatment efforts. Also, evaluate the patient's knowledge about nutrition to help structure your teaching plan, and guide the patient in appropriate dietary choices.

### Begin with diet history
Obtain a thorough diet history by asking the following types of questions:

**About food intake.** Because the patient may feel embarrassed and reluctant to talk about food intake, first establish a good rapport with

## Garren gastric bubble: A simple solution for obesity?
Although still experimental, the Garren gastric bubble is a promising new treatment for morbid obesity. The bubble—a durable balloon about 3″ in diameter—is inserted through a flexible plastic tube positioned in the stomach, then inflated with a syringe. Removal simply entails puncturing the bubble and withdrawing it through an endoscope.

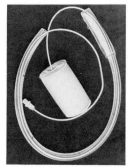

Like gastroplasty and gastric bypass, the gastric bubble reduces stomach volume, limiting food intake and promoting weight loss. However, insertion of the bubble is far simpler than the two surgical procedures. In fact, it may be performed on an outpatient basis, under sedation and with local anesthesia. After the bubble's in place, behavior modification, dietary restrictions, and exercise increase the likelihood of successful weight control.

him. Then ask him to describe a typical breakfast, lunch, dinner, or favorite snack. Find out what foods he likes to prepare, and explore his food preferences. Also ask about recent appetite changes and food allergies or restrictions.

About eating habits. When and where does the patient usually eat? Find out if he eats meals at the same time each day. Is eating usually hurried or relaxed? Does the patient snack? Does he have ill-fitting dentures or mouth pain that makes chewing or swallowing difficult?

About weight. Has the patient's weight changed recently? Was the change rapid or slow? Many obese patients alternate between crash diets and eating binges, causing marked weight fluctuations. Other patients may report poor appetite owing to disease or psychological disturbance, resulting in steady, and eventually hazardous, weight loss. Note the maximum and minimum weight that the patient can remember. Then obtain baseline weight to accurately evaluate the effectiveness of therapy.

About physical activity. Does the patient exercise daily? Less frequently? Have him describe the type of exercise he performs to help determine his energy demands.

About sociocultural background. Can the patient afford proper nutrition? Do cultural habits influence his diet? Note ethnic foods that the patient eats regularly. Also find out if he prepares his own meals and whether he enjoys or has difficulty doing so. For example, an elderly patient may no longer desire or be able to prepare nutritious meals.

About medication history. Find out what drugs the patient's taking and the dosage and schedule. Many drugs interfere with digestion, absorption, or use of nutrients. Also ask about chronic drug or alcohol abuse, which may cause malabsorption.

About medical history. Have the patient describe any illnesses requiring medical or surgical treatment. Note chronic GI disorders or GI surgery that may influence nutritional status. Also, recognize illnesses that may be confused with nutritional alterations. For example, diabetes may delay healing of skin lesions, as may nutritional deficiency.

About elimination. How frequently does the patient have a bowel movement? Have his bowel habits changed recently? Ask about diarrhea, steatorrhea, or bloody stools, which may indicate serious loss of electrolytes, fat and fat-soluble vitamins, or iron. Recognize that nausea and vomiting also contribute to nutrient depletion. Ask about constipation, which may indicate inadequate fluid intake or dietary fiber or thiamine deficiency.

## Perform the physical examination

Signs and symptoms of nutrient depletion or surplus are often subtle and nonspecific. The physical examination combines anthropometric measurements (see *Measuring skinfold thickness*) and general assessment of body systems to uncover clues about nutritional alterations.

## Measure height and weight

Height and weight are two of the most frequently used anthropometric measurements. To measure height, have the patient stand erect in his stocking feet with his feet together, his heels and back against the upright bar of the height scale, and his head held high, looking straight ahead. If the patient is unable to stand, try to learn his height from a family member or friend. To measure weight, have the patient wear light clothing without shoes, and weigh him on a beam or level scale. If the patient can't stand, use a bed or chair scale.

Compare the patient's actual weight with his ideal weight (see *Height and weight tables,* page 66). Use the formula: (actual weight ÷ ideal weight) × 100 to arrive at a percentage. A ratio of 80% or less usually indicates significant depletion of protein and fat reserves; a ratio of about 120% or more indicates obesity.

Also, determine the percentage of body weight change, when appropriate. Use the formula: usual weight − (actual weight ÷ usual weight) × 100. Remember that concurrent disease associated with fluid retention increases weight, making weight an unreliable index of nutritional status.

## Examine body systems

Complete the physical examination by assessing the hair, skin, nails, eyes, oral cavity, glands, and musculoskeletal and neurologic systems for signs of nutritional alterations.

Hair. Dull, dry, thin, and easily plucked hair that shows dyspigmentation may accompany protein-calorie malnutrition.

Skin. Loss of facial skin color, except for dark areas under the eyes, and nasolabial dermatitis may signal iron, protein, or B-complex vitamin deficiency. Dry, scaly, rough skin (follicular hyperkeratosis) may indicate vitamin A or fatty acid deficiency. Red, raised

# Measuring skinfold thickness

ecause subcutaneous fat accounts for about 50% of the body's adipose tissue, measuring skinfold thickness helps estimate total fat reserves. The triceps skinfold is most commonly measured. Although more reliable, the subscapular skinfold is less accessible for measurement. A skinfold thickness of at least 90% indicates no significant depletion of fat reserves; 60% to 90% indicates moderate to mild depletion; and below 60% indicates severe depletion.

When measuring skinfold thickness, you can also determine midarm circumference and midarm muscle circumference. The former reflects skeletal muscle and adipose tissue mass and helps evaluate protein and calorie reserves. The latter reflects skeletal muscle mass alone, providing a more sensitive index of protein reserves.

*To measure the triceps skinfold,* first locate the midpoint on the patient's upper arm using a nonstretch tape measure. Mark the midpoint with a felt-tip pen. Then, grasp the patient's skin with your thumb and forefinger about 1 cm above the midpoint. Place the calipers at the midpoint and squeeze them for about 3 seconds. Record the measurement registered on the handle gauge to the nearest 0.5 mm. Take two more readings, and average all three to compensate for any measurement error.

*To measure midarm circumference,* return to the midpoint that you marked on the patient's upper arm. Then, measuring at the midpoint, use a tape measure to determine the midarm circumference. *To calculate midarm muscle circumference,* multiply the triceps skinfold thickness (in centimeters) by 3.143, and subtract this figure from the midarm circumference.

*To measure the subscapular skinfold,* grasp the skin with your thumb and forefinger just

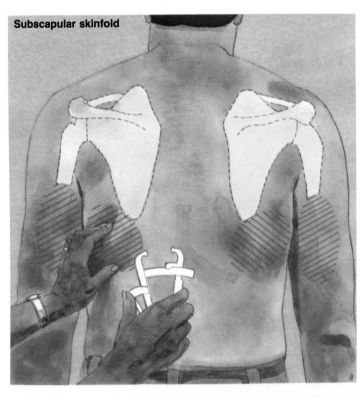

**Subscapular skinfold**

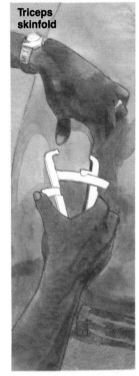

**Triceps skinfold**

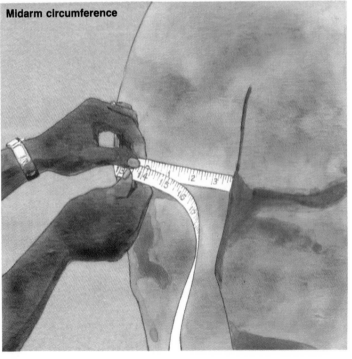

**Midarm circumference**

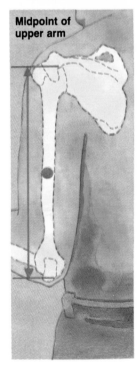

**Midpoint of upper arm**

below the angle of the scapula, in line with the natural cleavage of the skin. Apply the calipers and proceed as you would when measuring the triceps skinfold thickness.

## Height and weight tables

| Men | | | | | Women | | | |
|---|---|---|---|---|---|---|---|---|
| Height | Small frame | Medium frame | Large frame | | Height | Small frame | Medium frame | Large frame |
| 5' 2" | 128-134 | 131-141 | 138-150 | | 4' 10" | 102-111 | 109-121 | 118-131 |
| 5' 3" | 130-136 | 133-143 | 140-153 | | 4' 11" | 103-113 | 111-123 | 120-134 |
| 5' 4" | 132-138 | 135-145 | 142-156 | | 5' 0" | 104-115 | 113-126 | 122-137 |
| 5' 5" | 134-140 | 137-148 | 144-160 | | 5' 1" | 106-118 | 115-129 | 125-140 |
| 5' 6" | 136-142 | 139-151 | 146-164 | | 5' 2" | 108-121 | 118-132 | 128-143 |
| 5' 7" | 138-145 | 142-154 | 149-168 | | 5' 3" | 111-124 | 121-135 | 131-147 |
| 5' 8" | 140-148 | 145-157 | 152-172 | | 5' 4" | 114-127 | 124-138 | 134-151 |
| 5' 9" | 142-151 | 148-160 | 155-176 | | 5' 5" | 117-130 | 127-141 | 137-155 |
| 5' 10" | 144-154 | 151-163 | 158-180 | | 5' 6" | 120-133 | 130-144 | 140-159 |
| 5' 11" | 146-157 | 154-166 | 161-184 | | 5' 7" | 123-136 | 133-147 | 143-163 |
| 6' 0" | 149-160 | 157-170 | 164-188 | | 5' 8" | 126-139 | 136-150 | 146-167 |
| 6' 1" | 152-164 | 160-174 | 168-192 | | 5' 9" | 129-142 | 139-153 | 149-170 |
| 6' 2" | 155-168 | 164-178 | 172-197 | | 5' 10" | 132-145 | 142-156 | 152-173 |
| 6' 3" | 158-172 | 167-182 | 176-202 | | 5' 11" | 135-148 | 145-159 | 155-176 |
| 6' 4" | 162-176 | 171-187 | 181-207 | | 6' 0" | 138-151 | 148-162 | 158-179 |

Weights at ages 25 to 59 based on lowest mortality. Weight in pounds according to frame (in indoor clothing weighing 5 lb, shoes with 1" heels).

Weights at ages 25 to 59 based on lowest mortality. Weight in pounds according to frame (in indoor clothing weighing 3 lb, shoes with 1" heels).

pigmentation of exposed skin areas (pellagrous dermatosis) may indicate niacin or tryptophan deficiency. Petechiae and hyperpigmentation may reflect ascorbic acid, vitamin $B_{12}$, folic acid, or niacin deficiency.

**Nails.** Brittle, spoon-shaped nails with transverse ridges indicate iron deficiency.

**Eyes.** Paleness of the conjunctiva may indicate iron deficiency. Dull, soft corneas and Bitot's spots may reveal vitamin A deficiency. Red, fissured eyelid corners may indicate riboflavin, niacin, or pyridoxine deficiency.

**Oral cavity.** Redness, ulceration, and edema of the mouth and lips with angular stomatitis may indicate niacin or riboflavin deficiency. A red, edematous, and fissured tongue may accompany folic acid, niacin, vitamin $B_{12}$, or pyridoxine deficiency. Magenta discoloration or paleness of the tongue may indicate riboflavin or iron deficiency, respectively. Atrophy of the tongue's papillae may point to niacin, folic acid, vitamin $B_{12}$, or iron deficiency. Mottled tooth enamel may indicate fluoride excess, whereas caries may indicate fluoride deficiency. Spongy, receding gums that bleed easily characterize ascorbic acid deficiency.

**Glands.** Thyroid enlargement (goiter) may disclose iodine deficiency, whereas parotid enlargement may disclose protein deficiency or general malnutrition.

**Musculoskeletal system.** Muscle atrophy and dependent edema may accompany protein-calorie malnutrition. Thinness and softening of the skull bones, epiphyseal swelling, knock-knee, and bowlegs may signal vitamin D deficiency. Small bumps on the ribs may indicate vitamin D and calcium deficiency.

**Neurologic system.** Burning feet syndrome may indicate pantothenic acid deficiency. Tetany and neuromuscular irritability may indicate calcium deficiency. Apathy, confusion, and memory loss may reflect thiamine or niacin deficiency. Loss of tactile and vibration sense, particularly in the feet and ankles, and calf tenderness may indicate thiamine deficiency.

### Institute a weight loss program

In disorders of overnutrition, your nursing goals are to institute an effective weight loss program and to reform the patient's poor eating habits. When devising a diet program, consider the patient's present eating habits, activity level, and psychological state. Also, remember that caloric intake varies with age, sex, and physical activity level. Emphasize to the patient that permanent weight loss requires changed eating habits, not merely restricted caloric intake. Review the patient's present diet and let him discover its problem areas with minimum guidance. Above all, avoid being judgmental. Encourage the patient to suggest feasible changes in diet, thereby improving the prospect of compliance. Of course, offer nutritional advice, when necessary, to promote appropriate dietary choices. Offer suggestions, such as the following, to help the patient plan an effective program.

• Eat three meals a day.
• Substitute veal, fish, and poultry for beef and pork, which have more fat and calories.
• Season food with vinegar, lemon, pepper, and other spices and herbs.
• Choose low-calorie desserts like fresh or unsweetened canned fruits instead of pastry or cookies.
• Gradually eliminate sugar from coffee, tea, and other drinks and foods.
• Snack on low-calorie fresh vegetables or fruits.
• Thoroughly chew each mouthful.
• Watch for added fats, such as butter, salad dressing, and mayonnaise.
• Don't eat if you're not hungry.
• Avoid eating alone. Encourage conversation to slow eating and to reduce food intake.

Of course, you'll need to monitor the patient's body weight and caloric intake. Have him weigh himself weekly since losing several pounds is more encouraging than smaller daily weight losses. Provide emotional support and encourage the patient's family and friends to do the same. To motivate him, continually stress the benefits of weight loss: better health and better appearance. Refer the patient to local support groups or a hospital behavior modification program, if available. Encourage him to gradually increase his physical activity.

### Support the surgical patient

If the patient elects surgical treatment for obesity (gastric bypass or stapling), assist in determining his baseline health status preoperatively. This typically includes a physical examination; routine tests of cardiac, respiratory, and kidney function; and, possibly, endoscopy to rule out peptic ulcer. Explain to the patient that surgery will decrease the size of his stomach, limiting food intake. Warn him that he'll experience discomfort if he eats his accustomed amount of food. However, tell him the stomach is elastic and can be gradually stretched to hold additional food. Explain that he'll initially lose a large amount of weight but will then stabilize at a weight greater than average for his age and height. Also inform him that fluid and electrolyte imbalance may occur postoperatively until the GI tract adjusts to the surgery. Assure him that diarrhea is usually temporary.

Just before surgery, administer cleansing enemas and antibiotics, as ordered. After surgery, be alert for complications: respiratory complications, wound disruption and infection, and thromboembolism. Encourage coughing and deep-breathing exercises immediately. Splint the patient's abdomen to minimize incisional pain. Carefully inspect the wound site, and change the dressing frequently, observing aseptic technique. To help prevent thromboembolism, administer prophylactic low-dose heparin, as ordered, and ensure adequate hydration. Also, apply an antiembolic stocking, and encourage early ambulation. Typically, the patient is supported with intravenous fluids for several days postoperatively and is connected to low intermittent suction via a nasogastric tube until peristalsis returns. Because gastric bleeding is a potential complication, periodically check gastric secretions and stools for occult blood.

### Intervene to promote weight gain

Remedying the cause of undernutrition takes as much patience and ingenuity as managing obesity. If poor nutrition results from wasting disease or malabsorption, your approach is fairly direct and simple: intervene to fight the disease while providing an attractive, nutritious diet. However, if the cause is psychological, as in anorexia nervosa, you'll need to work with psychological counselors to uncover and resolve the fears and anxieties at the root of the disorder. If poor nutrition results from poverty, refer the patient to a social worker so he can take advantage of local assistance programs. If it results from social isolation or disability, encourage the patient to attend church or community-sponsored dinners and to share meals with friends and relatives, when possible. If it results from ignorance of nutritional needs, teach the patient about the four basic food groups, and note the number of servings required from each group per day. Contact the local dairy council and other educational groups for free or inexpensive visual aids to facilitate teaching. When introducing the patient to a nutritious diet, remember that food may visually or physically overwhelm him, especially if he's been eating meagerly for some time. Also consider the patient's current caloric needs, and then increase intake gradually. Initially offer small portions of attractive, yet bland and easily digested, food. Or offer dilute liquid food supplements, if necessary, and have the patient sip them slowly until tolerated. To help stimulate appetite, provide regular oral care, and ensure that the patient's room is tidy and odor-free at mealtimes. Suggest ways to increase caloric intake, such as the following:
• Eat dried fruits between meals to provide

# Detecting complications of intravenous hyperalimentation (IVH)

| Complication | Cause | Signs and symptoms | Treatment |
|---|---|---|---|
| Hyperglycemia | Overly rapid IVH delivery rate, lowered glucose tolerance, excessive total dextrose load | Glycosuria, nausea, vomiting, diarrhea, confusion, headache, and lethargy. Untreated hyperosmolar hyperglycemic dehydration can lead to convulsions, coma, and death. | Add insulin to the IVH solution. |
| Hypoglycemia | Excess endogenous insulin production after abrupt termination of IVH solution, or excessive delivery of exogenous insulin | Muscle weakness, anxiety, confusion, restlessness, diaphoresis, vertigo, pallor, tremors, and palpitations | If possible, give carbohydrates orally; infuse dextrose 10% in water or administer dextrose 50% in water by I.V. bolus. |
| Fluid deficit | Hyperglycemia, vomiting, diarrhea, fistula output, large burns, inadequate fluid replacement, electrolyte imbalance | Fatigue, dry skin and mucous membranes, wrinkled tongue, depressed anterior fontanelle (in infants), tachycardia, tachypnea, decreased urinary output, normal or subnormal temperature, decreased central venous pressure, weight loss, hemoconcentration | Increase fluid intake. |
| Fluid excess | Fluid overload, electrolyte imbalance | Puffy eyelids, peripheral edema, elevated central venous pressure, ascites, weight gain, pulmonary edema, pleural effusion, moist rales | Reduce fluid intake. |
| Hypokalemia | Muscle catabolism, loss of gastric secretions from vomiting, suction, or diarrhea; may occur when anabolism is achieved with its accompanying intracellular movement of potassium | Malaise, lethargy, loss of deep tendon reflexes, muscle cramping, paresthesia, atrial and ventricular dysrhythmias, decreased intensity of heart sounds, weak pulse, hypotension, and complete heart block | Increase potassium intake. A malnourished patient may require an initial dose of 60 to 100 mEq/1,000 calories. |
| Hypophosphatemia | Phosphate deficiency; infusion of glucose causes phosphate ions to shift at start of IVH or within 48 hours of inadequate phosphate intake | Serum $PO_4$ levels less than 1 mg/dl cause lethargy, weakness, paresthesia, glucose intolerance. Severe hypophosphatemia can cause acute hemolytic anemia, convulsions, coma, and death. | Add phosphates to the IVH solution. |
| Hypocalcemia | Increased doses of phosphates administered to correct hypophosphatemia, without supplemental calcium; hypoalbuminemia or excess free water | Nausea, vomiting, diarrhea, hyperactive reflexes, tingling at fingertips and mouth, carpopedal spasm, dysrhythmias, tetany, and convulsions | Add calcium to the IVH solution. |
| Hypomagnesemia | Inadequate intake of magnesium; exacerbated by severe diarrhea and vomiting | Lethargy, tremors, athetoid or choreiform movements, positive Chvostek's or Trousseau's sign, paresthesia, convulsions, and tetany | Add magnesium to the IVH solution. |
| Essential fatty acid deficiency | Absent or inadequate fat intake for an extended period | Alopecia, brittle nails, desquamating dermatitis, increased capillary fragility, indolent wound healing, reduced prostaglandin synthesis, increased platelet aggregation, thrombocytopenia, enhanced susceptibility to infection, fatty liver infiltration, lipid accumulation in pulmonary macrophages, notching of R waves in EKG, growth retardation (in children), triene to tetraene ratio greater than 0:4 | For the adult patient, infuse two or three bottles of 10% or 20% fat emulsion daily. |
| Zinc deficiency | Altered requirements associated with stress, the degree of intracellular zinc deficit, and induced zinc deficiencies from redistribution during anabolism | Diarrhea, apathy, confusion, depression, eczematoid dermatitis (initially in nasolabial and perioral areas), alopecia, decreased libido, hypogonadism, indolent wound healing, acute growth arrest, and hypogeusesthesia (diminished sense of taste) | Add zinc to the IVH solution. |
| Hypocupremia | Long-term IVH without addition of copper sulfate; infection, high-output enterocutaneous fistulas, and diarrhea predispose to copper deficiency | Neutropenia and hypochromic microcytic anemia | Add copper to the IVH solution. |

needed calories as well as minerals and vitamins. Also eat nuts or crackers and cheese between meals.
• Choose ice cream, canned fruits packed in syrup, or cheesecake for high-calorie, nutritious desserts.
• Add calories by using gravy and sauces, butter on vegetables, sour cream on potatoes, and cream in coffee.
• Avoid skipping meals.

### Administer supplemental feedings

When the undernourished patient is unable or unwilling to eat or when his energy requirements exceed oral caloric intake, enteral or parenteral nutritional supplementation is indicated. Enteral or tube feedings may be administered to patients with adequate bowel function. Prepare the patient for tube insertion, explaining the procedure step-by-step. Become familiar with the specific care steps for each type of tube feeding. For example, gastric gavage requires checking tube placement and residual stomach contents before each feeding. Also place the patient in semi-Fowler's position to prevent aspiration.

During tube feeding, monitor intake and output; weight; and blood urea nitrogen, serum and urine glucose, and serum electrolyte levels. Watch for signs of edema and dehydration. When starting therapy, dilute the feeding by half, and administer it slowly. Allow 4 to 5 days to achieve full-strength hyperosmolar solution in cases of serious nutrient depletion. Also, administer feeding at room temperature. Check for gastrointestinal upset, such as diarrhea, particularly when the feeding preparation isn't isotonic.

When administering IVH, one of your top priorities is preventing complications. (See *Detecting complications of intravenous hyperalimentation.*) Watch for subclavian artery injury after catheter insertion, thrombophlebitis, air embolism, pneumothorax, and endocarditis. Arrange for a chest X-ray after catheter insertion to rule out pneumothorax. Most important, observe strict asepsis when handling IVH solution and caring for the catheter site. Because the IVH solution is a good medium for bacterial growth and the central venous line gives systemic access, contamination and sepsis are always a risk. Strict surgical asepsis is required during solution, dressing, tubing, and filter changes.

During IVH, carefully monitor the rate of infusion to reduce the risk of hyperglycemia. Also monitor intake and output. Test for glucose and ketone in the urine every 6 hours, and notify the doctor when glycosuria is +2 or greater. Take vital signs every 4 hours, and watch for fever. Weigh the patient daily to evaluate therapy and to detect fluid imbalance. Also monitor laboratory data.

Slowly wean the patient from vein to oral feeding to minimize the risk of hypoglycemia. If hypoglycemia occurs, give orange juice or other simple sugar sources. As soon as possible, help the patient make the transition from parenteral to enteral feeding. Long-term parenteral feeding may cause atrophy of the small intestinal villi, resulting in malabsorption. Begin with simple food to prevent gastric upset and diarrhea. Then, as the gut begins to function normally, increase the amount and variety of food, as tolerated.

### Prepare the patient for discharge

A final evaluation of the patient's nutritional status before discharge verifies the effectiveness of therapy and helps outline follow-up care. Consider the patient's weight, laboratory data, and self-image in this evaluation as well as his understanding of dietary therapy.

Expect the patient's weight to change toward the norm or the limited goal set for him. Laboratory values—of serum albumin, lymphocytes, electrolytes, and glucose—should also show a corresponding return to normal or more acceptable levels. The patient's blood pressure should fall within the normal range.

Severe weight loss or obesity can distort the patient's self-image and concept of well-being. A return to normal body weight usually restores a healthy body image. However, if a distorted body image persists, suggest continued psychotherapy to prevent drastic weight changes after discharge. If the patient's happy about his new weight and nutritional status, he will probably cooperate to maintain them. Without this motivation to make a permanent behavioral change, he may slip back to customary eating patterns. Arrange follow-up care or contact community support groups to help the patient adhere to the prescribed diet.

Before discharge, have the patient plan menus on his own to familiarize himself with his diet and its practical applications. Include the patient's family in meal planning. Teach them the basics of good nutrition, using food models or pictures, when appropriate. Effective preparation will help ensure continual improvement in the patient's nutritional status after discharge and will reward your expert nursing care.

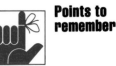

**Points to remember**

• Malnutrition results from deficiency or excess of nutrients. Physiologic, psychosocial, and environmental factors may contribute to its development.
• Basal metabolic rate and physical activity level are the two major factors influencing energy (caloric) demands.
• Treatment of obesity involves one or more therapies—dieting, exercise, drugs, surgery, and behavior modification.
• Treatment of undernutrition focuses on gradually increasing caloric intake. At times, tube feeding or intravenous hyperalimentation is necessary.
• Permanent weight loss or gain demands behavioral change, not merely altered caloric intake.
• Nutritional assessment, a key nursing responsibility, requires a thorough diet history and physical examination, including anthropometric measurements, and evaluation of laboratory test results.

# 5 MANAGING MALABSORPTION SYNDROMES

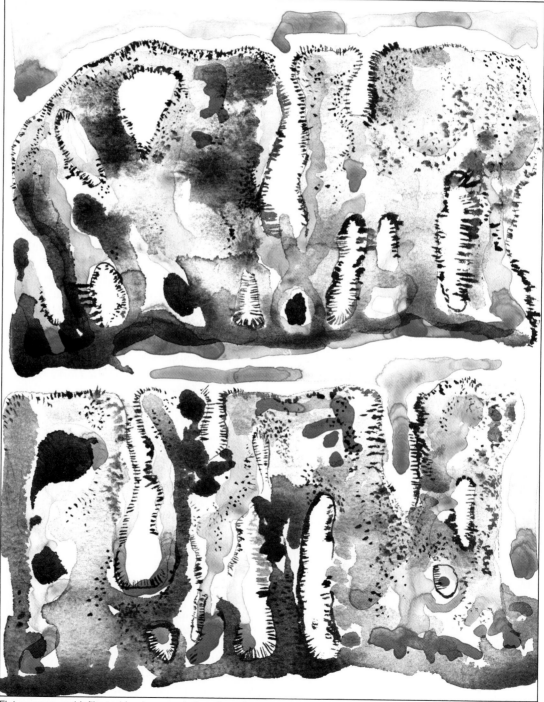

Flat mucosa and infiltrated lamina propria in celiac disease

n its mild and transient form, malabsorption produces nothing more serious than transient indigestion. But it isn't always so benign. For the many who seek medical help because of malabsorption, it's both severe and persistent, often leading to intractable diarrhea, nutrient deficiencies, and clinical starvation. Then, you're often called upon to help identify its often elusive cause by helping with diagnostic tests and specimen collection; to treat it by giving parenteral and enteral nutrition; to watch for significant changes in clinical status by continuous assessment; and to teach the patient how to change his diet and life-style to help restore and maintain optimal nutrition.

To perform these varied tasks well, from assessment and interpretation to patient support, you'll need a familiarity with the intricacies of normal digestion and absorption and an understanding of where and how various disorders can disrupt them.

## Many causes, many manifestations

The liver, stomach, pancreas, and small intestine regulate normal digestion and absorption. Any defect in one step of the digestive or absorptive process can impair the overall ability to obtain and use nutrients and may lead to overt malabsorption.

Such malabsorption has many possible causes and extensive clinical implications. These syndromes may result from primary small-bowel or pancreatic disease or may result secondarily from many systemic diseases. (See *Causes of malabsorption syndromes,* page 72.) Their effects may be selective, impairing absorption of a single nutrient, or broad, impairing absorption of many nutrients and creating widespread metabolic dysfunction.

The incidence of malabsorption syndromes varies according to the patient's age, sex, and ethnic origin. Lactose intolerance, the most common disorder, affects about 75% of American blacks and commonly appears in Asians and Greek Cypriots. Like most malabsorption syndromes, it's treated with diet therapy. The incidence of regional ileitis (Crohn's disease), an inflammatory bowel disorder that causes malabsorption of bile salts and many other nutrients, has been rising, mostly among Jews. This condition usually requires surgery and proves fatal in about 10% of patients.

Nontropical (celiac) sprue also seems to result from genetic predisposition since most patients with this disorder have the histocompatibility antigen HLA-B8. The highest incidence occurs among the British and Irish, among whom it affects 1 in 225 people. (The tropical form of sprue is, as its name implies, confined to certain tropical climates.) Nontropical sprue may be severe but often responds to diet therapy. Whipple's disease occurs most often in middle-aged males, rarely in females. Cystic fibrosis and abetalipoproteinemia appear in young children.

## PATHOPHYSIOLOGY

The fundamental mechanisms of malabsorption include biochemical and enzyme deficiencies, bacterial proliferation, mucosal disruption of the small intestine, disturbed lymphatic and vascular circulation, and loss of gastric or intestinal surface area.

### Biochemical and enzyme deficiencies

Decreased production or impaired usage of bile salts and enzymes produces malabsorption of the nutrients dependent on them for digestion and absorption.

**Bile salt deficiencies.** Secreted by the liver, bile salts are necessary for fat emulsification, hydrolysis, and absorption. (See *Fat digestion and absorption,* page 73.) Bile salt deficiency results in decreased formation of micelles, the compounds responsible for transporting digested fats to the intestinal mucosa for absorption. Deficient liver synthesis of bile, obstructed biliary channels, or disturbed bile salt reabsorption by the ileum leads to malabsorption of fats and fat-soluble vitamins.

Normally, the liver secretes 500 to 1,000 ml of bile salts daily, and the ileum reabsorbs about 80% for hepatic recycling. The rate at which bile salts return to the liver controls the synthesis rate. If the return rate decreases (bile salt deficiency), the liver compensates by increasing the synthesis rate. But, at a certain point, bile salt production can't keep up with reduced absorption: the bile salt pool size decreases, and up to 40% of fats are lost in the stool (steatorrhea). Unabsorbed bile salts, passing through the large intestine, cause irritative diarrhea.

**Disaccharidase deficiencies.** Located in the brush (microvillous) border of the intestinal mucosa, disaccharide enzymes split disaccharides into their component monosaccharides, rendering them absorbable. These enzymes include lactase, sucrase, maltase, and isomaltase. (See *Carbohydrate digestion and absorption,* page 74.)

*Lactase deficiency,* the most common disac-

## Causes of malabsorption syndromes

### Absorptive surface abnormalities

Biochemical and genetic abnormalities
  Abetalipoproteinemia
  Disaccharidase deficiency
  Hypogammaglobulinemia
  Nontropical (celiac) sprue

Inflammatory and infiltrative disorders
  Collagen disorders
  Lymphoma
  Nontropical (celiac) sprue
  Regional ileitis (Crohn's disease)
  Tropical sprue
  Ulcerative colitis

Massive bowel resection

### Cardiovascular disorders

Left ventricular failure

Mesenteric vascular obstruction

### Endocrine and metabolic disorders

Diabetes mellitus

Hypoparathyroidism

Zollinger-Ellison syndrome

### Enzyme and bile salt deficiencies

Pancreatic lipase deficiency or inactivation
  Exocrine pancreatic deficiency
    Chronic pancreatitis
    Cystic fibrosis
    Pancreatic tumor
  Zollinger-Ellison syndrome

Postgastrectomy malabsorption

Reduced bile salt concentration
  Drug precipitation of bile salts
    Neomycin administration
  Interrupted bile salt circulation
    Ileal resection
    Regional ileitis (Crohn's disease)
  Intestinal bacterial proliferation
    Blind loop syndrome
    Scleroderma
  Liver disease
    Intra- or extrahepatic cholestasis

### Lymphatic disorders

Lymphangiectasia

Lymphoma

Whipple's disease

charidase deficiency, precludes hydrolysis of dietary lactose and thus prevents its absorption. The unabsorbed lactose is metabolized by bacteria in the distal small intestine and large intestine and fermented to short-chain fatty acids, volatile fatty acids, lactic acid, hydrogen gas, and some carbon dioxide. These products cause osmotic diarrhea, cramps, discomfort, increased peristalsis, distention, and bloating. Lactase deficiency may stem from genetic causes or occur secondary to intestinal mucosal injury from viral hepatitis, bacterial infestation, or sprue.

Clinically significant deficiencies of other disaccharidases are rare, perhaps because nonlactase disaccharidases are less sensitive to mucosal injury than lactase.

**Pancreatic enzyme deficiencies.** Deficiencies of pancreatic enzymes, as occur in Zollinger-Ellison syndrome, cause maldigestion of carbohydrates, protein, and fat and malabsorption of vitamin $B_{12}$. Decreased pancreatic enzyme levels may follow destruction of pancreatic tissue, inadequate stimulation of the pancreas, or ductal obstruction. The resulting loss of pancreatic secretions means loss of trypsin, chymotrypsin, carboxypolypeptidase, pancreatic amylase, pancreatic lipase, and other digestive enzymes. Without these enzymes, as much as half the fat entering the small intestine and as much as one third of the protein and starch may remain unabsorbed, producing copious, fatty feces. (See *Protein digestion and absorption,* page 75.)

Chronic pancreatic enzyme deficiency also impairs absorption of vitamin $B_{12}$. To be absorbed, vitamin $B_{12}$ must combine with intrinsic factor, a glycoprotein synthesized and secreted by the stomach. This vitamin also binds to other glycoproteins, called R binders and found in saliva, gastric secretions, bile, and intestinal secretions, but these complexes aren't absorbable. In fact, pancreatic proteases degrade the R binders in the duodenum and permit vitamin $B_{12}$ to associate with intrinsic factor. Thus, the lack of pancreatic enzymes to degrade R binders leads to impaired $B_{12}$ absorption.

## Bacterial proliferation

Peristalsis normally prevents bacterial proliferation in the proximal small bowel by keeping intestinal contents mobile. Any abnormality that causes stasis of intestinal contents and bacterial overgrowth is called blind (stagnant) loop syndrome. The abnormality may be structural, as occurs with gastrectomy or enterostomy, or motor, as occurs with scleroderma or diabetic enteropathy.

An intestinal loop becomes blind when separated from the main GI tract or when intestinal contents can enter the loop but not readily exit. So stagnation occurs, causing bacterial breakdown (deconjugation) of bile salts. Reduced availability of bile salts inhibits micelle formation for lipid absorption, causing steatorrhea. Mucosal injury from the caustic

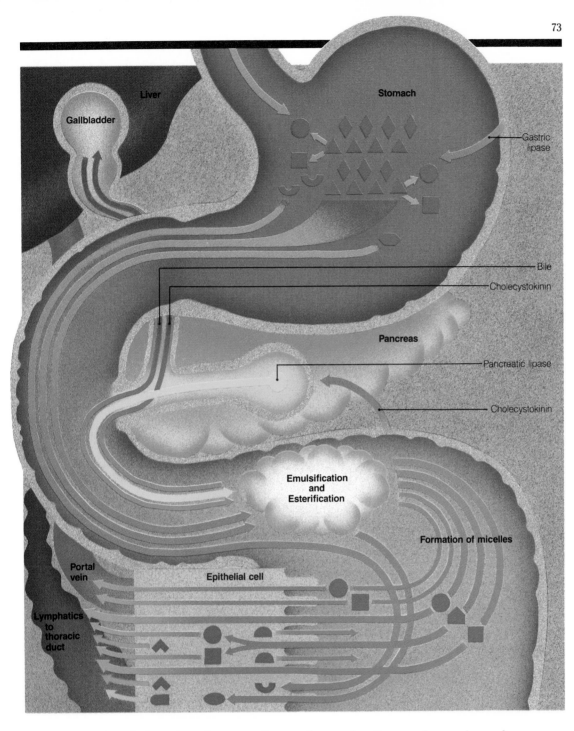

Liver

Gallbladder

Stomach

Gastric lipase

Bile

Cholecystokinin

Pancreas

Pancreatic lipase

Cholecystokinin

Emulsification
and
Esterification

Formation of micelles

Portal
vein

Epithelial cell

Lymphatics
to
thoracic
duct

## Fat digestion and absorption

Triglycerides (both long-chain triglycerides [LCT] and short-chain triglycerides [SCT]) make up almost all dietary fats.

In fat digestion, gastric lipase initiates SCT breakdown, a process continued by pancreatic lipase. Both intact SCTs and their end products pass into the intestinal mucosa and portal vein.

LCT digestion begins when the duodenum secretes cholecystokinin. This hormone stimulates bile release, which emulsifies the LCT molecules. Emulsification allows pancreatic lipase to cleave the fat into monoglycerides and some end-stage fatty acids and glycerol. These products join jejunal bile salts to form *micelles,* which release their fat content into the mucosa. The bile salts return to the intestine to transport additional fat products. Once deposited, fat products break down into fatty acids and glycerol and regroup into triglycerides. Forming *chylomicrons* by assuming a beta-lipoprotein coat to make them soluble, they pass into lymphatic circulation.

Cholesterol is absorbed similarly to LCTs, after hydrolysis from its ester form by pancreatic cholesterol esterase.

Fat malabsorption results from disorders of bile or lipase and from diseases of the jejunum and ileum.

**Key:**

- Fatty acids
- Long-chain triglycerides
- Short-chain triglycerides
- Glycerol
- Phospholipids
- Monoglycerides
- Bile salts
- Triglycerides
- Chylomicrons
- Cholesterol esters
- Cholesterol

products of bile salt deconjugation, as well as the bacteria and their breakdown products, also causes steatorrhea. Patchy mucosal lesions appear and further hinder fat absorption. Vitamin $B_{12}$ deficiency may occur secondary to bacterial ingestion of the vitamin.

### Mucosal disruption
Atrophy or infiltration of the villi lining the intestinal mucosa accounts for several malabsorption syndromes.

**Immune villous atrophy.** A genetically controlled defect or an immunologic injury in response to gluten ingestion may explain villous atrophy in nontropical (celiac) sprue, but the exact pathogenesis remains unknown. Clinical evidence suggests that gluten or its metabolites create a hypersensitivity reaction in the mucosa. Circulating antibodies to gliadin, a breakdown product of gluten, have been identified in patients with nontropical sprue. However, another theory suggests that absence of a certain peptidase may block hydrolysis of gluten into smaller peptides and amino acids, so that toxic peptides accumulate and damage the intestinal mucosa.

Classic changes shown in small-bowel biopsy are villous blunting and flattening, crypt elongation, and inflammatory infiltration of the lamina propria. Surface absorptive cells

## Carbohydrate digestion and absorption

Starch, sucrose, lactose, and D-xylose represent the major dietary carbohydrates. About 40% of the starch, a polysaccharide, hydrolyzes into the disaccharides maltose and isomaltose in the mouth and stomach through the action of the salivary enzyme, ptyalin. This action continues for several hours until all food has mixed in the stomach with gastric acid (HCl), whose low pH inactivates the enzyme. The remaining 60% of the starch is hydrolyzed in the duodenum by pancreatic amylase.

Ingested lactose and sucrose pass into the jejunum, along with maltose and isomaltose. There, the enzymes lactase, sucrase, maltase, and isomaltase split the four disaccharides into monosaccharides for absorption. They're absorbed through the portal vein into systemic circulation for metabolism and storage.

D-xylose, an existing monosaccharide, is absorbed intact from the jejunum.

Conditions that compromise the duodenum or jejunum, such as tropical or nontropical (celiac) sprue or duodenal or jejunal resection, also compromise absorption of the chief carbohydrates.

**Key:**

● D-xylose

▲ Lactose

■ Sucrose

◆ Starch

⬭ Isomaltose

⬡ Maltose

◆ Glucose

◗ Fructose

◡ Galactose

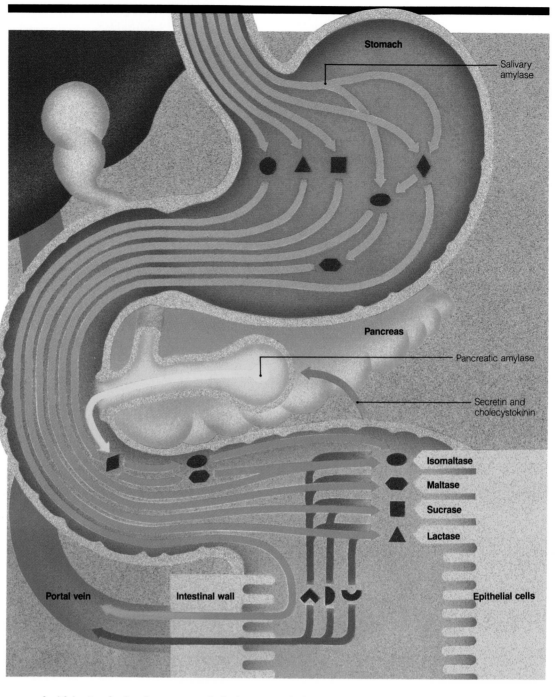

are cuboid instead of columnar, and their nuclei lack basal orientation. In addition, the mucosal epithelial cells renew themselves at a much higher rate than normal.

Malabsorption associated with mucosal damage results primarily from decreased uptake and transport of most dietary nutrients because of the marked loss of absorptive surface area and severe damage to the remaining villous cells. Also, alteration in mucosal permeability increases water and electrolyte secretion, and the loss of brush border enzymes commonly causes lactase and other disaccharidase deficiencies. In addition, impaired release of the hormones secretin and cholecystokinin, from the damaged duodenal and jejunal mucosa, may lead to bile salt and pancreatic enzyme deficiencies.

**Infectious villous atrophy.** An unidentified infectious agent, maybe bacteria, appears to cause villous atrophy in tropical sprue. The proximal small bowel usually shows mucosal abnormalities similar to those in nontropical sprue, but not usually including total villous atrophy. Early in the disease, villi are edematous—later, more characteristically leaf-shaped. Epithelial changes include villous broadening and shortening, crypt elongation, epithelial cell alterations, and infiltration by inflammatory cells. The ileum is affected more

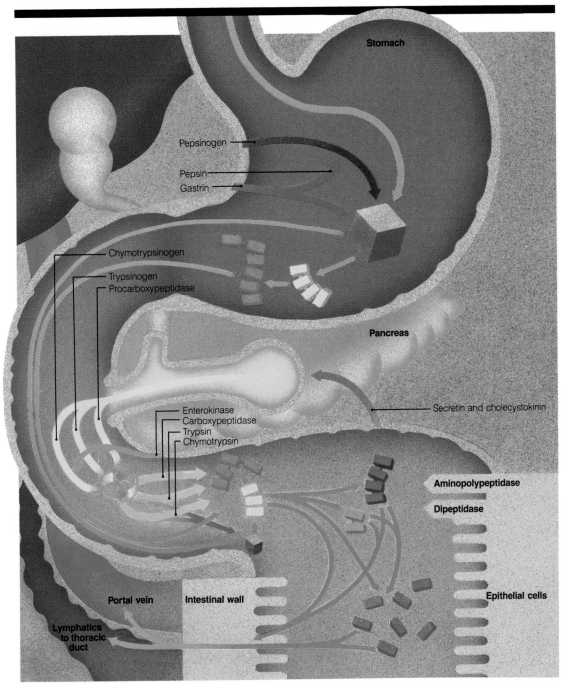

## Protein digestion and absorption

Dietary proteins are derived mostly from meats and vegetables. These proteins consist of long chains of amino acids linked by peptide compounds. Protein digestion involves hydrolysis of the peptides by highly specific enzymes.

Hydrolysis begins in the stomach with pepsin. Pepsin breaks down all types of dietary protein but is essential in reducing the connective collagen in meats, allowing other enzymes to digest the cell proteins. Pepsin needs the secretion of gastric acid (HCl) to work well: it works best at a pH of 2 (normal stomach pH) and is inactive at a pH of 5. This enzyme begins digestion by breaking proteins into constituent proteoses, peptones, and polypeptides.

In the duodenum and jejunum, the pancreatic enzymes trypsin, chymotrypsin, and carboxypolypeptidase reduce the three initial products to their basic peptides and end-stage amino acids.

In the lower jejunum and ileum, the enzymes aminopolypeptidase and dipeptidase hydrolyze the remaining peptides into amino acids. Then the amino acids are absorbed into the portal vein for metabolism and storage.

Protein malabsorption occurs in disorders that diminish gastric secretion of HCl, such as chronic atrophic gastritis, or inflammatory or infectious disorders involving the duodenum or jejunum, such as duodenal ulcer. Also, any resection of the stomach or duodenum and massive resection of the jejunum or ileum reduce protein absorption.

**Key:**

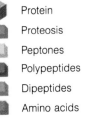

Protein

Proteosis

Peptones

Polypeptides

Dipeptides

Amino acids

---

often in tropical than in nontropical sprue, and changes are more widespread throughout the intestine, though not so severe as in nontropical sprue.

Malabsorption is similar to that in nontropical sprue, with fat malabsorption and steatorrhea; increased sodium and water secretion; and folic acid and vitamin $B_{12}$ malabsorption, causing megaloblastic anemia. Malabsorption probably results from bacterial infection and overgrowth via one of several pathogenic mechanisms. The offending bacteria may inhibit cellular metabolism of the intestinal mucosa; they may impede the enzyme activity needed for absorption; they may release an enterotoxin that deconjugates bile salts to cause steatorrhea and stimulates water and electrolyte secretion; or they may synthesize analogs to prevent folic acid absorption.

**Infiltrative lesions.** Several types of infiltrative lesions cause mucosal disruption that causes malabsorption. Intestinal mucosal inflammation, as occurs in regional ileitis (Crohn's disease), disrupts the absorptive surface, impairs ileal reabsorption of bile salts, and decreases micelle formation. Small-bowel neoplasms and mechanical obstructions also disrupt the mucosal absorptive capacity in sections. In disorders such as ulcerative colitis, protein exudation through

## Signs and symptoms of malabsorption

| Sign or symptom | Related pathophysiology |
| --- | --- |
| **General** | |
| Weakness, fatigue | Electrolyte imbalance, anemia, hypophosphatemia |
| Weight loss | Marked reduction in caloric intake or increased use of calories; decreased absorption of fats, proteins, or carbohydrates |
| **Skin, hair, nails** | |
| Anemia (pallor) | Iron, vitamin $B_{12}$, or folic acid deficiency |
| Dry skin and mucous membranes, poor skin turgor | Dehydration |
| Dermatitis | Niacin and other vitamin deficiencies, zinc deficiency, or fatty acid deficiencies |
| Ecchymoses, hemorrhagic tendency | Vitamin K deficiency inhibiting production of clotting factors II, VII, IX, and X; ascorbic acid deficiency |
| Brittle nails | Iron deficiency |
| Hair thinning and loss | Protein deficiency |
| **Head, eye, ear, nose, and throat** | |
| Night blindness, corneal dryness, swelling of lids | Vitamin A deficiency |
| Glossitis | Vitamin $B_{12}$, folic acid, iron, or niacin deficiency |
| Cheilosis | Riboflavin or iron deficiency |
| **Cardiopulmonary** | |
| Hypotension | Dehydration |
| Tachycardia | Hypovolemia, anemia |
| Peripheral edema | Protein malabsorption or enteric protein loss |
| **Gastrointestinal** | |
| Diarrhea, flatulence, borborygmi, distention | Impaired absorption of water, sodium, fatty acids, bile, or carbohydrates |
| Ascites | Hypoproteinemia |
| Malodorous, greasy stools | Steatorrhea |
| **Musculoskeletal** | |
| Bone pain (osteomalacia) | Vitamin D deficiency, hypocalcemia, hypophosphatemia |
| Muscle cramps | Hypokalemia |
| Muscle wasting | Protein malabsorption, reduced carbohydrate and fat sources for metabolic energy |
| **Neurologic** | |
| Altered mental state | Dehydration, vitamin $B_{12}$ deficiency (rare) |
| Paresthesias, ataxia | Vitamin $B_{12}$ deficiency |
| Tetany, Chvostek's sign, Trousseau's sign | Hypocalcemia, hypomagnesemia, vitamin D deficiency |

an ulcerated and inflamed mucosa, abnormal mucosal cell metabolism, and other mechanisms may produce protein loss. The severity of malabsorption varies with the severity of infiltration caused by the underlying disease.

**Disturbed lymphatic and vascular flow**
Two circulatory systems drain the small intestine: the lymphatic system and the portal venous system. Fat-soluble substances flow into the lymphatic system, which empties into systemic venous circulation; water-soluble substances drain into portal circulation, which leads to the liver.

**Lymphatic flow.** Any condition that impedes normal lymph flow from the mucosa through the abdominal lymphatic system to the thoracic duct and then to systemic circulation may promote the loss of lymph constituents (plasma proteins, chylomicron fat, and small lymphocytes). In turn, plasma protein loss is linked to excessive loss of minerals (iron, copper, and calcium); vitamin $B_{12}$; folic acid; and lipids. With disordered lymph flow, fat accumulation blocks the villous lymphatics, increases lymphatic pressure, and may rupture the lymph ducts, causing fat and protein loss into the intestinal lumen.

Intestinal lymphatic disorders may be congenital or secondary to other GI conditions. Secondary disorders include tumor, inflammation, radiation enteritis, regional ileitis, lymphangiectasia, lymphoma, and Whipple's disease. Also, cardiac conditions, such as congestive heart failure and constrictive pericarditis, may produce lymphatic obstruction, because elevated central venous pressure blocks lymphatic drainage through the thoracic duct.

**Vascular flow.** Any condition that compromises blood circulation to the intestinal wall, such as disease of the celiac or superior mesenteric arteries, causes malabsorption through intestinal ischemia. Impaired arterial blood supply can't meet postprandial metabolic demands, and the resultant abdominal pain discourages food intake. Malabsorption, probably related to impaired mucosal cell function, leads to steatorrhea and anorexia.

**Loss of gastric or intestinal surface area**
Iatrogenic factors, such as gastrectomy or intestinal resection, may also cause maldigestion and malabsorption via a decreased absorptive surface and increased motility.

**Gastrectomy.** Duodenal bypass in gastrectomy creates an afferent loop, which may

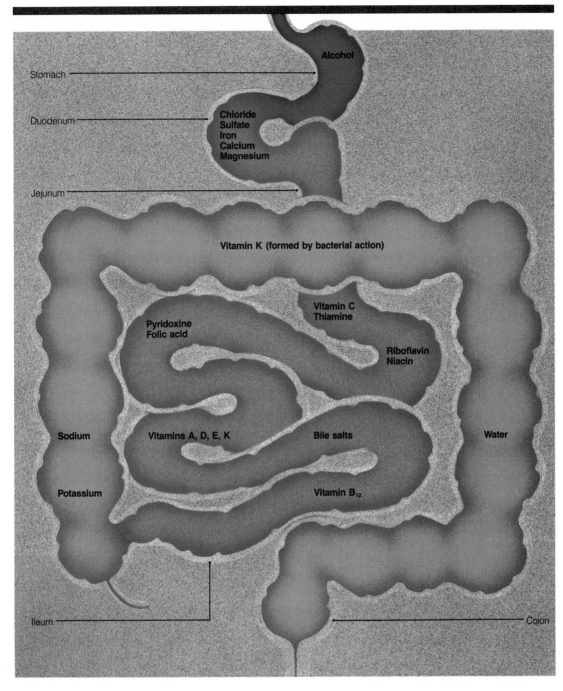

Stomach — Alcohol

Duodenum — Chloride / Sulfate / Iron / Calcium / Magnesium

Jejunum

Vitamin K (formed by bacterial action)

Vitamin C / Thiamine

Pyridoxine / Folic acid

Riboflavin / Niacin

Sodium

Vitamins A, D, E, K

Bile salts

Water

Potassium

Vitamin $B_{12}$

Ileum

Colon

## Other essential nutrients: Digestion and absorption

Specific sites in the GI tract absorb specific dietary nutrients. Most nutrient absorption takes place in the small intestine. Through enzyme action and mechanical means, nutrients pass into systemic circulation for metabolism and storage via either the portal vein or the lymphatic system and thoracic duct. By the time the chyme reaches the large intestine, it's devoid of nearly all nutrients except water, sodium, and potassium.

Logically, disorders involving the GI tract affect the absorption of nutrients specific for the involved area. Such disorders include resection and mucosal infection or inflammation, which decrease the absorptive surface area; insufficient enzyme activity due to an acute process or congenital lack of enzymes; and increased motility of intestinal contents, which prevents adequate mucosal exposure to nutrients.

For example, partial or total gastrectomy blocks absorption of calcium, iron, and other nutrients normally handled by the duodenum and reduces distal absorption of nutrients by speeding transit time. Also, regional ileitis (Crohn's disease) and resection of the involved distal ileum eliminate absorption sites for vitamin $B_{12}$ and bile salts.

In addition to diet therapy to avoid the specific malabsorption problem, treatment may involve supplements to replace lost vitamins, minerals, and pancreatic enzymes. (See *Vitamin, mineral, and pancreatic enzyme replacements*, page 78.)

---

promote bacterial overgrowth. By inhibiting duodenal release of cholecystokinin, bypass reduces the level of pancreatic enzymes and bile salts available for digestion and absorption and causes these digestants to be secreted out of phase with the bulk of the chyme, which is delivered directly to the jejunum. Loss of the stomach's reservoir function may shorten intestinal transit time, reducing the duration of contact between food and the intestinal surface. Finally, rapid food loading into the small intestine may unmask other subclinical malabsorption disorders, such as lactose intolerance (by sidestepping the duodenum, the major site of lactase activ-

ity) or nontropical sprue (by exposing the intestine to more gluten).

After gastrectomy, maldigestion may cause hypoproteinemia, vitamin $B_{12}$ deficiency, and calcium and iron deficiencies.

**Ileal resection.** Often done for regional ileitis and tumors, ileal resection causes loss of absorptive sites for vitamin $B_{12}$ and bile salts. Massive intestinal resection for tumors excises a large part of the absorptive intestine, causing severe nutrient malabsorption.

## MEDICAL MANAGEMENT
Clinical signs and symptoms of malabsorption are broad and variable and may be nonspe-

## Vitamin, mineral, and pancreatic enzyme replacements

### Water-soluble vitamins

**Folic acid**
Initial dose: 10 to 20 mg/day I.M. or I.V.
Maintenance: 5 to 10 mg/day I.M. or I.V.

**Vitamin $B_{12}$**
Initial dose: 30 to 60 mcg/day I.M. or S.C. for 5 to 10 days
Maintenance: 30 to 200 mcg/month I.M.
(Systemic disorder requires more intensive therapy.)

**Vitamin B complex**
P.O.: two or three multivitamin tablets daily, each containing the minimum daily requirement of niacin, riboflavin, and thiamine
I.M.: preparations available for general deficiencies

### Fat-soluble vitamins

**Vitamin A**
P.O.: oleovitamin A, 100,000 to 200,000 units/day in severe deficiencies; 25,000 to 50,000 units/day in moderate deficiencies

**Vitamin D (Vitamin $D_2$ [ergocalciferol])**
I.M. or P.O.: 30,000 units/day; dosage increased as needed to raise serum calcium levels to normal
(Dosage varies greatly according to response as determined by serum and urine calcium levels.)

**Combination A and D vitamins**
Concentrated A and D, USP (50,000 to 65,000 USP A units and 10,000 to 13,000 USP D units/gram) available instead of separate preparations

**Vitamin K**
P.O.: menadione, 4 to 12 mg/day; vitamin $K_1$ tablets, 5 to 10 mg/day
I.V. (for acute bleeding episodes): vitamin $K_1$, 10 to 50 mg over 10-minute period; repeated in 4 hours if needed

### Minerals

**Calcium**
P.O.: calcium gluconate, 1 to 5 g t.i.d.
I.V.: calcium gluconate, 10% solution for injection, 10 to 30 ml administered slowly according to response

**Iron**
P.O.: ferrous sulfate, 325 mg t.i.d.
I.M. or I.V.: iron dextran, calculated according to severity of anemia

**Magnesium**
P.O.: magnesium sulfate, 3 g every 6 hours for 4 doses
I.M.: magnesium sulfate, 1 g every 6 hours for 4 doses
I.V.: magnesium sulfate, 5 g added to 1,000 ml of dextrose 5% in water and infused over 3 hours

**Pancreatic enzyme supplements**
P.O.: pancreatin, 6,500 to 24,000 USP units of lipase activity with each meal
P.O.: pancrelipase, 4,000 to 32,000 USP units of lipase activity with each meal

cific. (See *Signs and symptoms of malabsorption,* page 76.) Clues to diagnosis appear through a complete history and a physical examination. Treatment is mostly dietary, after laboratory tests have determined specific causes.

### Blood and urine tests

Among more than a dozen different tests that can be done on blood and urine specimens, some screen for general digestive and absorptive malfunction, whereas others specifically indicate nutrient and enzyme deficiencies.

**Hematologic workup.** Lab tests on blood samples can suggest various malabsorption syndromes. Since red blood cell (RBC) production depends on dietary iron, vitamin $B_{12}$, and folic acid, malabsorption may cause deficiencies of these substances and associated anemias. RBC indices—mean corpuscular volume (MCV), mean corpuscular hemoglobin (MCH), and mean corpuscular hemoglobin concentration (MCHC)—help classify anemias. Decreased MCV, MCH, and MCHC indicate hypochromic microcytic anemia from iron deficiency. Increased MCV and variable MCH and MCHC indicate macrocytic (megaloblastic) anemia from vitamin $B_{12}$ and folic acid deficiency. Low serum iron levels indicate protein malabsorption occurring with insufficient gastric acid for ingested iron ionization.

Other blood studies may reveal:
• prolonged prothrombin time, reflecting inadequate synthesis of the clotting factor prothrombin (hypoprothrombinemia) due to malabsorption of vitamin K
• low cholesterol levels (hypocholesterolemia) from decreased fat digestion and absorption so that the liver cannot synthesize cholesterol
• low sodium, chloride, and potassium levels (hyponatremia, hypochloremia, hypokalemia), which can cause profuse diarrhea and electrolyte loss
• low calcium levels, indicating malabsorption of vitamin D and amino acids
• reduced levels of protein and albumin (hypoalbuminemia), reflecting protein loss
• decreased levels of vitamin A (retinol) and its precursor, carotene, suggesting bile salt deficiency and impaired fat absorption since vitamin A absorption requires both dietary fat and bile salts.

**Lactose tolerance test.** This screening test for disaccharidase deficiency involves serial blood samples taken after lactose administration. Patients with lactose intolerance usually will not achieve the normal 20% rise in blood glucose over the fasting level because of lactase deficiency or defective transport of monosaccharides across the intestinal mucosa. Development of diarrhea, gas, and cramps during the test and a drop in stool pH from 7 or 8 to 5.5 confirms lactase deficiency.

**Monosaccharide test.** This test may be performed to exclude the possibility that lactose intolerance results from poor absorption of monosaccharides rather than from lactase deficiency. Low serial blood glucose levels after ingestion of glucose and galactose suggest monosaccharide malabsorption as the primary cause, but a normal blood glucose curve confirms lactase deficiency.

**D-xylose absorption test.** This test screens for carbohydrate malabsorption and shows the absorptive integrity of the intestinal mucosa. D-xylose, a pentose sugar absorbed in the small intestine without the need for pancreatic enzymes, is carried intact through the liver and excreted in the urine. Since it's absorbed without digestion, measuring D-xylose levels in the blood and urine shows the small intestine's absorptive capacity. Low serum and urine D-xylose levels commonly result from nontropical sprue and other malabsorptive disorders that reduce the absorptive area of the proximal small intestine. But test results may be falsely low because of coexisting renal failure; ascites; bacterial overgrowth; hypothyroidism; and ingestion of certain drugs, such as indomethacin (Indocin).

**Urinary 5-HIAA.** Increased urinary excretion of tryptophan metabolites, specifically 5-hydroxyindoleacetic acid (5-HIAA), indicates abnormal metabolism of the amino acid tryptophan. This often accompanies protein malabsorption caused by nontropical sprue.

**Schilling test.** This three-stage test for vitamin $B_{12}$ absorption measures urinary excretion of the vitamin after standard radioactive and nonradioactive doses and can distinguish between intrinsic factor deficiency and various malabsorption syndromes. Stage one involves oral administration of radioactive $B_{12}$, followed by an intramuscular saturation dose of nonradioactive $B_{12}$. Normally, within 24 hours of ingestion, 8% to 40% of the radioactive dose appears in the urine, but patients with pernicious anemia and malabsorption syndromes show decreased urinary excretion. Stage two involves administering radioactive $B_{12}$ and intrinsic factor. Patients with pernicious anemia show normal urinary excretion, but those with sprue, blind loop syndrome, pancreatic deficiency, or ileal disease or re-

section still show decreased excretion. Stage three involves administering radioactive $B_{12}$ and antibiotics. Normal excretion points to malabsorption stemming from bacterial overgrowth. A change toward normal after a gluten-free trial diet confirms nontropical sprue and, after administration of pancreatic extract, indicates pancreatic deficiency.

### Breath tests
Two simple, noninvasive tests performed on breath samples provide quick and early evidence of common malabsorption disorders.

**Hydrogen breath test.** Breath analysis screens for lactose intolerance by measuring the hydrogen content of breath samples in the fasting state before and after ingestion of lactose. Because colonic bacterial action on unabsorbed lactose produces excess hydrogen and other gases in the breath, increased hydrogen content after lactose ingestion shows lactose intolerance. Two other tests, the lactose tolerance test and the monosaccharide test, may be used to find the main cause.

**Bile acid breath test.** This test requires inhalation of radiolabeled bile salts to assess the bile salt absorption rate in the small intestine. In ileal disease or resection, unabsorbed bile salts are deconjugated by colonic bacteria, releasing carbon dioxide. With normal bile salt absorption, patients finally breathe out radioactive carbon dioxide, but they do so more slowly than patients with bile salt malabsorption or bacterial overgrowth.

### Stool tests
Two tests on stool specimens may be used to see if GI distress stems from a disorder of fat digestion and absorption or from infestation by parasites or pathogenic bacteria.

**Fecal fat measurement.** Quantitative measurement of fecal fat in a 72-hour stool collection best detects steatorrhea. A nonspecific test of overall lipid digestion and absorption in the small intestine, pancreas, and liver, fecal fat measurement doesn't distinguish between maldigestion and intestinal mucosal disease as causes of fat malabsorption. Since about 94% of dietary fat is normally absorbed, the stool shouldn't hold more than 6% of the fat ingested during testing. Qualitative fat analysis in single stool specimens may be done, but it won't detect mild steatorrhea. Increased fecal fat shows malabsorption without giving differential diagnosis.

**Stool culture.** Bacteriologic examination of feces can isolate and identify pathogenic bac-

## Interpreting intestinal biopsies

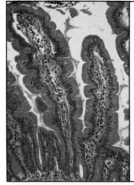

**Normal**
Longitudinal section of normal small intestinal folds shows regular, conically shaped villi with columnar epithelial cells. Within each villus lie a normal lamina propria with disbursed lymphocytes, a rich vascular network, and a central lymph vessel supported by smooth muscle that aids in villous motion.

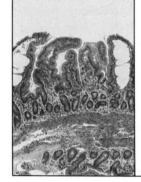

**Nontropical (celiac) sprue**
Characteristic mucosa in nontropical sprue displays atrophic villi with cuboidal epithelial cells, deepened crypts of Lieberkühn, and an expanded lamina propria heavily infiltrated by mononuclear cells.

**Lymphangiectasia**
Typical mucosal changes in lymphangiectasia reveal greatly dilated central lymph vessels, which broaden and distort the involved villi and lamina propria while leaving the submucosa and neighboring intestinal folds unaffected. Such dilation allows protein-rich lymphatic fluid to leak into the intestinal lumen.

teria, parasites, and (rarely) viruses that may be causing diarrhea, cramping, and other GI symptoms. Isolation of large numbers of a pathogen indicates infection and sometimes requires antibiotic sensitivity testing to guide drug treatment.

### Biopsy

Careful peroral biopsy of the small intestine is needed early in the diagnostic workup of malabsorption. The biopsy may be essential to diagnose certain diseases that affect the small bowel and to distinguish between maldigestion and malabsorption when they cause similar clinical signs. Biopsy may show characteristic changes in the villi, epithelial cells, crypts, lymphatics, and lamina propria. (See *Interpreting intestinal biopsies,* above.)

### Other studies

Ultrasound and computerized tomography scan are usually used before radiographic studies. Ultrasound can detect pancreatic or small-bowel tumors. GI X-rays may help to diagnose malabsorption or to rule out other GI disorders. Plain films of the abdomen may show pancreatic calcifications, suggesting chronic pancreatitis and resultant pancreatic deficiency as the causes of malabsorption. They can also identify congenital abnormalities, tumors, postsurgical changes, or any gross structural changes in the intestinal mucosa that affect nutrient absorption. Barium sulfate contrast studies of the stomach and small intestine may reveal anatomic defects as well as diffuse primary small-bowel disease. They can show the barium column breakup, mucosal fold coarsening, mucosal pattern disruption, and shortened intestinal transit time typical of nontropical sprue and other mucosal injuries.

### Treatment: Mainly dietary

Although surgery and drug therapy may help correct some malabsorption disorders, the primary treatment involves controlling diet to eliminate offensive ingredients and to replace lost nutrients. A low-fat diet may be ordered to avoid challenging below-normal function in gallbladder or pancreatic disease, severe steatorrhea, abetalipoproteinemia, cystic fibrosis, lymphangiectasia, scleroderma, and short-bowel syndrome. A high-protein, high-calorie diet with frequent feedings may be ordered after a total gastrectomy. Probably the most common diets prescribed are the lactose-free or lactose-restricted diet for lactose intolerance, and the gluten-free diet for nontropical sprue. (See *Lactose-free diet,* page 83, and *Gluten-free diet,* page 84.)

**Dietary supplements.** Medium-chain triglycerides, available in oil form, seem to be valuable in malabsorption disorders because they don't need bile salts or pancreatic lipase for absorption across the intestinal epithelium, and they pass rapidly through portal circulation rather than following the usual fat absorption route. Rapidly oxidized in the liver, they're an important source of calories and energy for patients with fat malabsorption from pancreatic enzyme or bile salt deficiency or lymphatic disorders such as lymphangiectasia.

Other supplements replace lost vitamins, minerals, and pancreatic enzymes in some malabsorption syndromes. (See *Vitamin, min-*

*eral, and pancreatic enzyme replacements,*
page 78.) For example, disorders of the intestinal absorptive surface require supplements of water-soluble vitamins, such as folic acid, vitamin $B_{12}$, and vitamin B complex; and important minerals, such as calcium, magnesium, and iron. A lactose-free diet requires calcium replacement. Bile salt deficiency and absorptive surface disruption require replacement of fat-soluble vitamins A, D, E, and K. Similarly, pancreatic deficiency requires supplements of pancreatic enzymes. Also, since hydration becomes important when malabsorption causes diarrhea, acute stages of malabsorption may require supplemental nutrition with intravenous hyperalimentation (IVH).

## Drug therapy: Sometimes helpful
Antibiotics and steroids may be used to treat various malabsorption syndromes.

**Antibiotics.** In tropical sprue, even though the pathogen has not yet been identified, treatment with antibiotics (usually tetracycline) is recommended for 3 to 6 months. In Whipple's disease, penicillin or tetracycline for 3 to 6 months usually destroys glycoprotein-containing macrophages and gram-negative bacilli that infiltrate the intestinal epithelium and lymphatics. Bacterial overgrowth from any cause responds to antibiotics such as tetracycline, usually in one 10-day course.

**Steroids.** In Whipple's disease, steroids are sometimes prescribed in combination with antibiotics when antibiotics alone prove ineffective. The patient is usually given prednisone or, if he's acutely ill, intravenous adrenocorticotropic hormone. When symptoms subside and the patient's weight normalizes, dosage can be decreased to maintenance level. Steroids are stopped when biopsy of the small intestine appears normal. In nontropical sprue, steroids (usually prednisone) may augment the gluten-free diet or replace it to overcome symptoms resulting from noncompliance. Steroids may not restore normal intestinal mucosa in nontropical sprue, but they usually provide clinical improvement within weeks.

## Managing underlying disease
Many disorders cause secondary malabsorption, which may respond to medical or surgical treatment of the underlying disease. Chemotherapy may control lymphoma or other tumors that disrupt the mucosa or impair blood or lymph circulation. Drug therapy to lower central venous pressure and resulting lymphatic back pressure may be effective in heart failure. Surgery may correct bacterial overgrowth caused by blind loop syndrome, strictures, fistulas, or diverticula. Partial resection of the small intestine may minimize malabsorption in regional ileitis, lymphangiectasia, and intestinal ischemia or obstruction. Treating the Zollinger-Ellison syndrome with cimetidine or gastrectomy to decrease excess gastric secretion reactivates pancreatic enzymes. Pericardiectomy to treat constrictive pericarditis may also reverse malabsorption due to lymphatic blockage. Medical or surgical elimination of biliary obstruction restores bile flow to the duodenum and corrects malabsorption due to bile salt deficiency.

## NURSING MANAGEMENT
Caring for the patient with malabsorption means understanding and meeting him on his own level so you can help him adapt to what's sometimes a permanent and inconvenient change in diet. The challenge begins with a probing history and physical examination. The thorough assessments required initially and during recovery test your skill in uncovering often hidden clues to the malady's origin.

## Phase one: Searching for clues
While taking the nursing history, keep in mind the patient's age, sex, and ethnic origin because these may help in differential diagnosis. Begin the history by asking about the patient's chief complaint. He may describe classic signs and symptoms of malabsorption, including anorexia, weight loss, abdominal distention, cramping, and passage of abnormal stools. Ask if the stools are gray, greasy, bulky, and malodorous. Ask about frequency of bowel movements and about associated borborygmus and flatulence. Do they occur 1 to 2 hours after meals? The patient may describe frequent bowel movements or, occasionally, only one bulky stool a day.

Explore the pattern and extent of weight loss. Has it been slow and progressive? Some patients may lose up to 30 lb before seeking medical help; others lose a few pounds in the first few months of illness, then stabilize at a less than ideal weight. Ask about food intake. Do symptoms develop after milk ingestion, suggesting lactose intolerance, or after a fatty meal, indicating bile salt deficiency? Anorexia and the need to avoid diarrhea and cramping may lead the patient to greatly reduce his intake, which only aggravates weight loss. Cramping is common in many malabsorption disorders, but severe pain is specific to certain ones, such as regional ileitis (generalized crampy pain), intestinal obstruction (acute periumbilical pain), intestinal ischemia (cramping pain 20 to 30 minutes after meals), and pancreatic disease (severe and radiating epigastric pain).

Inquire about general complaints that may be related to malabsorption, such as chronic fatigue, muscle weakness or cramps, and chronic depression. These are typically associated with carbohydrate malabsorption, protein deficiency, electrolyte imbalance, and anemia. Does the patient have frequent or recurrent respiratory infections? These signal impaired immunity and general malnutrition. Does the patient bruise easily or bleed copiously on slight injury? These indicate vitamin K malabsorption.

Next, explore the patient's medical history. Has he ever been diagnosed and treated for intestinal tumors, inflammation, or lesions such as diverticula? Does he have a history of gastric ulcers, pancreatitis, cystic fibrosis, or parenchymal or obstructive liver disease? Does he have predisposing conditions, such as diabetes mellitus or other endocrine disorders, scleroderma, cardiac problems, or vascular insufficiency? Has he had gastric or intestinal resection or received radiation therapy for cancer? All these conditions may cause malabsorption, as can certain drugs, such as calcium carbonate and cholestyramine, which cause malabsorption by blocking absorption of bile salts and vitamins.

**Psychosocial evaluation.** Since malabsorption syndromes tend to be chronic, and treatment may entail life-style changes, assess how the patient has coped with this and past illnesses. If coping mechanisms seem ineffective, explore possible support from family, friends, or community organizations.

**Physical assessment.** Early physical findings may be diffuse; however, dehydration, weight loss, muscle wasting, and systemic signs of nutrient deficiencies may be evident by the time the patient seeks medical attention. (See *Signs and symptoms of malabsorption,* page 76.) Usually, the patient appears cachectic and pale from malnutrition and anemia. Peripheral edema and dermatologic abnormalities may appear because of protein loss and vitamin deficiencies. Neurologic signs, such as paresthesias, tremors, and tetany, may be present in calcium and vitamin $B_{12}$ deficiencies. Peripheral lymphadenopathy may occur in malabsorption from lymphatic obstruction.

Abdominal assessment may be normal or

may show a tense, distended abdomen with hyperactive bowel sounds. With distention, you may find generalized abdominal tenderness on palpation. If you find a palpable liver below the right costal margin and hepatomegaly on percussion, malabsorption may stem from parenchymal liver disease or severe congestive heart failure. A right lower quadrant mass may stem from pathologic changes in ileal structure characteristic of regional ileitis. Remember, however, that in many patients with malabsorption the abdominal examination is unremarkable. You may find numerous other clinical manifestations characteristic of disorders underlying malabsorption syndromes during the physical examination.

### Phase two: Reversing malnutrition
When the history and physical examination have shown specific malabsorption, you're ready to form nursing diagnoses, to set goals, and to plan appropriate interventions. Your care plan will probably include these nursing diagnoses for malabsorption syndromes.

**Alteration in bowel elimination (diarrhea) related to malabsorption.** To decrease bowel movement frequency and passage of watery stools, first note the character, color, amount, and frequency of the patient's bowel movements, including liquid stool measurement and intake and output. Give antidiarrheal agents, such as diphenoxylate with atropine (Lomotil), deodorized tincture of opium (DTO), or kaolin with pectin (Kaopectate), as needed and ordered. Give psyllium (Metamucil), as ordered, to provide bulk and to decrease stool fluidity.

Treat the patient with an understanding attitude because he may be embarrassed. Give as much privacy as possible. Keep a commode or bedpan handy always, and empty it promptly after each use. Use a room deodorizer if stools are malodorous. Keep bed linen clean and dry. Consider inserting a rectal tube in patients with continuous, liquid diarrhea, but be sure to give good skin care and to change linen, as needed.

**Fluid volume deficit related to diarrhea.** To prevent dehydration and to maintain cardiovascular stability, note fluid balance trends and notify the doctor promptly if you see signs of dehydration or hypovolemia. Assess the patient at least every 4 hours for skin turgor, skin and mucous membrane dryness, tachycardia, hypotension, oliguria, light-headedness, and drowsiness. In acute illness, measure urine output and vital signs hourly, and

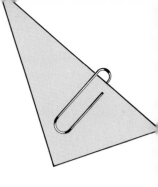

# Lactose-free diet

*Dear* _____

Your doctor has prescribed a lactose-free diet to to determine if lactose is the cause of your gastrointestinal symptoms. Lactose, the carbohydrate found in milk and milk products, is a common ingredient in many foods and medicines, so read all product labels carefully.

In planning meals, avoid milk, cheese, butter, margarine, and all products and dishes contain-ing them or containing lactose, curds, whey, casein, or dry milk solids. Because this diet may lack sufficient calories, calcium, iron, riboflavin, thia-mine, and vitamins A and D, be sure to include a soy milk sub-stitute, calcium-rich foods, or calcium tablets every day.

When appropriate, your doc-tor may allow you to begin add-ing foods containing lactose to your diet to test your ability to digest them. Add only one new food in small amounts each week. If you develop diarrhea, gas, intestinal discomfort, or other symptoms of intolerance, stop eating that food and notify the doctor. You may find that you can eat nearly everything but milk, ice cream, and Ameri-can and cottage cheese, so try adding these foods last.

| Foods allowed | Foods to avoid |
|---|---|
| **Beverages:** Ground coffee, tea, carbonated drinks, soy milk substitutes, cocoa made with water or milk substitute, fruit drinks without lactose, vegetable juice, wine | **Beverages:** Milk, instant coffee, soft drinks made from powder or tablet, Ovaltine, commercial hot chocolate, artificial fruit drinks with lactose, cordials, liqueurs |
| **Bread:** Homemade bread without milk; Italian, Vienna, or French bread prepared without milk; plain soda or graham crackers | **Bread:** Commercial breads, biscuits, crackers, muffins, pancakes, rolls, or sweet rolls with milk, lactose, or whey; packaged bread crumbs, breading mixes, and croutons |
| **Cereal:** Packaged or cooked cereals made without milk or milk products | **Cereal:** Dry cereals with milk, lactose, or whey; cream of rice; instant cream of wheat |
| **Desserts, sweets:** Homemade cake, cookies, and puddings made without milk; fruit ice; popsicles; gela-tin desserts; nondairy toppings without milk or milk products; sugar, honey, syrup; pure jam and jelly; hard candy; marshmallows; baking chocolate; choco-late chips and syrup made with cocoa | **Desserts, sweets:** Desserts containing milk or milk products; custard, ice cream, junket, sherbet; com-mercial toppings; lactose-based sugar substitutes; molasses; cream or milk chocolate; commercial candy containing milk or lactose; chewing gum |
| **Fats:** Milk-free margarine; nondairy coffee cream-er; vegetable oil and shortening; mayonnaise; salad dressing without cheese, milk, or milk products | **Fats:** Butter, margarine; cream, sour cream, powdered coffee creamer; salad dressing with cheese, milk, or milk products; commercial dips and spreads |
| **Fruit:** All fresh fruit; canned, frozen or dried fruit without lactose | **Fruit:** Canned, frozen, or dried fruit with lactose |
| **Protein:** Meat, fish, poultry, and eggs cooked without milk or milk products; lunch meat without milk addi-tives; kosher meat products; shellfish; nuts; peanut butter | **Protein:** Creamed or breaded meat, fish, or poultry; lunch meat with dry skim milk added; nonkosher frankfurters; sweetbreads, brains; cheese, yogurt |
| **Starch:** White and sweet potatoes, pasta, rice, and corn fixed without milk or milk products | **Starch:** Instant potatoes; packaged items with milk, lactose, casein, cheese, curds, or whey |
| **Soup:** Broths and broth-based soups | **Soup:** Cream soups, commercial soups containing milk or milk products |
| **Vegetables:** All fresh, frozen, or canned vegetables without milk or milk products | **Vegetables:** Vegetables prepared with cheese, milk, milk products, butter, or margarine |
| **Miscellaneous:** Salt, pepper, pure herbs and spices; catsup, mustard, olives, pickles, relish; vinegar; soy, steak, and tartar sauces; gravy without milk; popcorn without butter or margarine; plain potato or corn chips | **Miscellaneous:** All items containing monosodium glutamate extender and most dietetic and diabetic foods |

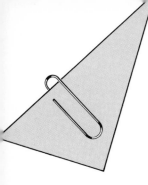

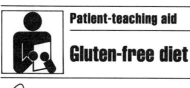

**Patient-teaching aid**

# Gluten-free diet

*Dear* _____

Your doctor has prescribed a gluten-free diet because you have trouble digesting gluten, a protein substance found in wheat, rye, oats, buckwheat, and barley. Be sure to read all product labels carefully. In planning meals, avoid all cereal and malt drinks and foods that are breaded or otherwise thickened or sauced with grain products other than rice, corn, soy, or gluten-free wheat flour. In time, you may find that you can add small amounts of gluten-containing products.

| Foods allowed | Foods to avoid |
|---|---|
| **Beverages:** Ground and decaffeinated coffee, tea; milk; hot chocolate; carbonated drinks; cocoa; fruit juice; vegetable juice; unfortified wine, rum | **Beverages:** Instant coffee with wheat; cereal drinks (Ovaltine and Postum); malted milk; root beer, ale, beer, gin, vodka, whiskey |
| **Bread:** Bread and other items made with corn, potato, rice, soybean, or gluten-free wheat flour | **Bread:** Bread, bread crumbs, crackers, pretzels, rolls, mixes, and other items made with wheat, rye, oat, buckwheat, or barley flour |
| **Cereal:** Packaged and cooked cereal made with corn or rice without malt flavoring or extract | **Cereal:** Cereal with wheat, rye, oats, buckwheat, or barley; wheat germ |
| **Desserts, sweets:** Baked goods made with gluten-free flour; homemade ice cream and sherbet; fruit ice; popsicles; custard; gelatin; meringues; pudding made with cornstarch, rice, or tapioca; sugar, honey, syrup, and molasses; jam and jelly; marshmallows; chocolate, cocoa; coconut; candy made with allowed foods | **Desserts, sweets:** Cake, cookies, crackers, doughnuts, pies, puddings, and candy made with wheat, rye, oats, buckwheat, or barley; commercial desserts, mixes, ice cream, and sherbet; ice cream cones; some pie fillings |
| **Fats:** Butter, margarine; cream; vegetable oil and shortening; pure mayonnaise; salad dressing thickened with cornstarch | **Fats:** Salad dressing thickened with wheat, rye, oat, buckwheat, or barley products |
| **Fruit:** All fresh, canned, frozen, or dried fruit | **Fruit:** Thickened or prepared fruit |
| **Protein:** Meat, fish, poultry, and lunch meats prepared without subject grains; cheese; eggs; nuts; peanut butter | **Protein:** Breaded meats, fish, and poultry; lunch and canned meats with cereal additives |
| **Soup:** Broth, clear soup; homemade soup made with allowed foods; cream soup thickened with cornstarch or potato starch | **Soup:** Commercial soup with wheat, rye, oats, buckwheat, or barley |
| **Starch:** Potatoes, corn, low-protein pasta, rice | **Starch:** Pasta, commercial stuffing mixes |
| **Vegetables:** All fresh, frozen, and canned vegetables | **Vegetables:** Vegetables prepared with cream or cheese sauces thickened with flour |
| **Miscellaneous:** Salt, pepper; pure herbs and spices; dry mustard; flavoring extracts; cider and wine vinegar; olives, pickles; baking powder; cornstarch, potato starch; sauces and gravies thickened with allowed foods; popcorn | **Miscellaneous:** Condiments made with wheat, rye, oats, buckwheat, or barley; distilled white vinegar; gravy mixes, malt flavoring extract |

monitor I.V. dextrose and saline solution replacement therapy. Monitor blood chemistry and other laboratory values daily for excessive loss of electrolytes, especially potassium, and notify the doctor promptly of abnormal levels. Give potassium replacement orally or I.V., as ordered.

**Alteration in comfort related to abdominal cramping and pain.** To ease abdominal cramping or pain, assess the patient for abdominal discomfort, especially after meals. Note nonverbal signs of distress, such as guarding, doubling over, change in affect, or withdrawal, as well as verbal complaints. Correlate the time of meals; the type of food or beverage ingested; and the evidence of flatulence, nausea, vomiting, or diarrhea accompanying the pain. Have the patient describe the exact location and type of pain. For cramping, give an anticholinergic, such as

Donnatol or belladonna, 15 to 30 minutes before meals, as ordered, and monitor its effect. Help the patient alternate rest periods with ambulation to stimulate peristalsis. Suggest diversionary activities, such as television and reading. For severe pain, possibly associated with an underlying pancreatic or liver disorder, cancer, or intestinal ischemia, give stronger pain relievers, such as narcotics, as ordered. For arthritic and sciatic pain associated with bone demineralization (as may occur with malabsorption of calcium and phosphorus in nontropical sprue), use comfort measures, such as frequent position changes and mild activity along with analgesics, as appropriate. Monitor calcium and phosphorus levels, and give their replacements, as ordered.

**Alteration in nutrition related to nutrient malabsorption and subsequent decreased oral intake.** To prevent or reverse nutrient deficiencies and to achieve and maintain appropriate body weight, remember that the patient may need nutritional buildup before maintenance therapy. Administer I.M. or P.O. vitamin and mineral supplements, as ordered.

If IVH is necessary, explain its benefits to the patient, and tell him about the insertion procedure and the frequent nursing checks involved. Help the doctor insert the central venous line, and afterwards carefully maintain the infusion at the prescribed rate. Use strict aseptic technique during dressing and tubing changes to prevent infection. Monitor intake and output, urine glucose levels, and serum electrolyte levels, as ordered.

Tell the patient on an oral diet to ingest frequent small amounts of high-calorie foods and high-electrolyte fluids. Suggest quick electrolyte replacements, such as Gatorade, meat broth, and bouillon. Remember that the patient with malabsorption may be anxious about eating because he's anticipating cramps and diarrhea. Encourage him to eat, and reassure him that antidiarrheal medication should reduce diarrhea and discomfort within 24 hours after the first dose. Provide a quiet, calm, and esthetically pleasing environment with few interruptions during meals.

If a special diet is needed, actively promote the diet to the patient. Work with the dietitian to help the patient fully understand the diet's benefits and rationale. Monitor the patient's diet trays while he is hospitalized, along with any food brought in by visitors. Record the patient's food and fluid intake and note his tolerance for specific foods. Compare weekly weights to note the weight trend.

**Knowledge deficit related to the disease process and nutritional therapy.** To help the patient and his family to understand the underlying physiologic mechanisms in his malabsorption syndrome and to understand the special diet prescribed for him, first assess their knowledge of the disorder and their expectations. Talk to them at their level of understanding, and review fundamental mechanisms of intestinal malabsorption, diarrhea, fluid loss, nutrient deficiencies, and diet therapy. In your teaching, be sure to include the person who does the shopping and cooking. Emphasize that diet therapy may require a lifetime commitment but that the reward is a healthy life. Provide written lists of foods to eat and foods to avoid, and teach the patient and his family to read labels to check for all forms of the offensive foods. Teach them to modify food preparation to avoid these products. (See *Lactose-free diet,* page 83, and *Gluten-free diet,* page 84.)

Teach the patient on a special diet to examine his intake if symptoms recur and to eliminate any new food that might have sparked the relapse. Tell him to notify the doctor if diarrhea persists for more than a few days.

Along with teaching sessions, give the patient and his family time to air their feelings and concerns about the illness and the therapy. Help them feel confident in their ability to follow the prescribed diet.

### Phase three: Evaluating your interventions

Consider your interventions successful if:
- the patient's bowel elimination doesn't exceed three to five semi-formed stools a day
- urine output exceeds 30 ml/hour
- skin turgor is good
- vital signs are stable
- no severe cramping occurs after meals, or pain is controlled with drugs
- weight gain is at least 1 lb/week
- no signs of vitamin, mineral, carbohydrate, protein, or fat malabsorption or deficiency appear
- the patient and his family understand the basic causes of his condition and follow the prescribed diet therapy.

### Nursing support: The turnaround

Your interventions try to set the patient with malabsorption on a firm path to recovery and to keep him comfortable in transit. Usually, the patient controls his recovery, but teaching and support can supply the means, desire, and confidence to remain well.

**Points to remember**

The liver, stomach, pancreas, and small intestine regulate normal digestion and absorption of nutrients.
- Any defect in digestion or absorption can lead to diarrhea, nutrient deficiencies, hypovolemia, or clinical starvation.
- The basic mechanisms of malabsorption include biochemical and enzyme deficiencies, bacterial proliferation, mucosal disruption of the small intestine, disturbed lymphatic or vascular circulation, and loss of gastric or intestinal surface area.
- Lactose intolerance is the most common malabsorption disorder, affecting about 75% of American blacks.
- Treatment for malabsorption disorders is largely dietary, eliminating or restricting intake of the offensive food constituents and supplementing diet with vitamin, mineral, and enzyme replacements. In secondary malabsorption, drug therapy, nutritional support, and surgery may be useful in treating the underlying disorder.
- The nurse's role in explaining the rationale for diet therapy and persuading the patient of its benefit is vital in encouraging lifelong compliance.

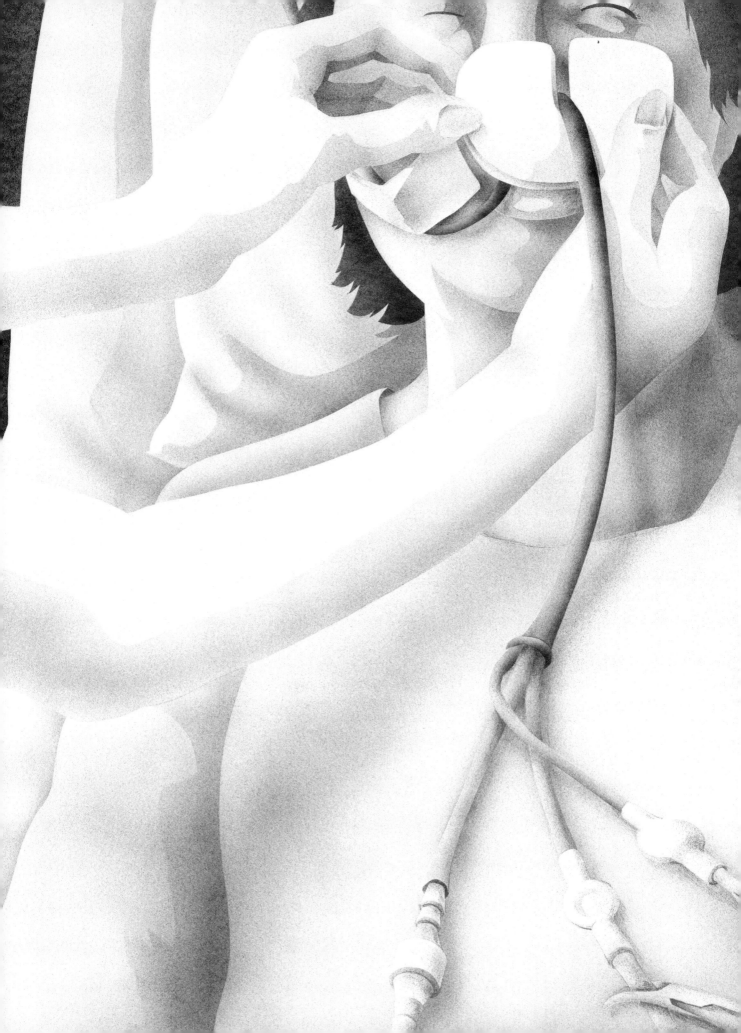

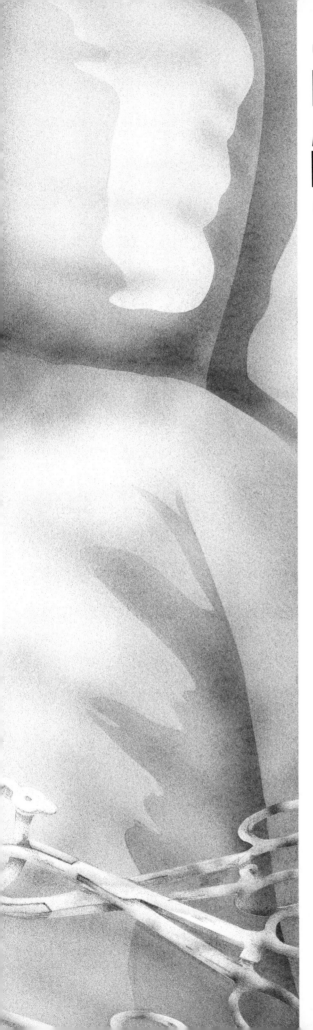

# INFLAMMATORY
# AND INFECTIOUS
# DISORDERS

# 6 INTERVENING IN UPPER G.I. INFLAMMATION

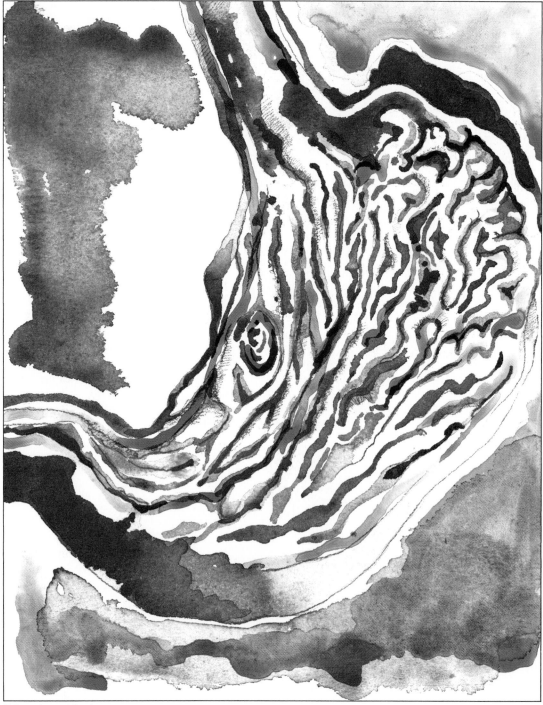

Subacute gastric ulcer

nflammation causes serious disorders throughout the upper GI tract. It commonly causes ulcers, which may lead to perforation and hemorrhage. Because even its milder forms can cause significant discomfort and impairment of lifestyle, you must understand how it develops, how to detect its sometimes subtle signs and symptoms, and how to prevent its serious complications.

### Barriers to cellular injury

The GI tract has several natural defenses against cellular injury. Mucus, secreted by mucous glands throughout the GI tract, provides one. In the mouth, mucus secreted by submaxillary glands mixes with a digestive enzyme to form saliva. Besides aiding in digestion, saliva dilutes, neutralizes, and removes irritating substances from the mouth. In the esophagus, a thick mucous layer protects the wall from mechanical and thermal trauma and protects against chemical trauma by diluting gastric acid reflux from the stomach. In the stomach, mucus lines the walls, protecting them from trauma and opportunistic organisms.

Another natural barrier to cellular injury is the stomach's acidic environment, which kills many foreign organisms. And still another barrier is provided by a balance of natural flora, which effectively retards the growth of opportunistic organisms by competing with them for space and nutrients.

Despite these defenses, microorganisms can invade the upper GI tract in several ways:
• They invade the mouth, parotid glands, esophagus, or stomach after a mechanical, chemical, or thermal injury weakens the wall. For example, bacterial esophagitis develops when a motor disorder called achalasia causes retention of food in the esophagus. The retained food decays, producing bacteria that invade the esophageal mucosa.
• They proliferate after ingestion of a caustic substance—such as a strong alkali. Caustic substances produce two kinds of damage: proliferation of infections, with possible perforation and peritonitis, and strictures and obstructions that form when the damaged tissue heals.
• They take hold when any change in the normal environment reduces resistance to foreign organisms. Reduced resistance gives way to the common virus that causes gastroenteritis every winter. The virus invades the GI tract, causing reversible lesions in the jejunum or stomach, resulting in impaired absorption, abdominal pain, nausea and vomiting, and diarrhea.
• They take hold when a change in the GI flora destroys the balance between organisms. Esophageal candidiasis, for example, causes esophagitis after oral antibiotics destroy the bacteria that normally check the proliferation of this fungus. With this infection, the esophagus becomes inflamed and swollen, and swallowing becomes painful and difficult.

### PATHOPHYSIOLOGY

In response to cellular damage, the body calls on its protective mechanisms—the immune system, the reticuloendothelial system, and the acute inflammatory response—to isolate, destroy, and remove the microbial invader. (See *The inflammatory response: Acute and chronic stages,* page 92.)

Vasodilatation and increased vascular permeability at the irritated site let fluid leak into the injured area. Fibrinogen from the edematous fluid forms clots to "wall off" the injured area. Within minutes, phagocytosis occurs as neutrophils and lymphocytes invade the damaged tissue to destroy any microorganisms present and to remove cellular debris. As a result, the collection of dead cells and necrotic tissue forms pus. After destruction and removal of cellular debris, healthy cells replace the destroyed and damaged cells in the normal tissue.

### Chronic inflammation destructive

Although acute inflammation serves an essential protective purpose in response to cellular injury, inflammation can become destructive. If an irritant persistently interferes with tissue repair, inflammation becomes chronic; and the edema, vasodilation, and other localized changes that accompany it interfere with normal activity.

Chronic stomach inflammation—chronic gastritis—usually produces diffuse, burning pain in the epigastric area, although it can be asymptomatic. Eventually, the inflammatory process damages the glands that secrete hydrochloric acid and essential gastric juices. Chronic gastritis initiated by immunologic factors causes destruction of parietal cells and leads to absence of intrinsic factor. Without intrinsic factor—essential for the absorption of vitamin $B_{12}$ from food—pernicious anemia results. In severe atrophic gastritis, intestinal metaplasia develops. In this condition, cells normally found in the small intestine replace

## Causes of upper GI inflammatory disorders

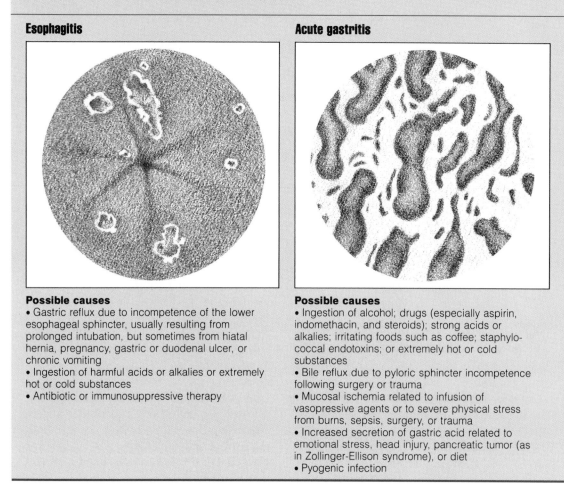

### Esophagitis

**Possible causes**
• Gastric reflux due to incompetence of the lower esophageal sphincter, usually resulting from prolonged intubation, but sometimes from hiatal hernia, pregnancy, gastric or duodenal ulcer, or chronic vomiting
• Ingestion of harmful acids or alkalies or extremely hot or cold substances
• Antibiotic or immunosuppressive therapy

### Acute gastritis

**Possible causes**
• Ingestion of alcohol; drugs (especially aspirin, indomethacin, and steroids); strong acids or alkalies; irritating foods such as coffee; staphylococcal endotoxins; or extremely hot or cold substances
• Bile reflux due to pyloric sphincter incompetence following surgery or trauma
• Mucosal ischemia related to infusion of vasopressive agents or to severe physical stress from burns, sepsis, surgery, or trauma
• Increased secretion of gastric acid related to emotional stress, head injury, pancreatic tumor (as in Zollinger-Ellison syndrome), or diet
• Pyogenic infection

normal gastric cells, and the stomach acquires the small intestine's absorptive capacity.

Eventually, ulceration may develop. The ulcer (called a *peptic ulcer* to indicate its location in the upper GI tract) can occur anywhere (see *Common sites of peptic ulcers*), but its most common site is the pyloric region of the duodenum. A peptic ulcer can develop at the site of chronic inflammation, particularly in infection or vascular obstruction.

*Gastric ulcers* probably result from a loss of mucosal resistance to normal levels of gastric acid especially when the protective mucosa is compromised following gastritis. This lowered resistance may develop because of three other pathophysiologic changes:
• First, gastric acid may diffuse back into the mucosa too quickly. (Normally, mucosal glands secrete gastric acid; afterward, the acid slowly diffuses back into the mucosa.)
• Second, lowered resistance may be due to mucosal damage by bile salts because decreased pyloric sphincter tone permits excessive reflux of bile salts into the stomach.
• Third, lowered resistance may be due to mucosal ischemia or mucous deficiency. This is probably the mechanism behind stress ulcers that develop secondary to severe burns, shock, acute trauma, and carcinoma.

*Duodenal ulcers* seem to result from overproduction of gastric acid in the stomach. Such overproduction may be due to an excessive number of parietal cells, which may be a *response* to excessive hormonal or neurologic stimulation of gastric secretion. Hormonal stimulation (by excess levels of gastrin) and neurologic stimulation (by the vagus nerve) may be responses to emotional stress.

Two other mechanisms may also lead to duodenal ulcers: first, a decrease in pancreatic secretions that normally protect the duodenum by neutralizing gastric acid; and second, abnormally rapid gastric emptying. Rapid emptying interferes with the buffering action of ingested protein, letting abnormally high levels of gastric acid into the duodenum.

## Common sites of peptic ulcers

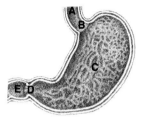

**Key**

**A** Esophagus

**B** Cardia

**C** Stomach

**D** Pylorus

**E** Duodenal bulb

### Chronic gastritis

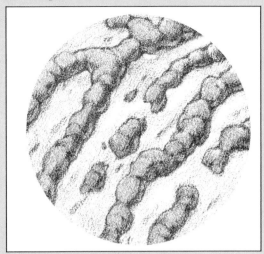

**Possible causes**
- Gastric stasis
- Bile reflux
- Repeated mucosal injuries
- Radiation therapy
- Immunologic factors (possibly destroying parietal cells, leading to pernicious anemia)
- Poor nutrition

### Peptic ulcer

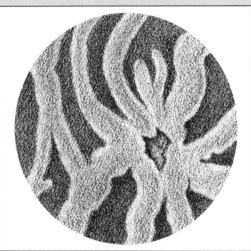

**Possible causes**
- Duodenal ulcer associated with hypersecretion of hydrochloric acid due to Zollinger-Ellison syndrome, stress-induced excessive vagal stimulation, genetic factors, or excessive intake of coffee
- Gastric ulcer associated with breakdown of mucosal barrier due to bile reflux; chemotherapy; or steroid, hormonal, aspirin, or indomethacin therapy

In all locations, peptic ulcers gradually erode the gastrointestinal wall. Erosion of the mucosal and submucosal walls causes slow bleeding (unless it involves a major vessel); interferes with gastric secretions, digestion, and absorption; and causes pain. Erosion of the muscularis mucosae leads to two major complications: hemorrhage and perforation. Slow hemorrhage from erosion of the gastric mucosa may go unnoticed. But erosion of a major blood vessel can cause hemorrhage manifested by hematemesis, melena, and hematochezia. With significant blood loss, hypovolemic shock may also occur. After perforation of the ulcerated wall, gastroduodenal contents leak into the peritoneum and may lead to peritonitis, hemorrhage, and septic or hypovolemic shock.

Complications of peptic ulcer include hemorrhage, perforation, penetration, and pyloric obstruction. Hemorrhage occurs when ulceration causes erosion of a major vessel. Mild episodes may cause occult blood in the stool;

severe episodes may cause hematemesis, melena, hypotension, weakness, tachycardia, and other signs and symptoms of shock. Perforation occurs when gastroduodenal contents empty into the abdominal cavity through a weakened gastric or duodenal wall, causing chemical peritonitis and, possibly, sepsis. Sudden onset of severe abdominal pain and signs and symptoms of peritonitis and shock follow perforation. Penetration occurs when an ulcer penetrates the structure and extends to surrounding structures; penetration usually remains sealed off, so contents do not spill into the peritoneum. Intractable pain and symptoms specific to other organs commonly accompany penetration. Pyloric obstruction occurs when tissue edema or overgrowth of fibrous scar tissue obstructs the pylorus. Vomiting (either with or without nausea) and pain are characteristic. In long-term cases of pyloric obstruction, dehydration and malnutrition also occur.

*(continued on page 94)*

# The inflammatory response: Acute and chronic stages

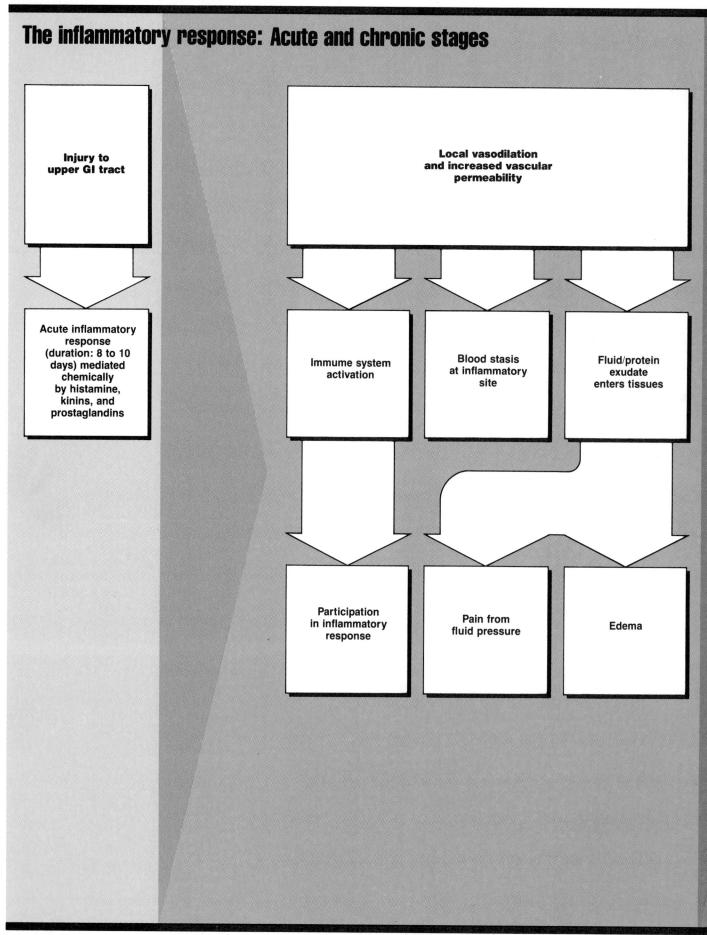

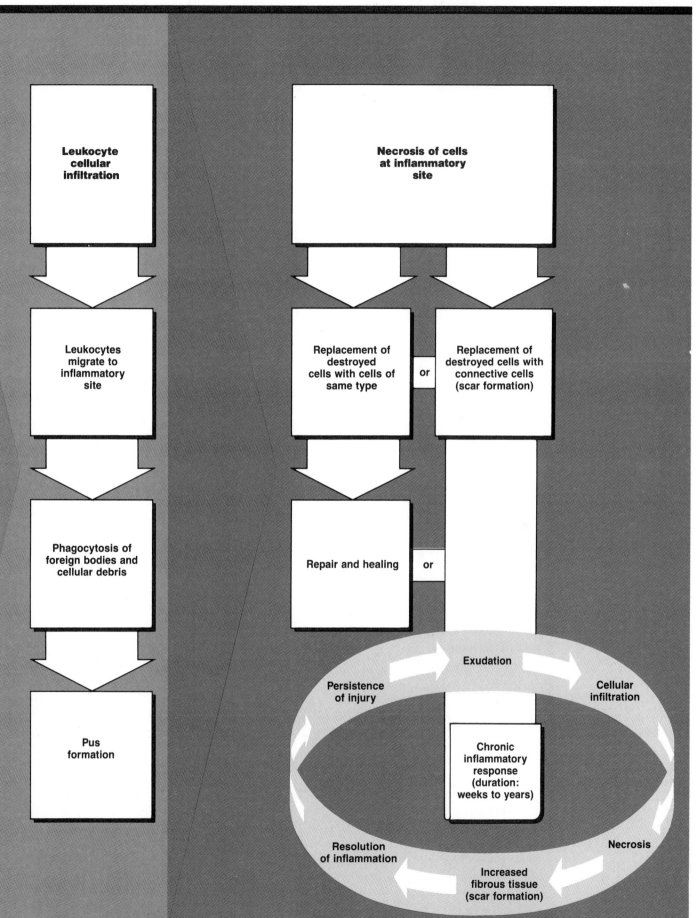

# Recognizing acute pancreatitis

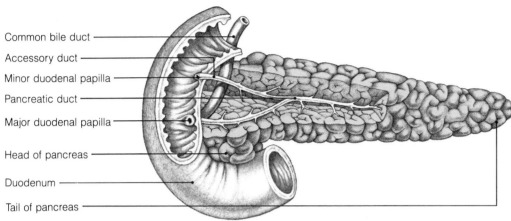

Common bile duct

Accessory duct

Minor duodenal papilla

Pancreatic duct

Major duodenal papilla

Head of pancreas

Duodenum

Tail of pancreas

An inflammation of the pancreas, acute pancreatitis occurs when enzymes normally excreted by the pancreas digest pancreatic tissue. This tissue destruction triggers the inflammatory response.

Acute pancreatitis frequently results from alcoholism. But it also results from biliary regurgitation; obstruction of the pancreatic ducts by a duodenal ulcer; infection; trauma; metabolic disorders; and such drugs as diuretics, steroids, and oral contraceptives. This time-limited disorder usually leaves the pancreas in normal functioning capacity following recovery.

### Getting a history
The chief complaint of the patient with pancreatitis is likely to be severe epigastric pain from distention or obstruction of the

pancreatic duct. The pain may radiate to the back and flanks, and it may intensify when the patient lies down. Vomiting may relieve the pain initially, but eventually it will increase ductal pressure and intensify the pain.

### Examining the patient
Observe the patient for mild jaundice from blockage of the common bile duct. Examine the abdomen: diminished or absent bowel sounds are likely because of ileus. Note tenderness, muscle rigidity, and guarding. Assess vital signs: low-grade fever, tachycardia, and hypotension are possible.

### Laboratory and diagnostic tests
A serum amylase level above 200 Somogyi units almost certainly indicates pancreatitis, especially if urine amylase and

serum lipase levels are also elevated. Serum glucose levels may be elevated because of malfunction of the pancreatic islet cell. Chest X-rays may show left pleural effusion and an elevated diaphragm; abdominal X-rays may show intestinal loop distention associated with ileus.

### Treatment goals
Medical and nursing goals include:
• *relieving pain* by giving analgesics and by teaching comfort measures such as sitting in a knee-chest position
• *restoring fluid and electrolyte balance* by replacing blood, fluids, and electrolytes; monitoring vital signs, intake and output, and laboratory values
• *resting the GI tract* with intravenous hyperalimentation, nasogastric suctioning, and antacids
• *managing complications*, such as hyperglycemia; mental changes from anoxia, sepsis, or alcohol withdrawal; breathing difficulties; and kidney failure
• *preventing secondary infection* through vigorous pulmonary hygiene
• *removing the cause*, if possible, to restore organ function
• *preventing subsequent attacks* by teaching the patient to avoid causative agents, to eat a balanced diet, and to recognize early signs of another attack
• *providing emotional support* and helping the patient work through his guilt (particularly if alcohol caused his pancreatitis).

## MEDICAL MANAGEMENT
In life-threatening emergencies like perforation or hemorrhage, successful medical management depends on immediate support of vital functions; replacement of blood, fluids, and electrolytes; and repair of the damage. In milder cases, however, diagnosis and treatment of an inflammatory or infectious disorder of the GI tract often depend on the patient's history and systemic signs and symptoms. The diagnosis of viral gastritis, for example, may depend on the presence of fever and nau-

sea and vomiting—particularly in a community where viral gastroenteritis is epidemic. And the diagnosis of chemical gastritis may be based largely on the patient's history of alcoholism.

The diagnosis may require several laboratory tests and diagnostic examinations.

### Tests for bleeding or infection
Several laboratory tests help detect and locate bleeding, infection, or inflammation in the GI tract.

• A *complete blood count* is likely to be the first test ordered. An elevated white blood cell count indicates the need for other tests to detect and locate infection or inflammation. Low hematocrit and hemoglobin levels strongly suggest bleeding and mandate additional tests (including examination of the stool for occult blood) to detect bleeding and any coagulation disorders.

• *Whole blood clotting time* and *clot retraction time tests* are ordered if a clotting disorder seems likely, and *serum calcium* measurements may be ordered to help determine a clotting deficiency, Zellinger-Ellison syndrome, or hypercalcemia.

• *Serum gastrin* levels are checked in suspected hypergastremic conditions such as atrophic gastritis.

• *Serum amylase* and *serum lipase* levels are measured to rule out acute pancreatitis, which may be caused by a peptic ulcer. (See *Recognizing acute pancreatitis.*)

## Diagnostic examinations locate injury

Locating the source and cause of any bleeding is difficult because bleeding can occur anywhere along the GI tract. (See *Common sites and causes of gastrointestinal bleeding.*) The most useful examination for locating bleeding is direct visualization of the upper GI tract with *endoscopy.* During this examination, a flexible tube passes through the mouth and esophagus into the stomach and duodenum. At each level, the examiner rotates and angles the endoscope to allow examination of the complete lining and any inflammation, ulcers, bleeding sites, or structural defects. During the examination, he can remove tissue speci-

## Common sites and causes of gastrointestinal bleeding

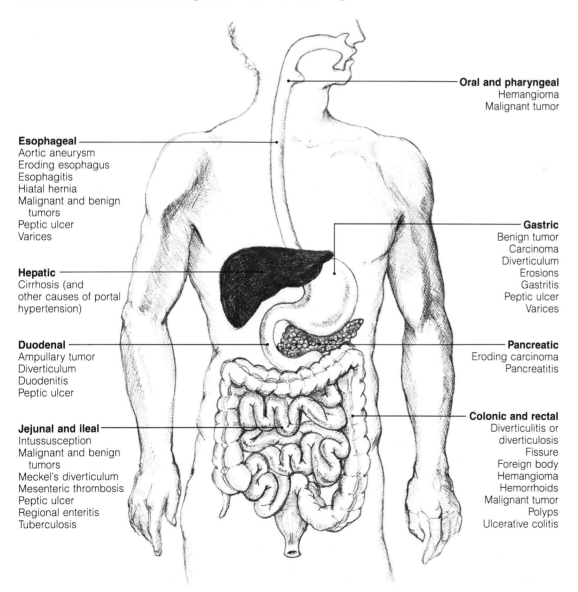

**Oral and pharyngeal**
Hemangioma
Malignant tumor

**Esophageal**
Aortic aneurysm
Eroding esophagus
Esophagitis
Hiatal hernia
Malignant and benign
  tumors
Peptic ulcer
Varices

**Gastric**
Benign tumor
Carcinoma
Diverticulum
Erosions
Gastritis
Peptic ulcer
Varices

**Hepatic**
Cirrhosis (and
other causes of portal
hypertension)

**Duodenal**
Ampullary tumor
Diverticulum
Duodenitis
Peptic ulcer

**Pancreatic**
Eroding carcinoma
Pancreatitis

**Jejunal and ileal**
Intussusception
Malignant and benign
  tumors
Meckel's diverticulum
Mesenteric thrombosis
Peptic ulcer
Regional enteritis
Tuberculosis

**Colonic and rectal**
Diverticulitis or
  diverticulosis
Fissure
Foreign body
Hemangioma
Hemorrhoids
Malignant tumor
Polyps
Ulcerative colitis

## Surgical procedures to treat gastric ulcer

### Vagotomy with gastroenterostomy

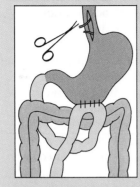

This fairly simple procedure involves resection of the vagus nerves and creation of a stoma for gastric drainage. It decreases motor activity and produces excellent clinical results in most patients. Possible complications include fullness after eating, dumping syndrome, and diarrhea.

### Vagotomy with antrectomy

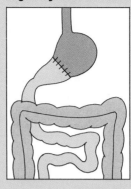

This procedure involves resection of the vagus nerves and removal of the antrum. It decreases motor activity and produces the lowest marginal ulceration rate (ulceration at operation site). Possible complications include fullness after eating, dumping syndrome, diarrhea, anemia, and malabsorption.

### Billroth I

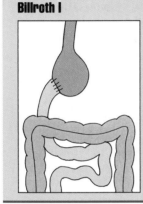

This partial gastrectomy involves gastroduodenostomy (anastomosis between the stomach and the duodenum) following removal of the distal 1/3 to 1/2 of the stomach. It reduces gastric secretion and helps to restore gastric emptying. Possible complications include dumping syndrome, anemia, malabsorption, weight loss, and marginal ulceration.

### Billroth II

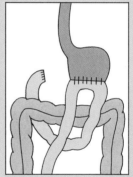

This partial gastrectomy involves gastrojejunostomy (anastomosis between the stomach and the jejunem) following removal of the distal segment of the stomach and antrum. It reduces gastrin secretion and helps to restore gastric emptying. Possible complications include dumping syndrome, anemia, malabsorption, weight loss, and marginal ulceration.

mens or cells for microscopic examination. And he can control localized bleeding by inserting an electrocautery or laser knife through the endoscope.

If the patient's having recurrent hemorrhages of unknown origin, selective *angiography* of the celiac, superior mesenteric, or interior mesenteric arteries may help locate their source. During the procedure, bleeding can be stopped temporarily by infusing vasopressin intraarterially to cause short-term vasoconstriction.

If the patient has an ulcer or obstruction, plain *abdominal X-rays* may show distention or perforation. And a *barium swallow test* may show strictures, varices, ulcers, or tumors.

Other diagnostic tests help rule out or confirm the involvement of other organs: *cholecystography* to evaluate gallbladder structure and function and to detect tumors; *endoscopic retrograde cholangiopancreatography* to evaluate pancreatic, biliary, and hepatic ducts; and *ultrasonography* and *computerized tomography scan* to identify structural abnormalities in all abdominal organs.

### Function tests check inflammation

If no anatomic basis for a patient's complaint of heartburn can be found, the doctor may order an *acid perfusion (Bernstein) test*. If the acid drip provokes recurrence of the patient's symptoms, he's likely to have esophagitis. Other tests are available to detect gastric reflux into the esophagus, bile reflux into the stomach, esophageal sphincter pressures, and peristaltic activity.

*Gastric analysis tests* also determine the amount of hydrochloric acid and other gastric juices the stomach secretes basally and when artificially stimulated.

### Two goals of treatment

Depending on the patient's clinical condition, initial treatment may aim to correct the cause of the disorder or to relieve the symptoms. If the patient has an ulcer, the doctor will probably try to reduce or neutralize stomach acids and to provide symptomatic relief with one or more of the following drugs:

• an antacid, which neutralizes excessive gastric acid, protecting the mucosal barrier

• cimetidine, which reduces gastric acid levels by blocking histamine (a powerful stimulant of acid secretion)
• an anticholinergic, which reduces gastric acid secretion and relaxes smooth muscles, slowing gastric emptying.

If the patient has a severe hemorrhage or medical treatment has failed to heal a chronic ulcer, surgery will be performed to control the bleeding and to try to prevent the ulcer's recurrence. Various surgical procedures may be used. (See *Surgical procedures to stop gastric bleeding.*) For example, a partial gastrectomy (removal of two thirds to three quarters of the stomach) may be performed to reduce the acid-secreting mucosa. A bilateral vagotomy may be performed to relieve ulcer symptoms and to eliminate vagal nerve stimulation of gastric secretions. A pyloroplasty may be performed to facilitate drainage and to prevent obstruction.

If the patient has gastritis or esophagitis caused by ingestion of a corrosive substance, medical treatment will include intravenous hyperalimentation (IVH) and tube feedings to allow the inflamed GI tract complete rest. After healing begins, frequent dilatation will help prevent strictures and obstructions from scar tissue.

If the patient has a bacterial or fungal infection, the doctor will order antimicrobial therapy. (Viral infections are usually self-limiting, requiring only symptomatic treatment, such as fluid and electrolyte replacement.)

## NURSING MANAGEMENT
Whether your patient has a GI tract infection or inflammation, nursing management begins with a thorough history and physical examination.

### Start with a thorough history
When you take a history, note any risk factors that predispose your patient to an inflammatory disorder of the GI tract.
• *Age.* The incidence of gastritis and peptic ulcer increases with age, with the incidence of both duodenal and gastric ulcers peaking after age 50.
• *Sex.* Women are more likely to develop chronic gastritis than men; and men are three to four times more likely to develop peptic ulcers than women.
• *Heredity.* A family history of peptic ulcer predisposes a patient to peptic ulcer; type O blood predisposes a patient to duodenal ulcer.

• *Life-style.* Cigarette smoking, spicy foods, alcohol, and coffee may predispose a patient to gastritis and peptic ulcer. (Alcohol is a leading cause of gastritis.)
• *Systemic disorders.* Sepsis, burns, trauma, head injuries, pulmonary disease, liver disease, pancreatitis, and endocrine disorders predispose a patient to peptic ulcer.
• *Emotional stress.* Chronic emotional stress may predispose a patient to gastritis or peptic ulcer.

Begin your initial interview by asking the patient to describe his symptoms, which may include pain, heartburn, a persistent feeling of fullness, nausea and vomiting, or a change in bowel habits. (See *Signs and symptoms of GI inflammation,* page 98.) Throughout the interview, keep in mind that GI symptoms are usually nonspecific and vary greatly among individuals.

**Ask about pain.** If your patient's chief complaint is pain, heartburn, or a feeling of fullness, ask him these questions.
• *What does the pain feel like?* Aching pain is likely with acute gastritis; gnawing or boring pain is likely with a hiatal hernia, gastric ulcer, acute pancreatitis, or duodenal ulcer. A feeling of fullness after eating is likely if inflammation is due to duodenal ulcer obstructing the GI tract. Heartburn is likely with a gastric ulcer or esophagitis from gastric reflux.
• *Where is the pain?* Severe epigastric pain is common with gastritis and peptic ulcer but varies among individuals. Pain in the midline most likely indicates gastritis; to the left of midline, gastric ulcer; and to the right of midline, duodenal ulcer. Epigastric pain that radiates to the scapulae and midback is common with pancreatitis. And substernal pain is common with esophagitis.
• *How severe is the pain?* Ask the patient whether the pain has interfered with any activities and where he'd place it on a scale of 1 to 10, with 10 being the most severe pain he's ever experienced. If the pain suddenly becomes more severe or decreases, consider the possibility of a medical emergency, such as hemorrhage, and take appropriate action.
• *When does the pain usually occur, and what, if anything, relieves it?* Pain from a peptic ulcer varies according to ulcer location but usually occurs 2 or more hours after eating and is relieved by food and antacids. Pain or fullness caused by eating is common with an obstruction; cramping pain after eating that intensifies when the patient bends over

## Signs and symptoms of GI inflammation

Look for combinations of signs and symptoms when assessing a patient with inflammation of the upper GI tract.

### Esophagitis
• Dysphagia
• Heartburn
• Odynophagia

### Acute gastritis
• Cramping, abdominal tenderness
• Epigastric discomfort
• Hematemesis/melena
• Nausea/vomiting

### Chronic gastritis
• Diarrhea
• Epigastric fullness/pain after meals
• Gastric ulcer symptoms, but no pain relief with hourly antacids
• Hematemesis/melena
• Intolerance to fatty/spicy foods

### Peptic ulcer
*Gastric:*
• Aching, burning, gnawing or cramping, usually within 1½ hours after meals; sometimes relieved by eating
• Fullness soon after beginning meals
• Nausea/vomiting
• Weight loss

*Duodenal:*
• Pain resembles that of gastric ulcer but usually occurs 2 to 4 hours after meals; relieved by eating; often recurs at night

or lies down may indicate hiatal hernia. Pain relieved by sitting in the knee-chest position may indicate pancreatitis. Pain that intensifies during swallowing probably indicates scarring from esophagitis; pain after swallowing is common with esophagitis from gastric reflux.

**Ask about nausea.** If your patient's chief complaint is nausea and vomiting, ask about its onset and frequency and about the appearance of the vomitus. Vomitus that contains food particles several hours after eating may indicate an obstruction from an ulcer near the stomach outlet. Vomitus that doesn't contain bile may indicate an obstruction proximal to the ampulla of Vater.

**Ask about a change in bowel habits.** If your patient's chief complaint is a change in bowel habits, such as diarrhea or constipation, start by asking about his normal bowel habits. These may vary from several stools a day to one or two stools a week. Follow up by asking how his bowel habits have changed, when the change occurred, and whether the appearance of the stool has changed.

**Ask about the patient's health history.** After the patient describes his chief complaint, ask about any other health problems. A sudden onset of fever and malaise suggests an infection. A gradual onset of fatigue and dizziness may indicate occult bleeding or pernicious anemia associated with chronic gastritis. Abdominal distention may indicate obstruction secondary to a peptic ulcer. An unpleasant taste in his mouth may result from gastric or esophageal reflux.

Also ask the patient about other disorders or medications that may influence his chief complaint. Has he been treated for gastritis or peptic ulcer? Does he have any neurologic disorders that might explain pain or difficulty in swallowing? Or diabetes, which might predispose him to infections? Is he allergic to any foods or medications? Has he been taking any drugs, such as aspirin, that might contribute to gastritis; an antifungal, which might cause nausea and vomiting; vitamins containing iron, which might cause nausea and black stools; or an antibiotic, which might predispose him to a fungal infection?

**Ask about his psychosocial history.** Has his job or personal life been a source of great stress recently? Does he have financial worries? Is he exposed to any toxic chemicals in his home or work environments?

Ask about eating, smoking, and drinking habits; and note excessive use of spicy foods, cigarettes, alcohol, and caffeine.

## Perform a physical assessment next

Thoroughly examine the patient, paying particular attention to the following:

**Skin.** Inspect the patient's skin and general appearance. Cold, clammy skin may be an indication of severe bleeding in the GI tract. If so, check the patient's vital signs, and take immediate action. Pallor, particularly of the mucosa, may indicate pernicious anemia associated with chronic gastritis.

**Mouth.** Inspect the patient's mouth for signs of general hygiene and health, and look for swelling and inflammation, which may indicate infection or a chemical burn.

**Abdomen.** Measure and record the abdominal girth if you suspect an obstruction or other cause of distention. Then auscultate all quadrants: high-pitched, tinkling sounds are likely proximal to an obstruction; a complete absence of sounds for at least 5 minutes is likely in a complete obstruction or ileus from a bacterial gastroenteritis. Next, percuss the abdomen, noting high-pitched, tympanic sounds, which indicate large collections of air. Finally, palpate the abdomen gently to detect tenderness and guarding.

**Vital signs.** Record your baseline findings; then note any trends, such as increasing heart rate accompanying a declining blood pressure, that might indicate developing shock from hemorrhage or dehydration from vomiting and diarrhea.

## Formulate nursing diagnoses

After assessing your patient on the basis of the history, physical examination, laboratory and diagnostic studies, and medical treatment plans, you're ready to formulate nursing diagnoses that reflect your patient's needs.

**Potential fluid volume deficit related to upper GI bleeding, vomiting, or diarrhea.** During the physical assessment, you will have noted any signs of dehydration, such as dry skin and mucous membranes, poor skin turgor, oliguria, or stupor. Assessment of the patient's vital signs may have indicated signs of hypovolemia from blood and fluid loss. Whatever these initial findings, use them as a baseline to evaluate your interventions.

To replace blood loss and to preserve adequate circulation, give whole blood, packed cells, or I.V. or oral fluids, as ordered.

Keep accurate records of intake and output, and report any discrepancies. Record weight daily, and watch for changes in the patient's condition that may indicate an increasing fluid deficit or continued GI bleeding: increasing heart rate and falling blood pressure, dry skin and mucous membranes, weight loss, continuing oliguria, changes in level of consciousness (which may indicate electrolyte imbalance), hematemesis, or bloody stools.

Your interventions are successful when your patient's vital signs and level of consciousness remain stable and his intake and output are balanced.

**Decreased cardiac output related to upper GI hemorrhage.** As you replace volume loss, offer cardiovascular and respiratory support, intervene appropriately to stop bleeding, and report any changes that might indicate a resumption of bleeding.

To provide cardiovascular and respiratory support, place the patient in a Trendelenburg position; give oxygen by mask, if appropriate; and keep the patient quiet to decrease oxygen consumption.

To stop gastric bleeding, administer iced saline lavage, or take other appropriate measures, as ordered.

To protect your patient from hypovolemic shock, monitor vital signs and total intake and output records every hour. Report any significant changes to the doctor immediately.

Your interventions are effective when your patient's vital signs are stable, all signs and symptoms of continued bleeding have disappeared, and urine output is at least 30 ml/hour.

**Alteration in comfort: Pain related to acute or chronic gastritis or to gastric or duodenal ulcer.** Document all pain for severity, duration, and location before and after administering antacids, anticholinergics, or a histamine blocker, as ordered.
• Give antacids every 30 to 60 minutes, as ordered, to relieve severe pain. If antacids are ordered after meals, give them 1 hour after meals to neutralize rebound acidity.
• Give anticholinergic drugs, as ordered. Tell the patient to report any side effects, such as visual disturbances, headache, dry mouth, or urinary retention.
• Give cimetidine, as ordered.

Help the patient rest and avoid stress by keeping his room lights low, teaching him muscle relaxation techniques to reduce tension, and encouraging him to discuss and resolve situations that are causing stress.

Your interventions are successful when your patient's restlessness and other signs of pain disappear and he tells you his pain is relieved.

**Alteration in elimination: Diarrhea related to eating contaminated food (acute gastritis).**
Document the consistency of every bowel movement, the number of bowel movements, and the relationship of food intake and diarrhea. If ordered, administer antidiarrheals to decrease peristaltic activity. Apply topical ointments to prevent or alleviate burning and skin breakdown.

Your interventions have been successful when your patient's stools return to their normal consistency and frequency.

**Alteration in nutrition related to dysphagia, food intolerance, and mouth soreness.** If the doctor orders IVH, infuse the feedings at the prescribed rate. If the patient's condition resulted from corrosive injury, you may be asked to help dilate the esophagus to prevent strictures and obstructions as healing progresses. As soon as the patient can eat solid food, help him choose a nutritionally balanced, calorically appropriate diet. Record weight daily.

Your interventions are successful when your patient's able to consume a nutritionally balanced diet, his weight returns to normal, and he's able to tell you the elements of a nutritionally balanced diet.

**Fear related to diagnosis and therapy.** Work to establish a personal relationship with your patient so he'll feel more comfortable admitting his fears. Offer information, reassurance, and encouragement frequently. Watch for nonverbal signs of fear and anxiety, and respond with reassurance.

You've succeeded when your patient becomes more relaxed and can relieve his fears by talking about them.

**Knowledge deficit about the disorder, therapy, self-care activities, and essential lifestyle changes.** Your initial interview with the patient helped you evaluate how well he understands his disease and its treatment. Based on this assessment, work with him to design and carry out a teaching plan.

Your interventions are successful when your patient has a basic understanding of his condition and how to care for himself after discharge.

## A final comment
Infection and inflammation of the upper GI tract require skilled nursing care to lead the patient toward recovery. Such care involves keen assessment skills to detect their sometimes subtle signs. But, most important, it involves thorough patient monitoring to maintain fluid balance, provide cardiovascular and respiratory support, and relieve pain.

**Points to remember**

• Upper GI infectious and inflammatory disorders range in seriousness from benign to potentially fatal.
• Signs and symptoms of these disorders are usually nonspecific and vary greatly among patients.
• Women are more likely to develop chronic gastritis than men, but men are three to four times more likely to develop peptic ulcer than women.
• Complications of peptic ulcer include hemorrhage, perforation, penetration, and pyloric obstruction.
• Treatment of upper GI inflammation aims to correct the underlying cause or to relieve symptoms.
• Thorough patient teaching helps prevent subsequent inflammatory attacks and helps reduce complications after surgery.

# 7 DEALING WITH LOWER G.I. INFLAMMATION

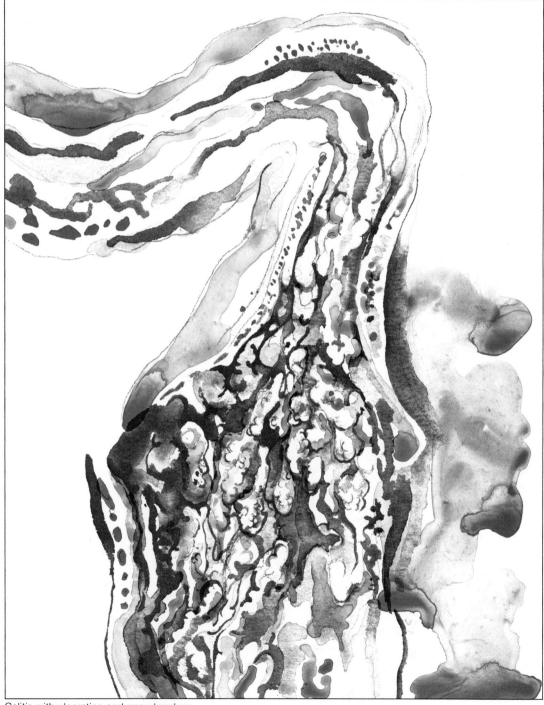

Colitis with ulceration and pseudopolyps

f you've ever dealt with lower bowel disorders, you know how difficult they can be to identify and manage. Their characteristic gastrointestinal symptoms—commonly, diarrhea, vomiting, rectal bleeding, and constipation—may signal any one of several different bowel disorders or may originate in other body systems. They can be transient and easily curable or stubbornly chronic and debilitating.

Caring for patients with these disorders—especially those with chronic inflammatory conditions such as Crohn's disease or ulcerative colitis—is singularly challenging. These patients tend to be nervous, demanding, and preoccupied with their health problems. They're often marked—fairly or unfairly—as difficult patients. Certainly, a strong psychosomatic component is involved in these conditions, the psychosocial costs of which are great. Understanding how lower bowel disorders develop and how they produce their effects can prepare you to recognize these sometimes elusive disorders and to manage them most effectively.

## CAUSES: INFECTION AND INFLAMMATION

The lower bowel contains bacteria and organisms which can cause superinfection from antibiotic therapy or can infect other systems if the bowel should rupture. However, most lower bowel disorders result from acute or chronic damage to the bowel lining, caused by bacteria, viruses, parasites, and various inflammatory and dietary factors. For convenience, these disorders are broadly classed as infectious or inflammatory.

### Common infections

Infectious disorders are further classified according to the pathogens involved: bacteria, viruses, or parasites. (See *Lower bowel pathogens,* page 102.) Infection may result from direct person-to-person or person-to-object contact or from ingestion of contaminated food or water. Acute infectious diarrheas range from slightly annoying to fulminant and life-threatening. They tend to affect very young, elderly, or debilitated patients most seriously.

**Bacterial diseases.** These include salmonellosis, shigellosis (bacillary dysentery), botulism, and pseudomembranous enterocolitis.

*Salmonellosis* results from infection by the gram-negative organism *Salmonella.* Of some 1,700 known *Salmonella* serotypes, 10 account for most cases of salmonellosis in Americans; of these, *S. typhimurium* is the most common, accounting for abut 24% of all isolates.

*Shigellosis,* also known as bacillary dysentery, results from infection by any one of four species of the gram-negative bacteria *Shigella: S. sonnei, S. flexneri, S. dysenteriae,* and *S. boydii.* Since 1960, *S. sonnei* has been the most common isolate in the United States, except among American Indians, who are more frequently infected by *S. flexneri. S. dysenteriae* and *S. boydii* can be introduced into the United States by visitors or returning travelers.

*Botulism,* a severe food poisoning, results from ingestion of food contaminated by an exotoxin produced by the gram-positive, anaerobic bacillus *Clostridium botulinum.* The mortality from botulism is about 25%; death is most commonly caused by respiratory failure during the first week of illness. Other clostridial strains, such as *C. perfringens* and *C. difficile,* usually produce a milder, self-limiting intestinal enteritis, especially among adults. The same is true of such bacteria as *Escherichia coli, Campylobacter fetus,* and *Yersinia enterocolitica.*

*Pseudomembranous enterocolitis* is an acute inflammation and necrosis of the small and large intestines that usually affects the mucosal lining. It may extend into the submucosa and, rarely, other layers. The exact cause of this disease is unknown, but recent work implicates a toxin or toxins produced by *C. difficile.* Marked by fulminating diarrhea, this rare condition is usually fatal in 1 to 7 days because of severe dehydration and toxicity, peritonitis, or perforation of the gut. This disease commonly results from superinfection. (See "Superinfection" on page 104.)

**Viral diseases.** These include endemic diarrhea from *rotavirus,* which mainly affects children aged 6 to 24 months, and *Norwalk virus,* which causes about a third of the viral gastroenteritis epidemics in the United States, attacking persons of any age. Although *poliovirus, coxsackievirus, picornavirus, echovirus,* and others have been associated with gastroenteritis in humans, it's not yet clear whether they are the specific pathogens.

**Parasitic diseases.** These include amebiasis or amebic dysentery, which results from infection by *Entamoeba histolytica,* and giardiasis, which results from the nonamebic protozoan *Giardia lamblia.* Another cause of bowel infection is the flagellate *Dientamoeba fragilis,* which creates mild intestinal upset. Amebiasis and giardiasis infect 1% to 5% of Americans annually.

## Lower bowel pathogens

| Pathogen | Method of transmission | Incubation period | Clinical features | Duration of illness |
|---|---|---|---|---|
| **Bacteria** | | | | |
| *Salmonella* | Ingestion of contaminated food or water | 8 to 24 hours | Nausea and vomiting, abdominal pain, diarrhea with mucus or blood | 2 to 5 days |
| *Shigella* | Direct anal-oral transmission | 24 to 48 hours | Abdominal pain, bloody or mucoid diarrhea | 4 to 7 days |
| *Clostridium botulinum* | Ingestion of contaminated food or water | 12 to 72 hours | Dry mouth, sore throat; nausea and vomiting; diarrhea; neuromuscular disturbances; diplopia, weakness, impairment of cranial nerves followed by descending paralysis | Weeks |
| *C. perfringens* | Ingestion of contaminated food or water | 6 to 24 hours | Diarrhea, abdominal cramping | < 24 hours |
| **Viruses** | | | | |
| Rotavirus | Direct anal-oral spread | 1 to 3 days | Diarrhea, vomiting, fever | Usually 5 to 8 days |
| Norwalk virus | Direct anal-oral spread | 1 to 2 days | Diarrhea, vomiting, fever, abdominal cramps, headache, malaise | Usually 1 to 2 days |
| **Parasites** | | | | |
| *Entamoeba histolytica* | Ingestion of cysts in contaminated food or water, direct anal-oral spread | As short as 4 days | Abdominal pain, flatulence, bloody diarrhea, fever (many infections are asymptomatic) | Weeks to months |
| *Giardia lamblia* | Ingestion of cysts in contaminated food or water | 9 to 15 days | Abdominal pain, flatulence, diarrhea stools that are pale and contain mucus (many infections are asymptomatic) | Days to months |

### Inflammation

Inflammatory disorders are divided into inflammatory bowel diseases (ulcerative colitis and Crohn's disease) and other lower bowel disorders, including appendicitis and diverticular disease of the colon. Inflammatory bowel diseases are most common in developed countries, such as the United States, Great Britain, and those in northern Europe.

**Ulcerative colitis.** This disease affects the mucosa and submucosa of the colon. It usually begins in the rectum and sigmoid colon, often extending upward to involve the entire colon; it rarely affects the small intestine. It results in congestion, edema, and ulcerations that eventually progress to abscesses. The disease primarily affects adults aged 15 to 30, especially women; it is also more prevalent among Jews and higher socioeconomic groups. Incidence of ulcerative colitis in the United States among white adults is 4 to 6 cases per 100,000; overall incidence is 40 to 100 cases per 100,000 and is rising.

**Crohn's disease.** Also known as regional enteritis or granulomatous colitis, this disease can affect any part of the gastrointestinal tract and involves all layers of the intestinal wall. It may also involve regional lymph nodes and the mesentery. Although its cause is unknown, it's thought to start in the submucosal lymphatic system of the intestine. This disease most commonly affects adults aged 30 to 60; it's two to three times more common among Jews and least common among blacks. About 100,000 Americans have Crohn's disease, and an estimated 10,000 new cases are reported every year. Worldwide incidence is estimated at 0.5 to 6.3 cases per 100,000; and prevalence, at 10 to 70 cases per 100,000.

**Etiologic theories.** The exact cause of inflammatory bowel disease is still unknown. Crohn's disease and ulcerative colitis may be different manifestations of the same disease, sharing a number of common features. Six etiologic theories have been proposed.

• *Infection.* Since inflammatory bowel disease

produces mucosal changes in the colon similar to those in infectious diarrhea, many suspect bacteria, viruses, and their metabolites, but no consistent pathogen has yet been identified.

• *Immune reactions.* Support for this idea stems from the presence of immunologically mediated conditions (such as iritis and systemic lupus erythematosus) in some patients and of immune-related disorders (such as autoimmune hemolytic anemia and erythema nodosum) in others. Support also stems from the effectiveness of adrenal corticosteroids in some patients. But, no definite ties between the disease and the various immune mechanisms have yet been established.

• *Food allergies.* Studies suggesting that ulcerative colitis may result from a gut allergic reaction to food substances, especially cow's milk proteins, have not been substantiated.

• *Heredity.* Multiple familial occurrences of inflammatory bowel disease have been documented in 15% to 40% of patients, including monozygotic and dizygotic twins. The disease may occur in family members who are born in widely separated areas or who live apart for long periods. Its prevalence among Jews, its reported association with ankylosing spondylitis, and a possible connection with the presence of certain human leukocyte antigen (HLA) histocompatibility antigens all hint at some genetically mediated cause, probably acting in tandem with external agents and deficient host defense mechanisms.

• *Prostaglandins.* These hormones are thought to be mediators of the inflammatory response in inflammatory bowel disease. Elevated prostaglandin levels have been found in rectal biopsy tissues of patients with ulcerative colitis, and drugs that inhibit prostaglandins (such as sulfasalazine and prednisolone) are most effective in treating this disease.

• *Psychosomatic causes.* For years, ulcerative colitis was thought to result from psychosomatic factors, such as severe emotional stress or obsessive/compulsive behavior. But these emotional problems are now thought to *result* from the disease, not cause it.

## Appendicitis
This is the most common major surgical disease—affecting from 7% to 12% of Americans. It usually results from an obstruction of the intestinal lumen by kinking, a fecal mass, stricture, calculus, tumor, parasite, foreign body, or viral infection. It's most common in adolescents and young adults, with peak inci-

dence between ages 15 and 24. If untreated, this disease is invariably fatal; however, with the availability of antibiotics, its mortality and incidence have declined.

Appendicitis is most prevalent in urban populations, especially where low-fiber, high-meat diets are common. Interestingly, vegetarians have a comparatively lower incidence of the disease, which supports the suspicion that a dietary deficiency of crude fiber may be a major etiologic factor.

## Diverticular disease
Like appendicitis, this disease is also common in urban populations subsisting on diets low in fiber and high in refined carbohydrates. In diverticular disease, bulging pouches (diverticula) in the gastrointestinal wall push the mucosal lining through the surrounding muscle. The most common site for diverticula is the sigmoid colon, but they may develop anywhere from the proximal end of the pharynx to the anus.

Diverticular disease has two clinical forms. In *diverticulosis,* diverticula are present but do not cause symptoms. In *diverticulitis,* the inflamed verticula may cause potentially fatal obstruction, infection, or hemorrhage. (See *Distinguishing diverticular disorders,* page 113.) Diverticulitis occurs in about 10% of Americans, and its incidence rises with each decade of life, peaking in the 50s. It affects more men than women.

## PATHOPHYSIOLOGY
Lower bowel disorders result from invasion and infection of the intestine by bacteria, viruses, or parasites; from inflammatory processes; or from a combination of these factors. Except in botulism, they cause pathologic changes in the intestinal lining, and most result in diarrhea (abnormally frequent passage of loose stools or blood, or both).

## Bacterial effects: Ulceration or toxicity
Bacteria that survive ingestion affect the GI tract in two ways. One group of bacteria, including *Salmonella, Shigella, Yersinia,* and *C. perfringens,* colonizes and attacks the epithelium then penetrates to the mucosa, causing superficial ulcerations in microvilli tips. The resulting acute inflammation stimulates the bowel to secrete copious mucus, water, and electrolytes, causing diarrhea, which may be bloody because of ulceration.

The second group, including enterotoxic strains of *E. coli* and *Vibrio cholerae,* does not destroy tissue but adheres to epithelial cell surfaces and releases endotoxins. These endotoxins stimulate release of mucosal adenylate cyclase, resulting in massive secretion of fluid and electrolytes into the bowel lumen. This process, which peaks in a matter of hours, produces a profuse, watery diarrhea.

*C. botulinum* also secretes an endotoxin (botulin). When this powerful substance is absorbed by the gastrointestinal tract, it affects peripheral nerve endings within 24 hours. It causes abnormal GI motility (diarrhea or, in infant botulism, constipation) and widespread neurologic dysfunction, including fatigue, visual disturbances, dysarthria, dysphagia, and descending muscle paralysis, which is fatal in about 25% of patients.

### Viral effects: Inflammation and atrophy
Although some viruses cause mucosal inflammation, the mechanism involved is unclear. Apparently, the virus particles are most abundant in the small bowel, where they inflame the epithelial cells of villi, causing them to shorten and eventually, to atrophy. This increases loss of fluid and electrolytes to the intestinal lumen and leads to diarrhea and malabsorption. Fortunately, viral enteritis is usually benign and self-limiting.

### Parasitic infections
Amebiasis and giardiasis are frequently spread by fecal contamination, especially in countries with poor sanitation and no water filtering, such as India.

In amebiasis, *E. histolytica* infects the mucosal surface, feeding on intestinal bacteria and exfoliated epithelial cells. When encapsulated as cysts, amoebas pose no threat, but as mobile trophozoites, they multiply rapidly and invade the submucosa, producing small, discrete, superficial erosions. Once embedded in the submucosa, the trophozoites secrete cytolytic enzymes, which allow them to burrow even deeper into the intestinal wall, where they spread laterally. This activity causes flask-shaped ulcers, which can lead to extensive mucosal loss. The involved tissue becomes highly inflamed, causing bloody diarrhea. Without treatment, amebiasis may involve the peritoneum, the enteric vascular system, and eventually the liver (possibly via the portal vein), where the disease causes abscesses, hepatic enlargement, and even complete destruction of the organ. (See *Amebiasis: From person to person.*)

In giardiasis, *G. lamblia* is ingested in its encysted form and infects the duodenum and proximal small intestine. The cysts become free-swimming trophozoites and, with sucking disks, they attach themselves in clusters to the bowel mucosa. These trophozoites encyst again, travel down the colon, and are excreted. The pathogenesis of diarrhea associated with giardiasis is unknown, but it may involve inflammation, mucosal damage, and excessive mucosal secretion. The disease causes malabsorption and increased transit time through the intestine.

### Superinfection
Reinfection with the same bacteria, virus, or parasite often results in pseudomembranous enterocolitis, which frequently occurs in debilitated patients who undergo abdominal surgery or have been treated with broad-spectrum antibiotics.

Whether antibiotic therapy triggers pseudomembranous enterocolitis is debatable. Some investigators, having found such bacteria as *C. difficile* and *Staphylococcus aureus* in patients' stool, are convinced that antibiotics alter the normal intestinal flora, encouraging normally small bacterial populations to grow and produce endotoxins. The toxins cause a granular, hyperemic mucosa; in advanced cases, yellow patches of exudate coalesce to form a membrane containing leukocytes, mucus, and fibrin. As inflammation progresses, the mucosa becomes edematous and congested and, in extreme cases, ulcerative and necrotic. Diarrhea is the primary symptom.

### Inflammatory bowel disease
Ulcerative colitis and Crohn's disease regularly cause diarrhea, but appendicitis and diverticulosis don't. This can be explained pathophysiologically. (See *Inflammatory bowel disease: Two forms,* pages 106 and 107.)

**Ulcerative colitis.** This condition produces continuous involvement of the colonic mucosa and submucosa. It usually begins in the rectosigmoid and may extend proximally into the transverse colon and sometimes as far as the ileum. Its early inflammatory lesions commonly develop at the base of the *crypts of Lieberkühn,* located between the bases of the villi. As the inflammation progresses, it damages the crypt epithelium, stimulating polymorphonuclear lymphocytes to invade the crypt lumen and to form an abscess. If multiple abscesses form, they may coalesce and develop into ulcerations; these eventually de-
*(continued on page 108)*

# Amebiasis: From person to person

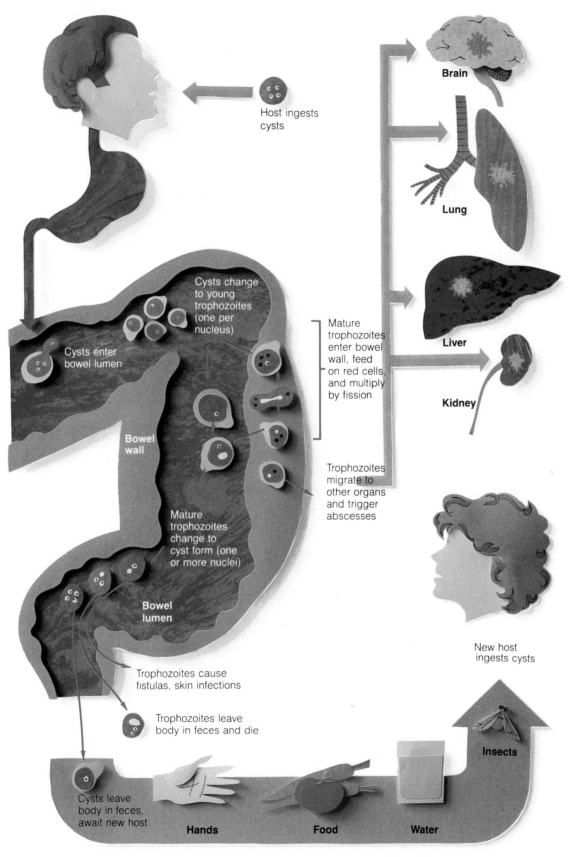

Host ingests cysts

Brain

Lung

Liver

Kidney

Cysts change to young trophozoites (one per nucleus)

Cysts enter bowel lumen

Bowel wall

Mature trophozoites change to cyst form (one or more nuclei)

Bowel lumen

Mature trophozoites enter bowel wall, feed on red cells, and multiply by fission

Trophozoites migrate to other organs and trigger abscesses

Trophozoites cause fistulas, skin infections

Trophozoites leave body in feces and die

Cysts leave body in feces, await new host

New host ingests cysts

Insects

Hands          Food          Water

Human beings are the main host of *Entamoeba histolytica,* the protozoan responsible for amebiasis. In most cases, cysts are ingested by eating or drinking feces-contaminated food and water. They may also be ingested in other ways, for example, through oral sex.

As shown, the ingested cysts pass unchanged into the small intestine, where the nuclei convert to active trophozoites. The young trophozoites quickly mature, multiply by fission, and invade the intestinal tissue. Here they produce enzymes that cause small flask-shaped ulcers with tiny surface openings. These ulcers progressively undermine the tissue surface, eventually causing the edges to collapse and to form a large ulcer with ragged overhanging edges.

If the trophozoites penetrate the mesenteric vein, they may reach and infect the liver. And if they get into general circulation, they may infect other organs, including the lungs, kidneys, and brain.

# Inflammatory bowel disease: Two forms

These views detail characteristic pathologic changes in the bowel in ulcerative colitis and Crohn's disease.

In *ulcerative colitis*, inflammation is confined to the intestinal mucosa and submucosa; lesions spread continuously without passing over healthy bowel tissue.

In early stages, the mucosa becomes granular; in later stages, the inflammation penetrates to the muscularis propria, and strips of inflamed, undermined mucosa form pseudopolyps.

In chronic disease, the bowel mucosa becomes pale and granular (see top far right), and normal vascular and glandular patterns are lost. The bowel lumen narrows, and the sigmoid colon shortens, with loss of haustra.

In *Crohn's disease,* all bowel wall layers are involved. This inflammatory bowel disease spreads from one bowel segment to another, sometimes skipping over healthy areas.

The disease inflames the intestinal wall, resulting in a tortuous membranous covering, with thickened exudative strands. Enlarged lymph node chains are commonly found in the thickened mesentery. Mesenteric fat advances on the intestine, sometimes wrapping itself completely around the bowel wall (bottom far right).

Lymphatic swelling also thickens the intestinal wall. The mucosa is swollen; red; and covered with aphthous, linear, and other ulcers. Because of ulcers and transverse fissures, the mucosa has a cobblestoned look.

In acute disease, plasma cells and lymphocytes infiltrate all bowel layers. Ulcers penetrate into the submucosa, and fissures extend from these through the bowel wall, causing fistulas and abscesses.

The accompanying chart details other distinguishing features of these two disorders.

## Comparing ulcerative colitis and Crohn's disease

| Characteristic | Ulcerative colitis | Crohn's disease |
|---|---|---|
| Usual disorder site | Rectosigmoid and left colon | Right colon |
| Distribution | Continuous | Segmental |
| Course | Remissions and relapses occur | Slow, progressive |
| Depth of involvement | Mucosal and submucosal | Transmural |
| Small bowel involvement | Rare | Common |
| Bowel lumen size | Normal | Narrow |
| Rectal bleeding | Common | Rare |
| Anorectal fistulas | Rare | Common |
| Anal abscesses | Rare | Common |
| Crypt abscesses | Common | Rare |
| "Cobblestoning" of mucosa | Rare | Common |
| Inflammatory masses | Rare | Common, extensive |
| Toxic megacolon | Rare | Rare |
| Pseudopolyps | Common | Rare |
| Granulomas | Absent | Common |
| Strictures | Absent | Common |
| Shortening of bowel | Common | Rare |
| Mesenteric fat/lymph involvement | Absent | Common |
| Carcinoma | Risk increases 10% with each decade | Increased risk |
| Diarrhea | Common | Common |
| Hematochezia | Common | Rare |
| Steatorrhea | Rare | Common |
| Tenesmus | Severe | Rare |
| Fever | During acute attacks | Common, often persistent |
| Abdominal pain | Rare | Common |
| Weight loss | 20% to 50% of cases | 60% to 70% of cases |

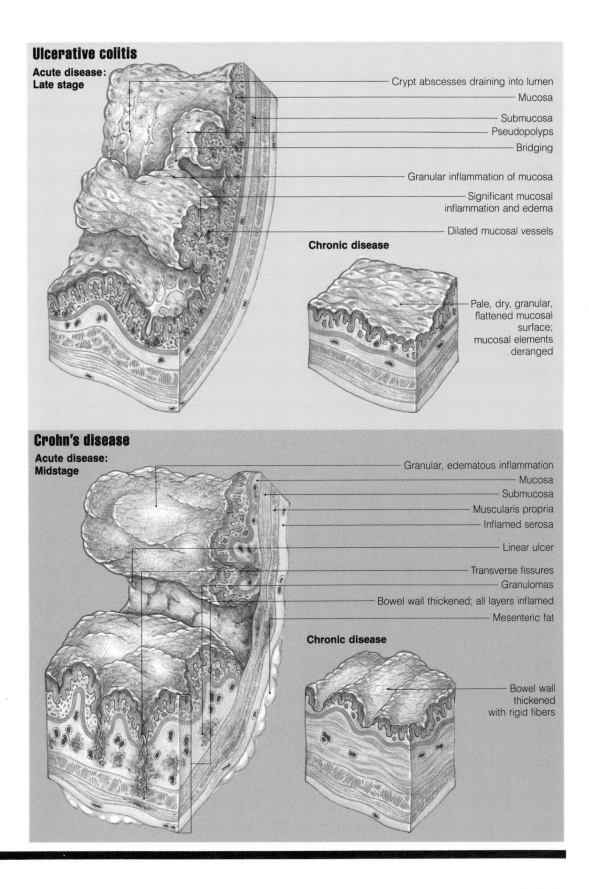

## Ulcerative colitis

**Acute disease:
Late stage**

Crypt abscesses draining into lumen

Mucosa

Submucosa

Pseudopolyps

Bridging

Granular inflammation of mucosa

Significant mucosal inflammation and edema

Dilated mucosal vessels

**Chronic disease**

Pale, dry, granular, flattened mucosal surface; mucosal elements deranged

## Crohn's disease

**Acute disease:
Midstage**

Granular, edematous inflammation

Mucosa

Submucosa

Muscularis propria

Inflamed serosa

Linear ulcer

Transverse fissures

Granulomas

Bowel wall thickened; all layers inflamed

Mesenteric fat

**Chronic disease**

Bowel wall thickened with rigid fibers

stroy the mucosal epithelium, causing bleeding and diarrhea, this disease's symptoms.

Ulcerative colitis may cause two types of diarrhea. In pseudodiarrhea, rectal inflammation causes repeated urges to defecate (tenesmus), but the patient passes only small amounts of blood and pus. In true diarrhea, colonic mucosal destruction reduces water and sodium absorption, increasing the volume of excretion; in addition, inflammation results in decreased colonic motility, reducing the colon to a passive conduit for secretions. Decreased absorption, increased excretory volume, and decreased retention result in abundant, watery diarrhea.

As diarrhea progresses, anemia, dehydration, and fluid and electrolyte imbalances occur. Anemia results from chronic loss of blood, which is passed in the stools; dehydration results from recurrent loss of blood, fluid, and protein; and electrolyte imbalance results from losses of sodium and potassium. Chronic malabsorption of nutrients leads to weakness, fatigue, and severe debilitation.

Pseudopolyps develop in ulcerated areas; granulation tissue develops, forming a base for epithelialization; and the mucosal musculature becomes thickened, shortening the colon. At the same time, other symptoms of the disease may appear, including arthritis; eye changes, such as uveitis and retinitis; and erythema nodosum, characterized by nodules on the face, arms, and legs.

Remission and relapses are common; the fewer the attacks, the better the patient's chances for successful treatment and remission.

**Crohn's disease.** This disease usually involves the right colon and small intestine at the terminal ileum, duodenum, or jejunum, but it can occur anywhere in the GI tract. It causes patchy rather than continuous inflammation and eventually involves all bowel layers; resulting fistulas may penetrate the bowel wall and extend into adjoining bowel segments. In severe cases, regional lymph nodes are enlarged. As this disease progresses, the affected bowel permanently fibroses and thickens, and the lumen narrows. In Crohn's disease, diarrhea may or may not be bloody. Other symptoms include weakness, fatigue, anorexia, and fever. If concentrated in the terminal ileum, this disease may cause right lower quadrant pain and obstructive symptoms, such as nausea, vomiting, and distention.

Because Crohn's disease affects the small intestine, it can interfere with absorption of vital nutrients and may cause malnutrition. Thus, duodenal inflammation may cause malabsorption of calcium, iron, and folate, whereas terminal ileum inflammation may cause bile salt and vitamin $B_{12}$ malabsorption.

Early complications may include enterocutaneous fistula, perirectal ulcers, or abscesses. Skin disorders, joint problems, and liver disease may also occur.

### Appendicitis
The vermiform appendix, obstructed by kinking, swelling, or a fecal mass, undergoes spasm, edema, ischemia, bacterial proliferation, and mural inflammation. Eventually, the appendix fills with pus, and microabscesses develop along its surface. Bowel loops, peritoneal folds, or the peritoneum itself may adhere to the appendix, and abscesses may develop at or near it.

Typical symptoms of appendicitis include constipation and steady, well-localized lower right quadrant pain, worsened by movement, coughing, and deep breathing. If undetected, the inflamed appendix may burst, resulting in peritonitis and septicemia.

### Diverticulitis
Abnormal diverticular pouches become inflamed after perforation. If the perforations are small, the inflammation may be confined to the affected diverticulum. If they're large, an abscess may involve or even surround the colon. Occasionally, complete perforation of a diverticulum may cause diffuse peritonitis. (See *Complications of diverticulitis,* page 110.)

Because diverticula form mostly in the sigmoid colon, a common symptom of the disease is constant left lower quadrant pain. Other symptoms include bloating and flatus, alternating periods of constipation and diarrhea, fever, and leukocytosis.

### MEDICAL MANAGEMENT
Infectious disorders, diverticulitis, and appendicitis yield readily to careful diagnosis and treatment; however, correct diagnosis of ulcerative colitis and Crohn's disease is more difficult because of their many similarities and poorly understood mechanisms. Treatment includes surgical removal of affected tissues and drug therapy to control symptoms.

Reliable diagnosis of infectious and inflammatory lower bowel disorders requires various blood and stool tests, as well as radiographic and endoscopic tests. Where appropriate, biopsy is part of an endoscopic examination.

## Blood tests

In infectious disorders, a *complete blood count (CBC)* may be taken, but results usually are normal. In acute intestinal inflammation, there may be a slight increase in white blood cells (WBCs), but this increase is not diagnostic. In chronic inflammatory disorders, however, the CBC is a useful tool. For example, in patients with ulcerative colitis, Crohn's disease, and diverticulitis, the CBC typically shows anemia from bleeding, iron or folate deficiency, or chronic disease. The CBCs of these patients will show low hematocrit levels. *WBC counts* will be mildly elevated. Significant WBC elevation suggests an intraabdominal abscess, perforation, or toxic megacolon.

*Serum electrolytes,* such as potassium, magnesium, and sodium, may be abnormally low in both infectious and inflammatory conditions because of excessive vomiting and diarrhea.

*Serum protein electrophoresis* may reveal hypoalbuminemia in ulcerative colitis or Crohn's disease from protein loss or inadequate oral intake.

## Stool tests

Blood, which is usually bright red, appears in the stool in ulcerative colitis, Crohn's disease, or diverticulitis from inflammation and ulceration. But, a *fecal occult blood test* may reveal fecal blood in some infectious disorders, such as amebiasis or bacterial enteritis.

*Stool cultures* are the most useful diagnostic tool for identifying bacterial and parasitic disorders, but they may not provide conclusive information about viral disorders. When giardiasis is suspected but stool cultures are inconclusive, *duodenal aspiration* provides more accurate information.

## Radiologic studies

Barium enema studies are especially useful in diagnosing inflammatory disorders; depending on the severity of the inflammation, these tests can demonstrate various filling defects characteristic of these disorders.

In *ulcerative colitis,* barium studies may show inflammation that appears granular, with small ulcerations. The colon is narrowed and shortened and may show pseudopolyps and loss of haustration.

In *Crohn's disease,* barium studies may show barium reflux into a narrowed terminal ileum, bowel wall irregularity and thickening, and fistula tracks between bowel segments. Appearance of ulcers indicates active disease.

In *diverticulitis,* the rectosigmoid colon may show pouches, distortions, and narrowing of the lumen.

Barium enema studies are contraindicated in acute inflammatory conditions in which intestinal perforation is possible (for example, appendicitis or diverticulitis).

*Abdominal X-ray films* may demonstrate the accumulation of air or fluid in the GI tract. In *ulcerative colitis,* X-rays show a tubular, gas-filled colon with absent haustra. In *Crohn's disease,* the bowel wall shows asymmetrical inflammation and segmentally distributed ulcerated lesions.

A plain X-ray film may reveal air under the diaphragm, indicating perforation in appendicitis or diverticulitis.

## Endoscopy

Endoscopic procedures allow the doctor to see abnormalities directly, to locate bleeding sources, and, if needed, to get a biopsy specimen for cytologic or histologic exam.

*Sigmoidoscopy* involves direct observation of the rectum, sigmoid colon, and attendant mucosa; it allows the doctor to locate rectal or colonic bleeding and to detect the inflammation. In active ulcerative colitis, sigmoidoscopy reveals inflamed, profusely bleeding mucosa and colonic ulcerations. In diverticulitis, this examination reveals an inflamed or swollen diverticular mucosa.

*Colonoscopy,* which allows direct observation of the entire colon, may be used instead of sigmoidoscopy to diagnose Crohn's disease. Characteristic patchy inflammation rules out ulcerative colitis, but sometimes a biopsy may be needed to confirm Crohn's disease.

*Rectal biopsy* can be done with or without an endoscopic exam to confirm the type of inflammatory bowel disease. Granulomas in the specimen confirm Crohn's disease.

Endoscopic procedures carry the risk of intestinal perforation, so they may be contraindicated in patients with any type of active inflammatory disease.

## TREATMENT

Treatment of lower bowel disorders should prevent or reduce tissue damage, promote healing, and restore normal bowel function through drugs, replacement therapy, diet, and, if necessary, surgery.

## Drug therapy

Use of antibiotics for specific infectious disorders is controversial because they may foster and prolong the symptoms of salmonellosis

## Complications of diverticulitis

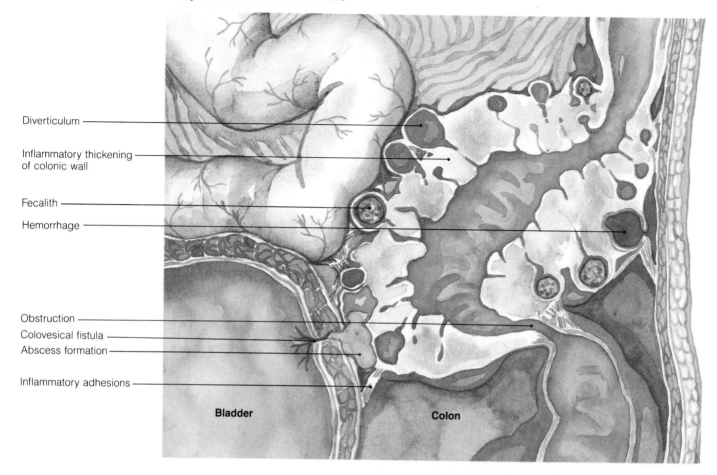

Diverticulum

Inflammatory thickening of colonic wall

Fecalith

Hemorrhage

Obstruction
Colovesical fistula
Abscess formation

Inflammatory adhesions

**Bladder**

**Colon**

and other bacterial infections, for example, by causing bacterial overgrowth.

The amebicide metronidazole (Flagyl) is the drug of choice for amebiasis and giardiasis. Chloroquine phosphate (Aralen) or emetine hydrochloride is used to treat liver abscesses resulting from amebiasis.

Sulfasalazine (Azulfidine) is widely used for treating ulcerative colitis and Crohn's disease. If this is ineffective or if the disorder is severe, corticosteroids such as prednisone (Deltasone) may be used. All these drugs reduce mucosal inflammation, relieve fever, and halt diarrhea.

As a last resort, immunosuppressive drugs such as azathioprine (Imuran) may be prescribed for ulcerative colitis. Although this drug's action is unclear, it seems to reduce inflammation by preventing lymphocytic migration.

### Symptomatic treatment
If the patient has had vomiting or severe diarrhea for over 24 hours and is dehydrated, intravenous fluids and electrolytes—such as 0.9% normal saline solution, dextrose 5% in

water, and supplemental sodium and potassium—are given. Blood or plasma expanders, such as Plasmanate, may be indicated in severe cases to prevent hypovolemic shock from blood loss.

Blood loss may lead to anemia, which, in patients with inflammatory disorders, usually means iron deficiency anemia. This condition is confirmed by a hemoglobin level below 11 g/dl or a hematocrit level below 33%. Such values usually suggest treatment with iron supplements.

### Nutritional support
Diarrhea and malabsorption quickly debilitate patients with inflammatory disorders. To compensate, they're often put on low-residue elemental diets, such as Ensure or Vivonex, which provide 1,500 to 2,400 calories/day to help establish a positive nitrogen balance. These oral supplements are absorbed in the upper bowel, thus reducing the flow through inflamed lower bowel segments.

To avoid cramping and diarrhea, patients with lactase deficiency from ileal inflammation should avoid all dairy products.

**Intravenous hyperalimentation.** Patients who can't maintain adequate oral nutrition can benefit from intravenous hyperalimentation (IVH) with a hypertonic solution of glucose; nitrogens (amino acids and polypeptides); and other nutrients, such as multivitamins and electrolytes. IVH solutions contain dextrose 20% to 50%; a liter bottle of dextrose 20% solution contains about 1,000 calories and 6 g of nitrogen. For IVH to restore nitrogen balance, to rebuild body tissues, and to promote weight gain, the patient should receive 2,500 to 3,000 calories/day.

IVH is often used to rest the bowel and allow inflammation to heal. It's also given to improve the patient's nutritional status before major intestinal surgery. IVH therapy requires special care to avoid contamination, rapid infusion, and air embolism.

## Surgical cure possible

Inflammatory bowel disorders that relapse frequently, with persistent perforation, severe uncontrollable hemorrhage, obstruction, and abscesses or fistulas, require surgery to remove the damaged bowel section. Total proctocolectomy with construction of a permanent ileostomy cures intractable ulcerative colitis. Surgery for Crohn's disease preserves as much small bowel function as possible, to avoid malabsorption and other nutritional problems. For example, if the entire distal ileum is removed, bile salt may be malabsorbed, causing diarrhea and vitamin $B_{12}$ deficiency. Usually, part of the distal ileum and right colon are removed, and a permanent ileostomy is formed. Surgery for Crohn's disease may not be curative, since inflammation can recur elsewhere in the intestine.

Appendicitis is cured by appendectomy; if the appendix is perforated, abscesses may require drainage.

Uncomplicated diverticulitis needs segmental colonic resection. If perforation causes widespread sepsis, a temporary loop colostomy may be needed. If sepsis is controlled after 6 to 8 weeks, the colostomy can be closed.

## NURSING MANAGEMENT

Reviewing the pathophysiology of lower bowel disorders should help you take a relevant patient history and perform a thorough physical examination. After collecting the subjective and objective data, you can use it to form nursing diagnoses, to set care goals, and to plan and evaluate your interventions.

## Get a patient history

Begin your assessment with a thorough patient history. Try to elicit the patient's chief complaint. What does he mean when he mentions diarrhea or loose or bloody stools? For instance, when he says "loose stools," how often does he experience this symptom each day? Are his "bloody stools" flecked with reddish color, or are they bright red?

**Ask the patient to describe his symptoms in detail.** How long has he had diarrhea? Has it affected his appetite or eating habits? Has he vomited or experienced nausea? Do any of his family, friends, or co-workers also have diarrhea? Has the patient or any of his family or acquaintances recently traveled abroad? If so, where did they go and what did they do? (Some countries are more notorious for "travelers' diarrhea" than others.) Also, determine if the patient has had diarrhea from any previous disorder. Has his weight changed, or has he felt unusually weak or fatigued? These symptoms may result from chronic diarrhea or poor intake.

Determine when his diarrhea occurs (before, during, or after meals); ask whether he's seen mucus or pus in his stools. Does he experience abdominal pain or tenesmus?

**Evaluate the patient's psychosocial status.** Has his disorder restricted his social life? Has he recently endured severe stress, as in bereavement, loss of his job, or divorce? Such stress can aggravate a developing inflammatory bowel condition or cause changes in eating habits.

**Get a medication history.** If the patient has been taking antibiotics, he may show signs of drug-induced enteritis (diarrhea, fever, abdominal pain, leukocytosis). Prolonged or excessive use of laxatives or antacids may also induce diarrhea.

## Perform the physical examination

Continue your assessment with a physical examination. Obtain vital signs and weight to use as baseline data. Compare the patient's weight with previous weights, if possible, to check for loss.

If your patient is an adolescent, pay special attention to his growth and development. Be sure to compare his height and weight with established norms; he may be smaller than normal if he has ulcerative colitis or Crohn's disease. He may also lag in sexual maturation.

**Check the patient's skin and musculoskeletal system.** Erythema nodosum, erythema multiforme, aphthous mouth ulcers, and tender, swollen, or deformed joints may accompany ulcerative colitis and Crohn's disease. Pale skin and mucous membranes may indicate anemia, possibly associated with GI blood loss.

Because diarrhea compromises fluid and electrolyte status, the patient may be dehydrated. In mild dehydration, he may have dry mucous membranes; in severe dehydration, his skin will be dry and lack normal turgor.

**Check the patient's eyes.** Look for reddened conjunctivae or iritis, since both occur with ulcerative colitis and Crohn's disease. If pupillary response is sluggish and the patient complains of blurred vision, suspect botulism.

**Check respiration.** Increased pulse and dyspnea on exertion may result from compromised oxygenation stemming from anemia, possibly indicating ulcerative colitis, Crohn's disease, or diverticulitis.

**Inspect the abdomen.** If it's distended, the bowel may be filled with gas, a sign of appendicitis or diverticulitis. (See *Distinguishing diverticular disorders,* page 113.) In thin patients you may see peristalsis, which may indicate an obstruction.

*Auscultate the abdomen.* In diarrhea resulting from infectious or inflammatory disorders, you may hear hyperactive bowel sounds. Absent bowel sounds may indicate a perforated appendix or diverticulum or peritonitis. High-pitched "tinkling" sounds suggest intestinal fluid and air under tension in a dilated bowel.

*Percuss the abdomen.* You'll hear high-pitched tympanic sounds over areas of the bowel filled with gas and dull sounds over areas filled with fluid or stool. Gas may suggest appendicitis or diverticulitis; fluid suggests ascites.

*Palpate the abdomen.* In ulcerative colitis and diverticulitis, tenderness occurs in the area over the sigmoid colon; in appendicitis, it occurs over the right lower quadrant at the cecum. If the appendix is in its normal position, tenderness can be localized to McBurney's point, which is one third the distance between the anterior superior iliac spine and the umbilicus. Right upper quadrant tenderness may indicate Crohn's disease or ileitis.

Rebound tenderness anywhere in the abdomen may indicate peritoneal inflammation. If inflammation is localized, rebound tenderness is localized accordingly.

**Examine the rectum.** Digital examination may reveal blood or pus and, in Crohn's disease, anal canal ulceration. Inspect the perianal region for abnormalities, such as fissures, fistulas, abscesses, or inflammation.

## Formulate nursing diagnoses

By integrating subjective data from the interview and objective data from the physical examination, you can formulate appropriate nursing diagnoses to help you set workable goals and plan effective interventions. Unless the patient is gravely ill, involve him in your care plan, and be flexible in adjusting it to meet his needs.

**Diarrhea related to inflammation of bowel mucosa.** Your goals are to reduce the frequency of abnormal bowel movements, to reestablish a normal elimination pattern, and to maintain integrity of perianal skin.

To achieve these goals, you must first evaluate the severity of the diarrhea. Accurate input and output records are essential. Be sure to measure and document all the patient's stools.

To avoid or reduce perianal skin irritation, wash, dry, and powder the perianal region after each bowel movement. Apply petrolatum or an emollient, such as A and D ointment, as needed.

If the patient's diarrhea is profuse and watery, guard against dehydration. Replace fluid losses orally if the patient isn't nauseated or vomiting. Give tepid fluids since hot or cold fluids may stimulate the bowel. Withhold milk and solid foods until diarrhea stops. With severe fluid losses, give I.V. fluids, as ordered.

Give antidiarrheal drugs, as ordered. For severe diarrhea, this usually means diphenoxylate hydrochloride with atropine sulfate (Lomotil). Antispasmodics, such as propantheline bromide (Pro-Banthine), and tranquilizers, such as diazepam (Valium), may also be required to help relieve symptoms.

When diarrhea has subsided, provide a bland, low-fat, low-carbohydrate diet for 2 or 3 days. Encourage the patient to rest, and emphasize the importance of avoiding stresses that could trigger a relapse.

Your care measures are effective if the patient's stool production returns to normal, he's adequately hydrated and comfortable, and his perianal skin is intact.

**Fluid and electrolyte deficit related to profuse and frequent diarrhea and vomiting.** Your goal is to help the patient maintain adequate hydration, as evidenced by good skin turgor and adequate urine output.

To achieve these goals, weigh the patient every day. Sudden weight loss may indicate fluid loss and potential dehydration. Assess the patient's mouth for dryness. Assess his skin, including turgor, for signs of dehydration.

Note whether he complains of thirst or seems disoriented. If the patient isn't vomiting, administer fluids (such as Pedialyte or Gatorade) orally, as ordered, to replace electrolytes. Monitor intake and output; watch for urine output below 30 ml/hour and urine specific gravity above 1.030, which indicate dehydration.

If oral rehydration is ineffective (fluid loss exceeds 10% of body weight and other signs of dehydration are present), administer I.V. fluids (such as Ringer's lactate), as ordered. Carefully monitor sodium and potassium levels and report abnormal levels to the doctor. Check the patient's vital signs every 2 to 4 hours—if his temperature and pulse rise, blood pressure declines, and breathing becomes dyspneic or labored, he may be headed for shock.

Your interventions are effective if the patient has good skin turgor, moist mucous membranes, adequate urine output (above 30 ml/hour), urine specific gravity below 1.030, stable vital signs, and normal sodium and potassium levels.

**Anemia related to blood loss from chronic colonic ulceration accompanying ulcerative colitis or Crohn's disease.** Your goal after reaching this diagnosis is to foster adequate tissue perfusion, as evidenced by pink mucous membranes, normal respiratory function, and stable vital signs.

Assess your patient for signs and symptoms of blood loss and anemia. Look for pale skin, nail beds that don't blanch, and pale conjunctivae. Report bloody or tarry stools (melena) to the doctor.

If blood loss is severe, the patient will complain of headache, dizziness, and fatigue. Monitor vital signs for evidence of impending shock, such as hypotension, tachycardia, tachypnea, and anxiety.

Monitor hematocrit and hemoglobin levels; hematocrit levels below 30% and hemoglobin levels below 10 g/dl indicate anemia or acute or chronic blood loss. Administer blood transfusions, as ordered, for severe anemia and hemorrhage. Monitor the patient's response, and watch for transfusion reactions. If the doctor suspects iron deficiency anemia, ad-

## Distinguishing diverticular disorders

| Disorder | Infection signs | Symptoms | Bowel activity | Clinical findings |
|---|---|---|---|---|
| Diverticulosis (uncomplicated diverticulum) | • None; temperature and white cell count normal | • Most patients asymptomatic<br>• May cause nonspecific symptoms resembling irritable bowel syndrome<br>• Pain usually in left lower quadrant; diffuse abdominal pain occurs less often; may be chronic or intermittent; affected by eating or bowel evacuation | • Constipation may alternate with diarrhea; usually associated with fecal impaction within diverticula | • Abdominal, rectal, and proctoscopic exams usually negative, but may reveal lower quadrant tenderness and hypertrophic sigmoid<br>• Barium enema confirms diagnosis |
| Diverticulitis (inflamed diverticulum) | • Fever, leukocytosis with shift to the left | • Left lower quadrant pain; nausea, vomiting | • Constipation common; obstinate constipation results from increasing pericolitis, reflects partial or complete colonic obstruction | • Abdominal and rectal exams reveal left lower quadrant tenderness and palpable sigmoid<br>• Abdominal plain film may show ileus, pelvic soft tissue mass, or, with perforation, free air<br>• Proctosigmoidoscopy without air insufflation must be done to rule out other lesions |
| Free perforation of inflamed diverticulum | • Fever, leukocytosis with shift to left from septicemia | • Sudden onset of severe abdominal pain | • Constipation with rectal tenderness | • Barium enema identifies perforation by presence of barium outside the lumen<br>• Abdominal distention from paralytic ileus or peritonitis<br>• Abdominal and proctoscopic examinations reveal tenderness, spasm; rebound present; left lower quadrant findings soon cross midline and become generalized<br>• Abdominal plain films show free air |

# The continent ileostomy: A new choice

Until recently, patients with ulcerative colitis who needed surgery had only one choice: a conventional ileostomy, which drains continuously into an ostomy pouch. But today patients may opt for an often more desirable procedure, the *continent ileostomy*, in which drainage is automatically controlled by a stoma valve. Patients who already have a conventional ileostomy may switch if they're willing to undergo another operation.

As shown here, a continent ileostomy consists of an intraabdominal pouch surgically constructed from the terminal ileum, which usually escapes involvement in ulcerative colitis. Solid waste collects in the nipple-valved pouch until the patient drains the pouch through the stoma with a catheter.

If your patient's scheduled for a continent ileostomy, monitor his fluids for several days before surgery. Turn him frequently, and if he already has an ostomy, provide appropriate care.

After surgery, a catheter is inserted through the patient's stoma and into the pouch about 2″ (5 cm) from its posterior side. The catheter is connected to low intermittent suction for the next 2 to 6 weeks to keep the pouch empty, thus preventing rapid distention of the pouch and allowing suture lines to heal. Regularly check the catheter for patency, and irrigate it with 20 to 30 ml of normal saline solution every 2 to 4 hours to prevent obstruction.

If all goes well, about 2 to 4 days after surgery, the color of drainage from the pouch should change from blood-tinged to greenish brown, indicating the return of peristalsis. The patient will then be started on clear liquids and gradually advanced to low-residue solids.

A day or so before the catheter is to be removed, it will be clamped for 3- to 4-hour periods, except during the night, when continuous drainage is al-

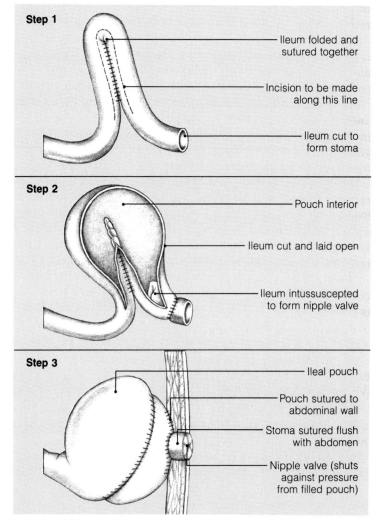

**Step 1**
- Ileum folded and sutured together
- Incision to be made along this line
- Ileum cut to form stoma

**Step 2**
- Pouch interior
- Ileum cut and laid open
- Ileum intussuscepted to form nipple valve

**Step 3**
- Ileal pouch
- Pouch sutured to abdominal wall
- Stoma sutured flush with abdomen
- Nipple valve (shuts against pressure from filled pouch)

lowed. After catheter removal, you'll need to teach the patient how to empty the pouch by inserting a lubricated #28 catheter through the stoma. Some patients prefer to sit while draining their pouches, but standing usually yields better results. Drainage can also be quickened by having the patient increase his intraabdominal pressure and contract his abdominal muscles.

Pouch capacity will determine how often it must be drained. Immediately after surgery, the pouch will hold about 70 to 100 ml of fluid. A month later it will hold about 200 ml; 6 months later, about 600 ml. At that time, it need be emptied only three

or four times daily.

Your patient will need to carry a catheter with him wherever he goes. Between intubations he'll cover his stoma with a small gauze square to keep his underclothes from being soiled by mucus. Before applying the gauze, he should wash the stomal area with warm water and then dry it completely.

You'll also need to teach your patient how to irrigate his pouch. This should be done weekly—or more often if undigested food causes a drainage block. To prevent blocks, suggest the patient avoid fibrous foods, such as corn, mushrooms, nuts, lettuce, celery, peas, and citrus fruits.

minister iron supplements, as ordered. Usually, these are given parenterally because oral supplements tend to irritate an already inflamed mucosa. To lower the anemic patient's oxygen requirement and to reduce the strain on his heart and lungs, encourage him to rest and to observe scheduled nap times.

Your interventions are effective if your patient has stable vital signs, normal hemoglobin and hematocrit values, and healthy skin and mucous membrane coloration.

**Inadequate nutrition related to inflammation and decreased nutrient absorption.** Your goal in this diagnosis is to help the patient achieve good nutrition, as evidenced by his ability to maintain normal weight.

Teach your patient the importance of increased caloric and protein intake. If he dislikes the prescribed diet, suggest that he eat smaller portions more often. If he's scheduled for bowel surgery, remind him that improving nutrition will improve surgical outcome.

Check the patient's weight and take calorie counts daily to monitor progress. If the doctor orders oral protein supplements in the form of elemental diets, give them 300 to 350 ml at a time; instruct the patient to drink them slowly. Administer vitamin supplements (for example, vitamin $B_{12}$ or folic acid), as ordered. IVH may be ordered if the patient can't maintain his weight on daily meals.

Your interventions are successful if the patient's weight stabilizes at an acceptable level, skin turgor is good, and he's gained strength from the diet.

**Knowledge deficit related to drug therapy for inflammatory bowel disease.** Your goal is to enable the patient to understand the rationale for drug therapy and its expected effects. To help him acquire this knowledge, begin by teaching him the names of the drugs. Explain what each drug is for, when he should take it, and what the dosage is. Discuss possible side effects and interactions, and tell him how to recognize and deal with side effects. If appropriate, supply a handwritten schedule to guide drug therapy. Also give him printed information about each drug, if possible. After effective teaching, the patient should understand the prescribed drug therapy, its side effects, potential complications, and expected benefits.

**Knowledge deficit related to ileostomy or colostomy procedures.** Your goals are to help the patient accept his changed bowel condition, to prepare him mentally for the surgery, and to ensure compliance in ostomy care procedures.

To achieve these goals, teach the patient about the procedure, including its advantages and disadvantages. Begin by considering the patient's age, physical condition, and ability to comprehend the information. Before the operation, thoroughly explain the procedure, its possible complications, and expected benefits. (See *The continent ileostomy: A new choice.*) Discuss selection and use of ostomy appliances; if possible, show him the actual appliances. Teach him how to measure stoma size and shape to ensure proper fit. Supply printed information for him to read, and answer all his questions as completely as you can. If your community has an ostomy association, encourage the patient to join. Sometimes a visit from someone who has adjusted to life with an ileostomy may help him get used to the idea.

After the operation, teach the patient how to apply a protective skin barrier and how to manage his appliance. Remind him that skin care is important; to prevent excoriation, teach him how to properly cleanse the stoma site whenever he changes his appliance. Advise him to follow his doctor's advice if he detects redness, blisters, or ulcerations around the stoma. Instruct the patient in odor control; he can use odor-proof appliances or ostomy deodorants, which can be placed in the bottom of the appliance. Proper diet is vital for patients with an ileostomy. Encourage your patient to avoid foods, such as corn or peanuts, that can plug the stoma. Tell him if he chews his food well, it will pass through his ileostomy in 4 to 6 hours. Reassure the patient that after surgery he should be able to lead a near-normal life; usually, the ileostomy does not restrict normal social or physical activities, including sports or sex.

Your interventions are successful if the patient shows that he understands the procedure and what it will mean to his life and can discuss the situation intelligently. He'll also demonstrate the ability to care for his stoma and appliance, keeping them free of excoriation, odors, and other problems. His self-confidence will be restored as he goes about the activities of daily living.

## A SPECIAL CHALLENGE
Today, improvements in prevention, diagnosis, and treatment of lower bowel disorders are allowing many patients to live longer and more productive lives. As a result, effective nursing care and patient teaching have become increasingly important.

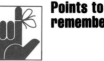

**Points to remember**

- Infectious lower bowel disorders are caused by bacteria, viruses, or parasites. Inflammatory bowel disorders have less precise origins; infectious agents, immune reactions, food allergies, heredity, prostaglandins, and psychosomatic factors may all play a role.
- Abdominal pain and diarrhea are symptoms common to all infectious disorders and to ulcerative colitis and Crohn's disease.
- Diarrhea accompanied by blood loss and malabsorption poses a major threat that must be treated with fluid, electrolyte, and nutritional replacement.
- Use of antibiotics to treat infectious bowel disorders is controversial since the drugs may prolong, rather than shorten, an infection's course, possibly resulting in drug-induced enteritis.
- Surgery is the treatment of last resort and may be ordered for patients with inflammatory bowel disorders. Patients who have ostomy procedures can lead near-normal lives with good nursing care and postoperative counseling.

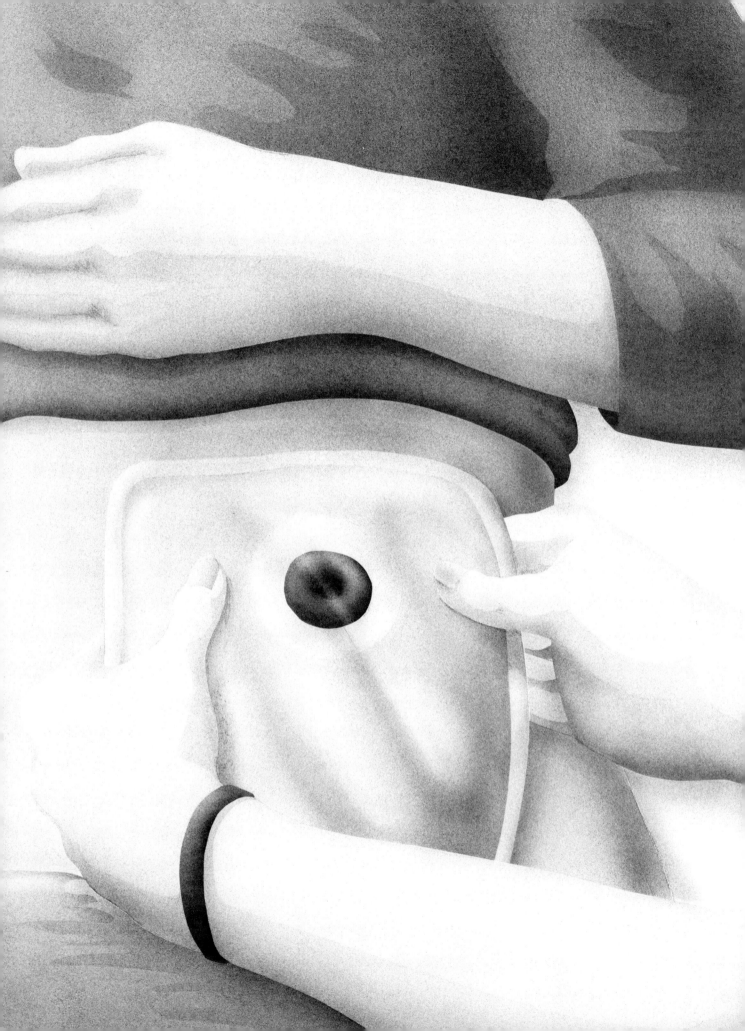

# OBSTRUCTIVE DISORDERS

# 8 DETECTING UPPER G.I. OBSTRUCTIONS

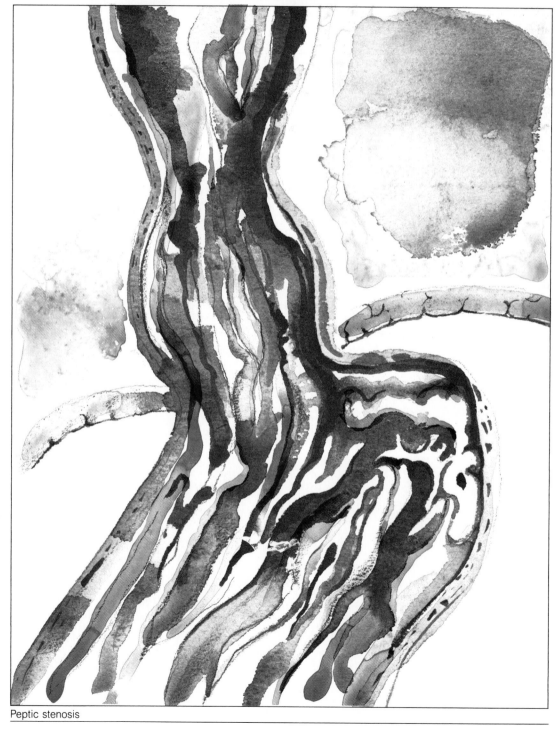

Peptic stenosis

anking among the most common disorders, upper GI disorders severely disrupt the patient's quality of life. These disorders' mild forms often require patients to live with severe dietary restrictions and to cope with recurring malaise; persistent dysphagia often prevents them from enjoying meals; and severe forms are life-threatening.

To care effectively for patients with upper GI disorders, you must be ready to assess quickly and to intervene appropriately in situations that range from life-threatening hemorrhage to transient discomfort. Upper GI disorders often need long-term and follow-up care, and whether your patient has a serious and painful condition or one causing only mild discomfort, one of your main roles should be teaching him to ease his anxiety and cope with his disease. The way to do this is to ensure that the patient understands what's happening to him. In other words, teach him the fundamental physiologic mechanisms of his disease.

## PATHOPHYSIOLOGY

Upper GI disorders may be classified as obstructive or disruptive. In either case, they deprive the entire GI system and other body systems of normal nutrition.

### Obstructive disorders

Upper GI obstructions may result from motor (functional) abnormalities or structural (mechanical) impairment.

**Motor disorders.** These disorders cause functional obstruction and are due mostly to nerve impairment or destruction. Defective innervation causes muscle atony and dysfunction through loss of normal motor activity. In the esophagus, for example, impaired innervation stops normal food propulsion through the esophagus and into the stomach.

Such motility failure may stem from neuromuscular disease such as occurs in myasthenia gravis and amyotrophic lateral sclerosis, in which changes occur in the submucosa and muscular layers of many tissues and organs. In these disorders, impaired voluntary and autonomic motor activities cause dysphagia and abnormal esophageal transit.

*Achalasia* and *esophageal spasm,* for example, are associated with abnormal esophageal innervation. Diffuse esophageal spasms, characterized by multiple, repetitive, and uncoordinated peristaltic waves, commonly occur simultaneously in the smooth muscle part

(mid and lower) of the esophagus. These spasms cause all esophageal segments to contract, making movement of food ineffectual. What causes esophageal spasms is unknown, but they may be related to degeneration of afferent vagal nerve fibers and fibers of the intrinsic nerve plexuses.

Achalasia (formerly called "cardiospasm") is marked by the absence of coordinated peristaltic waves and the failure of the lower esophageal sphincter (LES) to relax normally. It also involves a possible degeneration of vagal and intrinsic plexus nerve elements. And, in achalasia, the LES is hypersensitive to gastrin, which increases LES contractions.

In achalasia and esophageal spasm, the lack of muscle tone, the failure of the LES to relax, and the pressure of food cause the esophagus to dilate. Since, in achalasia, the LES pressure is elevated and the esophageal lumen is dilated, muscle may hypertrophy around the sphincter. Peristaltic waves may be absent (aperistalsis) or may become erratic and ineffectual. Commonly, the esophageal muscle wall hypertrophies, particularly in patients with diffuse esophageal spasms.

**Effects of motor obstruction.** These disorders often cause dysphagia and substernal pain (esophageal colic), which may range from slight discomfort to excruciating pain resembling that of myocardial infarction. Such pain may radiate to the back, neck, jaw, and arms. Another effect of obstruction is food and fluid retention in the esophagus, causing esophagitis. Frequent regurgitation of tasteless, mucoid fluid or undigested food retained in the esophagus is common in upper GI obstruction and may cause aspiration pneumonia if it occurs during sleep.

Motor dysfunction tends to be chronic with progressive dysphagia and weight loss. *Stagnant esophagitis* may stem from the retained food residue and cause stricture formation and hemorrhage. Esophagitis that persists for years may cause secondary carcinoma.

Acute gastric dilatation, an uncommon but serious motor disturbance, may obstruct the passage of food. The dilatation may occur postoperatively, after trauma or application of a whole body cast, or during pregnancy. Hiccups, a common symptom, appears early.

**Structural disorders.** These produce mechanical obstruction through pathologic tissue changes from within or without the GI tract that partially or completely obstruct passage of food and fluid. *Extrinsic tumors* may cause obstruction by compressing a portion of the

# Major esophageal structural disorders

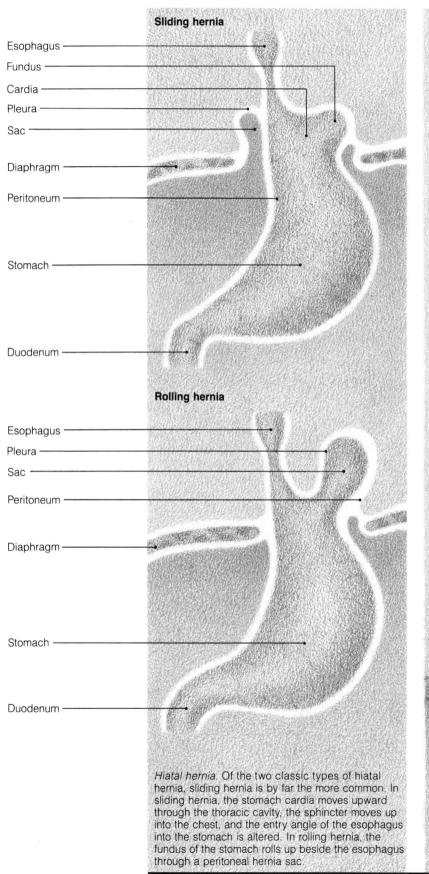

**Sliding hernia**

Esophagus
Fundus
Cardia
Pleura
Sac
Diaphragm
Peritoneum
Stomach
Duodenum

**Rolling hernia**

Esophagus
Pleura
Sac
Peritoneum
Diaphragm
Stomach
Duodenum

*Hiatal hernia.* Of the two classic types of hiatal hernia, sliding hernia is by far the more common. In sliding hernia, the stomach cardia moves upward through the thoracic cavity, the sphincter moves up into the chest, and the entry angle of the esophagus into the stomach is altered. In rolling hernia, the fundus of the stomach rolls up beside the esophagus through a peritoneal hernia sac.

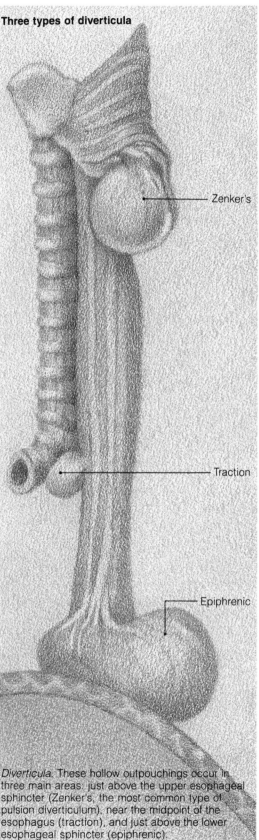

**Three types of diverticula**

Zenker's
Traction
Epiphrenic

*Diverticula.* These hollow outpouchings occur in three main areas: just above the upper esophageal sphincter (Zenker's, the most common type of pulsion diverticulum), near the midpoint of the esophagus (traction), and just above the lower esophageal sphincter (epiphrenic).

GI tract to the point of occlusion. *Intrinsic tumors* may develop within the GI tract's muscular wall or in the lumen itself. *Leiomyoma* is the most common benign esophageal tumor. *Squamous cell carcinoma* is the primary malignant tumor; it's usually found in the lower esophagus.

*Gastric volvulus* and *adult pyloric stenosis,* two rare conditions, also produce upper GI obstruction. In volvulus, the stomach is twisted; in adult pyloric stenosis, the pyloric musculature is hypertrophied either from a tumor involving the pylorus or from a peptic ulcer that scarred it.

*Esophageal rupture* may be complete (Boerhaave's syndrome) or partial (Mallory-Weiss syndrome). Usually, it follows forceful or prolonged vomiting, often associated with alcohol intoxication. During vomiting, the upper esophageal sphincter (UES) usually relaxes to allow ejection of its contents. When the UES fails to relax, the closed pharynx becomes an obstructive force that raises esophageal pressure, causing the mucosa to tear at its weakest point. This often occurs during intoxication with impaired consciousness. Other causes of esophageal wall perforation include retching, coughing, severe straining, and, occasionally, blunt chest trauma.

Because the esophagus has no serosal layer with strengthening collagen and elastic fibers, it's less resilient than the rest of the GI tract and consequently ruptures at a lower pressure than any other part of the alimentary tract. During vomiting, the lower esophagus may suddenly enlarge to five times its normal size. It also enlarges rapidly when a large food bolus is swallowed. Another factor that makes the esophagus especially vulnerable to tears and rupture is that pressure within the thoracic cavity is less than atmospheric, while esophageal intraluminal pressure is greater than that within the thoracic cavity.

*Complete rupture* most frequently occurs through the left lateral wall of the lower esophagus. Then, regurgitated gastric contents and swallowed air leak into the mediastinum, producing subcutaneous emphysema in the neck region. Such rupture may also affect the pleural cavity, producing pneumothorax, pleural effusion, and inflammation.

In *Mallory-Weiss syndrome,* small linear ulcerations appear in the mucosa, usually at the gastroesophageal junction. These produce a singular, longitudinal mucosal or submucosal tear that does not totally perforate the esophagus and does not communicate with the mediastinum. Incomplete rupture may be from mild vomiting episodes. However, incomplete rupture causes more massive bleeding than complete rupture: in partial rupture the blood vessel lumen remains open, whereas complete rupture causes vessel retraction and lumen constriction, which reduces bleeding. An esophageal tear extending into the stomach is associated with massive bleeding because of the cardia's rich submucosal blood supply. This area is involved in about 60% of esophageal tears, and its involvement may cause severe shock and death.

### Esophageal diverticula

Esophageal diverticula, outpouchings in the esophageal wall, usually appear in weakened muscular areas.

*Pulsion diverticula* may be associated with other esophageal diseases, such as esophageal spasm, achalasia, and hiatal hernia, in which intraesophageal pressure is elevated. These diverticula are called pulsion diverticula because they are pushed out by increased intraesophageal pressure. Pulsion diverticula may become large enough to trap food and produce dysphagia at a low esophageal level. Many pulsion diverticula are asymptomatic and become significant only with food and fluid retention.

*Zenker's diverticula,* the most common type of pulsion diverticulum, occur in the posterior hypopharyngeal wall, a weak area just above the cricopharyngeal muscle border and the UES. Normally, during swallowing, the pharynx closes, the UES opens, and food is moved from the oropharynx to the esophagus. But if UES pressure is elevated, swallowing makes intrapharyngeal pressure stop at the weakest area, the posterior hypothorax. This type of diverticulum usually causes the most marked symptoms. At first, saliva and food particles are regurgitated, especially after eating. The throat is irritated and must be cleansed repeatedly after eating. Gurgling sounds may be heard in the neck area. Later, as the pouch enlarges, food particles are retained for several days, and halitosis and hoarseness develop. At this time, regurgitation may occur during sleep with resulting aspiration pneumonia and infection. The pouch may become so large that it compresses the esophagus and causes dysphagia. Untreated Zenker's diverticula can completely obstruct the esophagus.

*Traction diverticula* develop near the esophageal midpoint at the bifurcation level of the trachea from scar tissue, adhesions, or chronic inflammation. They usually involve all tissue layers, have a wide mouth, are less sacular than Zenker's diverticula, and are typically asymptomatic. *Gastric diverticula* are uncommon and, usually, asymptomatic.

### Three types of hiatal hernia

Hiatal hernia (esophageal or diaphragmatic hernia) occurs when the diaphragm opening encircling the distal esophagus and stomach weakens or enlarges to allow part of the stomach to protrude through the opening into the thoracic cavity. This condition may stem from congenital weakness, trauma, loss of muscle tone from aging, or increased intraabdominal pressure.

Types I and II are the classic forms of hiatal hernia. In type I, or sliding hiatal hernia (the most common), the stomach cardia moves upward through the hiatus into the thoracic cavity. The sphincter moves up into the chest, changing the entry angle of the esophagus into the stomach to impair the mechanism for preventing reflux, and esophageal motor dysfunction follows.

In type II, a paraesophageal or rolling hernia, the fundus of the stomach rolls up beside the esophagus through a peritoneal hernia sac. Type II hernias can become large enough to accept almost the entire stomach. Type III hernias mix the features of types I and II.

Hiatal hernia is common and causes symptoms in about 50% of persons with it. But when it causes symptoms, they are multiple and often severe and may cause serious complications. Heartburn (pyrosis) from gastric reflux is the most common symptom. Others include eructation and bloating due to increased swallowing from trying to remove acid from the esophagus. Regurgitation or reflux may cause aspiration pneumonia.

When a portion of the stomach slides into the thoracic cavity in a hiatal hernia, intrathoracic pressure increases, causing pain, shortness of breath, and tachycardia. Accompanying esophageal spasm may cause severe pain resembling angina pectoris, radiating into the back, shoulder, or arm. This pain is not relieved by nitroglycerin and may be aggravated by lying down.

Hiatal hernia symptoms are intensified by eating large meals, raw fruits, and spicy foods and by drinking alcoholic or caffeine-containing beverages. They can also be aggravated by reclining within 2 or 3 hours of eating and by lifting heavy objects and bending.

Associated reflux may cause esophagitis, scarring, strictures, and narrowing of the esophageal lumen. Herniation that pinches the stomach can cause chronic gastritis. Hemorrhage is rare, but it may occur from esophagitis and erosions; and chronic blood loss may cause anemia. Incarceration of a stomach part is a rare and serious complication that occurs with severe substernal pain and signs of upper GI obstruction. It needs immediate surgery. Strangulation is often associated with paraesophageal hernia. Apparently, the size of the herniation does not determine the intensity of clinical effects.

### Strictures and foreign bodies

Esophageal stricture or stenosis, which makes the esophageal lumen too narrow for a food bolus, may be congenital or acquired. Congenital esophageal stricture is rare and tends to occur with other birth defects. Acquired stricture may stem from caustic chemical ingestion; disorders such as scleroderma, postoperative fibrosis, and adhesions from thoracic surgery; or irritation from chronic gastric reflux or prolonged nasogastric (NG) intubation.

Foreign bodies also partially or totally occlude the lumen. They usually lodge in the esophagus just below the UES, near the aortic arch, and just above the LES, where the lumen diameter is normally narrow. But they may lodge anywhere the lumen is narrow from stricture, invasive tumors, or structural abnormalities such as a lower mucosal (Schatzki) ring. In adults, foreign bodies come from food, usually a piece of meat or bone. Elderly persons with dentures, all persons who don't chew adequately, and small children who are likely to swallow objects are susceptible to a retained foreign body. Once a foreign body reaches the stomach, it may pass through the remaining GI tract without difficulty. But long, sharp objects or open safety pins may perforate the esophagus, stomach, or intestine. Large objects may cause gastric obstruction, ulceration, and bleeding. Whatever their size or shape, foreign objects are most dangerous when they lodge in the esophagus. If they lodge in the pharynx, they can occlude the respiratory tract. In any part of the upper GI tract, they provoke an inflammatory response with associated edema, which aggravates the obstruction and may also cause respiratory distress. The attendant irritation may cause an esophageal abscess.

The effects of an obstructing foreign body

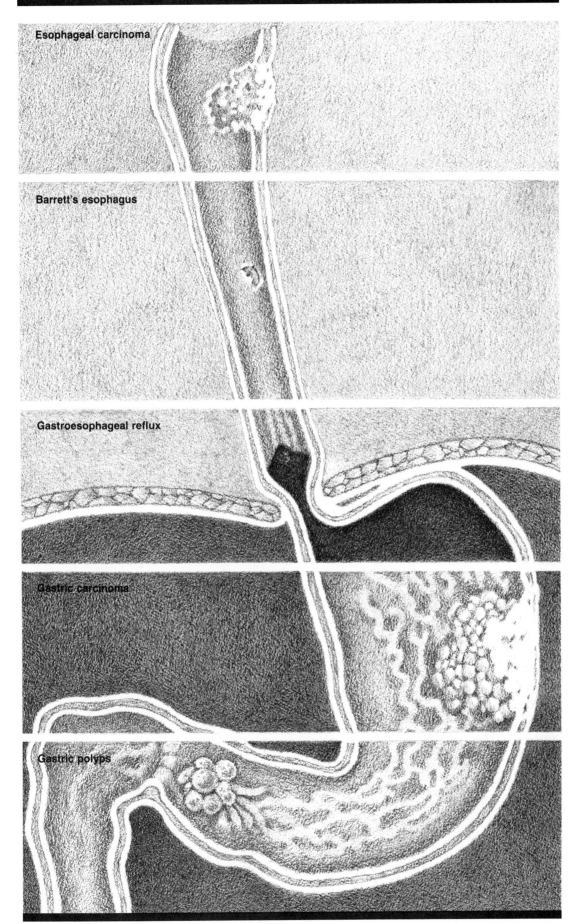

Esophageal carcinoma

Barrett's esophagus

Gastroesophageal reflux

Gastric carcinoma

Gastric polyps

# Disorders of the epithelium

Epithelial abnormalities from such disorders as esophageal carcinoma, gastroesophageal reflux, Barrett's esophagus, gastric carcinoma, and gastric polyps disrupt upper GI function.

*Esophageal carcinoma.* Ninety-five percent of these tumors are epidermoid and can occur equally at the proximal, middle, or distal third of the esophagus.

*Gastroesophageal reflux.* In this disorder, decreased lower esophageal sphincter pressure allows stomach contents to regurgitate into the esophagus. The resulting exposure to acidic stomach contents causes hyperemia, friable mucosa, and mucosal ulcerations.

*Barrett's esophagus.* In this complication of chronic gastroesophageal reflux, the columnar epithelium is potentially premalignant, with increased risk of adenocarcinoma.

*Gastric carcinoma.* Most neoplasms are adenocarcinomas arising from normal or metaplastic mucous cells.

*Gastric polyps.* There are three types of gastric polyps—hyperplastic, adenomatous, and hamartomatous. Both hyperplastic (the most common) and adenomatous (the second most common) polyps can be either sessile or pedunculated and are found in the antrum. Hamartomatous polyps (the least common) are seen as part of polyposis syndrome. Gastric polyps are rarely malignant; adenomatous polyps are premalignant, especially if they are over 2 cm; but hamartomatous polyps are not premalignant.

depend on its location and the degree of obstruction. So effects may range from no symptoms or mild dysphagia to complete inability to swallow. Marked dysphagia is a classic sign of esophageal stricture. Severe shock may mean perforation and hemorrhage.

### Disruptive disorders

Two disruptive disorders involving blood vessels of the GI tract include esophageal and gastric varices and gastric bleeding from peptic ulcer.

*Esophageal varices* occur in the lower esophageal submucosa and result from portal hypertension, which dilates collateral circulation of the vessels that lie between the two venous systems (the left gastric vein that drains the abdominal esophagus and the thoracic veins that drain the rest of it). Although esophageal varices are usually associated with liver disease, they may result from hepatic vein thrombosis, which also increases pressure in the portal system. These varices become grossly distended, and the vessel walls become weak, attenuated, and prone to massive hemorrhage with concomitant disruption of normal blood supply to vital body parts.

Bleeding from varices may be provoked by increased abdominal venous pressure from coughing, lifting, straining, vomiting, trauma, and physical exertion. Moreover, *gastric varices* have developed by the time esophageal varices become evident, and these may also bleed. Besides disrupting the esophageal and gastric walls, bleeding varices cause anemia and possible damage to other body tissues from shock.

*Peptic ulcer disease* is another common source of bleeding with scarring and stenosis. Such scarred tissue often interferes with normal function, disrupting normal gastric secretion and motility. Associated bleeding may be mild and chronic or massive and acute and follows wall erosion. Massive bleeding is life-threatening in itself, but progressive erosion through the gastric wall causes additional complications. When erosion progresses to perforation, gastric contents spill into the peritoneum, causing peritonitis and shock.

### Abnormal epithelium

Conditions involving abnormal epithelium may also disrupt upper GI function. These include polyps, tumors, gastroesophageal reflux, and Barrett's esophagus. The epithelium may also be damaged if the LES is incompetent with reflux of gastric contents.

*Polyps* are usually benign tumors arising from the epithelium of the stomach mucosa. They tend to develop after prolonged epithelial irritation. Gastric polyps are generally rare; they tend to be solitary and located in the antrum. Most gastric polyps are nonneoplastic and hyperplastic and do not become malignant. Neoplastic polyps, called "adenomas," have a greater potential for malignancy.

*Gastric cancer*, abnormal epithelial growth arising from the stomach's mucous membrane, may be characterized by an intestinal epithelium made up of goblet cells rather than chief and parietal cells. Gastric polyps and cancer occur more often in patients with pernicious anemia associated with gastric atrophy and achlorhydria. *Esophageal cancer* usually consists of squamous cell carcinoma arising from squamous mucosa typical of normal structure and, sometimes, of adenocarcinomas arising from distal esophageal mucous glands.

All these conditions affecting the epithelium may cause ulcerated mucosa with associated clinical signs of *gastroesophageal reflux,* including pyrosis as the major symptom. It appears after meals and is exacerbated by bending over or lying down. It may awaken the patient early in the morning. Complications of gastroesophageal reflux may include aspiration pneumonia, esophagitis, esophageal stricture, and deep esophageal ulcers. *Esophagitis* stems from chronic mucosal irritation by hydrochloric acid and digestive enzymes, sometimes occurring with stricture. Its effects include dysphagia; mucosal erosions; regurgitation of bitter, sour-tasting gastric contents; hoarseness; throat clearing; and a sensation of pressure at the back of the neck. Regurgitation may occur with incompetence of the upper and lower esophageal sphincters. Laryngeal aspiration of regurgitated material may produce spells of coughing and choking. Erosion causes shallow ulcers and blood loss, which is usually not life-threatening but which may become severe after excessive alcoholic intake.

When reflux causes severe esophageal ulceration, the squamous epithelium may be replaced with the columnar epithelium, causing *Barrett's esophagus,* or Barrett's syndrome. In this condition, the characteristic gastric epithelium replaces the squamous epithelium, probably because the former is more resistant to peptic digestion. Patients with Barrett's esophagus are at increased risk of developing esophageal adenocarcinoma. In such patients, ulcers in the epithelium appear as typical gastric ones and may cause stricture. They may bleed more profusely than other esophageal ulcers and may perforate into the thoracic cavity.

## Neoplasms: Esophageal and gastric

*Esophageal neoplasms* initially cause dysphagia with solid foods, gradually progress to difficulty in swallowing liquids, and occur with weight and strength loss. In advanced stages, bleeding occurs and metastasis to nearby structures is possible. Cough, hoarseness, or vocal-cord paralysis may follow as esophageal cancer spreads to the recurrent laryngeal nerve.

Signs of *gastric neoplasms* are vague and insidious at first but may reflect progressive ulceration. Later, anorexia, weight loss, dysphagia, eructation, regurgitation, indigestion, nausea and vomiting, hematemesis, melena, and anemia occur. Gastric carcinoma metastasizes readily to adjacent structures such as the esophagus and duodenum. It may spread by lymphatic invasion to the liver, peritoneum, and cervical lymph nodes. Most gastric cancers are adenocarcinomas. Because its early symptoms are so vague, gastric carcinoma is usually in an advanced stage before diagnosis.

## MEDICAL MANAGEMENT

With upper GI disorders, the results of the routine physical examination may be negative unless a mass is palpable, but signs of malnutrition, poor skin turgor, and muscle wasting may be significant. Visual examination of the pharynx may show swallowing problems. But the general scarcity of early clinical signs makes a careful history the major basis for early diagnosis, which may be lifesaving. Of course, suspected upper GI disorders require confirmation by special diagnostic tests.

### Radiography and imaging

X-ray studies include abdominal and chest films in the upright and supine positions. Films in the upright position may show obstructive masses. Either upright or supine position films may show abnormal placement of upper GI tract areas from enlarged adjacent organs or masses. Signs of an enlarged esophagus and absence of the normal gastric air bubble suggest achalasia. The supine position film may show hiatal hernia. Free air below the diaphragm may mean perforation.

**Cineradiography.** This rapid-sequence X-ray study can give details about the pharyngo-esophageal area. It's useful for studying the swallowing mechanism, strictures, and the effects of masses. It can also detect achalasia.

**Barium swallow.** The barium contrast study can help assess esophagus size, patency, filling capacity, and position. As the patient swallows the barium, the radiologist watches the barium column as it passes through the esophagus. A narrowing of the column may mean stricture, tumor, or varices. Para-esophageal tumors may cause extrinsic esophageal compression, which may be revealed as a narrowed barium column. Intrinsic compression by an esophageal tumor may also cause a narrowed barium column or a filling abnormality. Abnormal contour of the barium column indicates a motor disorder. Leakage of the barium detects esophageal perforation. With the patient in Trendelenburg's position, barium swallow may demonstrate a hiatal hernia and gastroesophageal reflux.

**Upper GI study.** This barium contrast study can detect anatomic malposition, obstructive tumors, and ulcerations of the lower esophagus, stomach, and duodenum.

**Splenoportography.** This rarely used invasive procedure may be necessary sometimes to diagnose portal hypertension associated with esophageal varices.

**Gastroesophageal scintiscan.** This test uses a nonabsorbable isotope in a tubeless technique to detect reflux. After the patient ingests the isotope, scintillation is counted over the lower esophagus and stomach with a gamma camera. Scintillation that appears over the esophagus confirms reflux.

### Endoscopy for a direct look

Esophagoscopy allows direct esophageal visualization. When varices and tumors are too small for detection by routine radiographic procedures, this method provides a way to view mucosa and check for such causes of upper GI dysfunction as polyps.

Gastroscopy, another endoscopic procedure, directly visualizes the stomach and duodenum. It's performed in association with esophagoscopy if ulcers, polyps, mucosal inflammation, or tumors are suspected. With endoscopy, biopsies can be taken from masses or abnormal mucosa, as visualized in the esophagus or stomach. Washings of the area are obtained for exfoliative cytology study. Thus, endoscopy with biopsy provides differential and usually accurate diagnosis of benign and malignant conditions.

## Laboratory studies

A complete blood count helps detect anemia that may result from upper GI tract bleeding and may show decreased hemoglobin and hematocrit levels in patients with reflux esophagitis, ulcerating tumors, Mallory-Weiss syndrome, esophageal varices, and gastric ulcers. Cardiac enzyme studies to rule out possible myocardial infarction are recommended for patients with pyrosis, chest pain, and vomiting before assuming the presence of an upper GI disorder.

**Manometry/esophageal motility studies.** Manometry studies measure upper GI sphincter and LES pressures and graphically record esophageal motility. In achalasia, these studies show increased sphincter pressure. They show decreased pressure if the LES is incompetent, as in gastroesophageal reflux. In diffuse esophageal spasm, they reveal simultaneous high-pressure recordings in several areas of the esophagus. Manometry may also help evaluate other disorders, such as scleroderma, that affect esophageal motility.

**Esophageal acidity tests.** These tests evaluate intraesophageal pH and LES competence.

*The acid clearing test* assesses esophageal motility. Normally, hydrochloric acid drops are cleared from the esophagus in fewer than 10 swallows. A greater number of swallows suggests decreased esophageal motility.

*The acid perfusion (Bernstein) test* determines if instillation of hydrochloric acid into the esophagus causes pain or discomfort similar to the patient's usual symptoms. Recurrence of the symptoms after instillation of the acid (a positive test) indicates an esophageal disorder such as esophagitis.

*The acid reflux test* is performed with a pH probe placed above the LES to measure esophageal pH during various movements that increase intraabdominal pressure. Esophageal pH of less than 4 on three or more different occasions confirms gastroesophageal reflux.

## Conservative treatment: At first

Unless the patient's life is at risk, treatment begins with conservative medical support while a complete diagnostic workup proceeds. Medical support alone controls some upper GI disorders and is a valuable adjunct to acute care and surgical intervention.

**Medical support.** In many patients with upper GI tract disorders, the common clinical signs include dysphagia; hyperacidity; pyrosis; regurgitation; vomiting; halitosis; anorexia; weight loss; epigastric, substernal, or retrosternal pain; and occult-to-mild bleeding. In such patients, therapy is a bland diet with small feedings to minimize irritation.

*Bland diet* is still important and often routine even though its effectiveness has recently been questioned. Nevertheless, most clinicians agree on the following points.
• Milk stimulates gastric secretion, as does eating frequent meals.
• Alcohol damages gastric mucosa.
• Caffeine stimulates acid secretion (so does decaffeinated coffee).
• Highly seasoned and spicy foods and foods known to cause symptoms should be avoided.
• Bedtime snacks should be avoided because they stimulate acid secretion after the patient lies down.
• Patients with gastroesophageal reflux should not eat for several hours before retiring.
• Smoking should be stopped because of its relationship to cancer and the high incidence of cancer in upper GI tract disorders and because nicotine has a marked anticholinergic effect and markedly reduces LES pressure.

*Positioning may help.* Patients with gastroesophageal reflux usually benefit from having the head of the bed raised 6″ to 8″ (15 to 20 cm). Infants with severe gastroesophageal reflux should be elevated 30°. Both children and adults in the upright position benefit from the effect of gravity. Patients with esophageal motor or structural defects find that an upright position may help relieve dysphagia. Patients with motor disorders may find that throwing the shoulders back, arching the back, and extending the neck aids the passage of food into the stomach. Valsalva's maneuver increases intrathoracic pressure and may help in the passage of food, but it's contraindicated in patients with cardiac problems.

*Antacids* help neutralize the acidity that causes pyrosis and dyspepsia in gastric ulcer, hiatal hernia, and gastroesophageal reflux. Antacids with lowered sodium content are recommended. Sodium bicarbonate is not recommended for use as an antacid because of its systemic effect, the possibility of rebound hyperacidity, and its potential for causing metabolic alkalosis and hypernatremia.

*Cholinergic drugs* such as bethanechol offer some assistance in gastroesophageal reflux because they increase LES pressure and hasten gastric emptying. *Anticholinergic drugs* inhibit acetylcholine action, decrease acid and pepsin secretion, relieve smooth muscle spasm, and delay gastric emptying. But their

# Esophageal tubes and their advantages

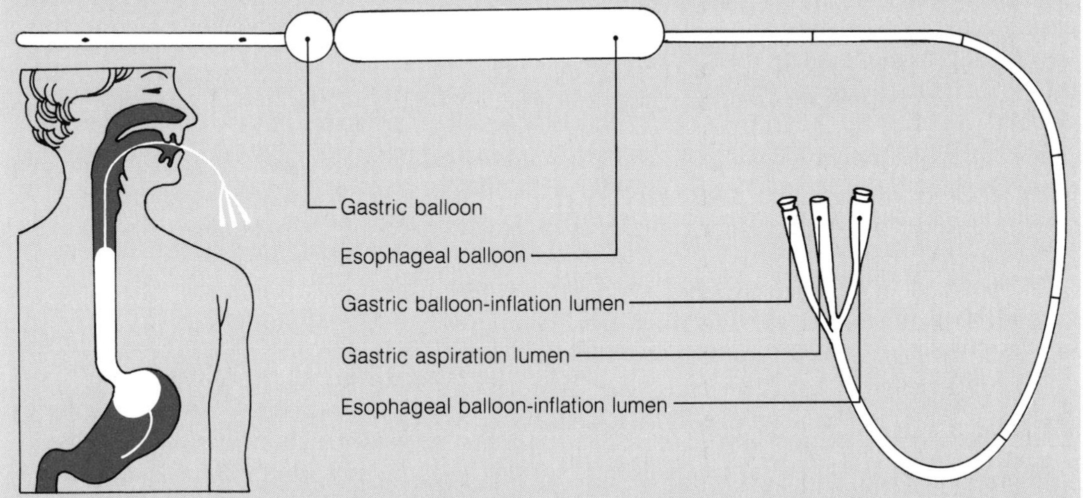

Gastric balloon

Esophageal balloon

Gastric balloon-inflation lumen

Gastric aspiration lumen

Esophageal balloon-inflation lumen

**Sengstaken-Blakemore tube**
This three-lumen, double-balloon tube provides a gastric aspiration port that allows drainage from below the gastric balloon and also can be used for instilling medication.

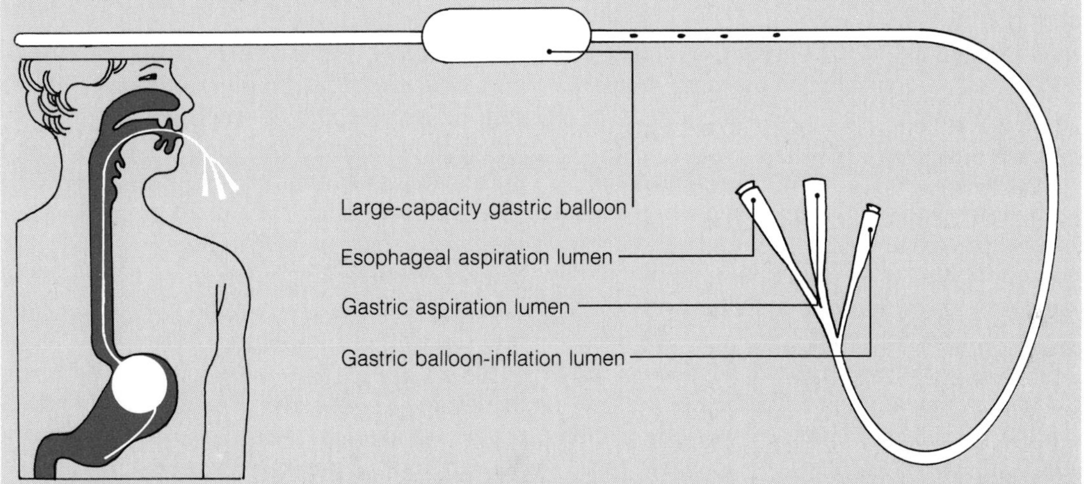

Large-capacity gastric balloon

Esophageal aspiration lumen

Gastric aspiration lumen

Gastric balloon-inflation lumen

**Linton tube**
This three-lumen, single-balloon tube provides ports for esophageal and gastric aspiration and reduces the risk of esophageal necrosis because it doesn't have an esophageal balloon.

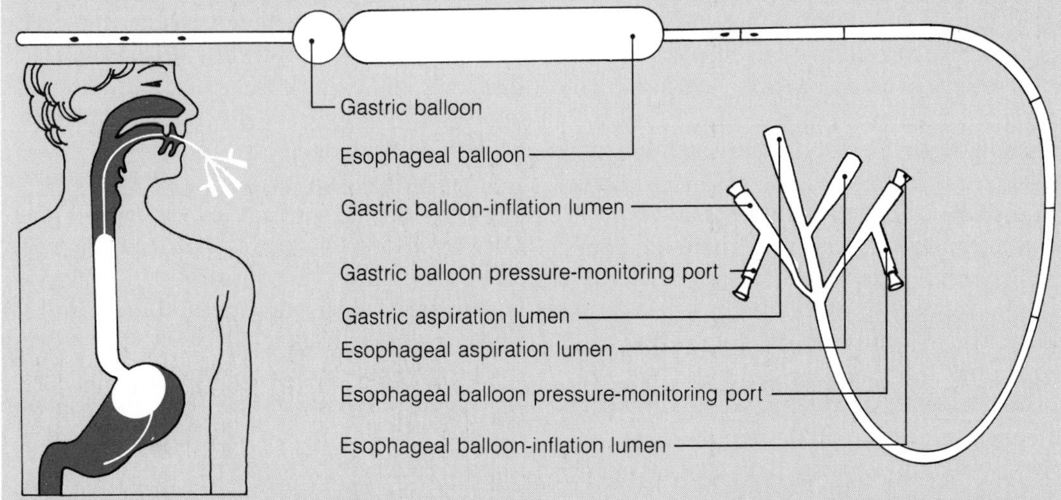

Gastric balloon

Esophageal balloon

Gastric balloon-inflation lumen

Gastric balloon pressure-monitoring port

Gastric aspiration lumen

Esophageal aspiration lumen

Esophageal balloon pressure-monitoring port

Esophageal balloon-inflation lumen

**Minnesota esophago-gastric tamponade tube**
This four-lumen, double-balloon tube provides pressure-monitoring ports for both balloons without the need for Y connectors.

value in promoting ulcer healing is now in question because effective dosage is high and may cause marked side effects. Anticholinergics are also ineffective for treating motor disorders such as achalasia. In some centers, the calcium blocking agent nifedipine is used to treat achalasia through its effect on decreasing LES tone.

*Anti-inflammatory agents,* such as aspirin, phenylbutazone, and indomethacin, should be avoided because of their tendency to cause bleeding and ulceration.

*Cimetidine,* a histamine $H_2$ antagonist, is not an anticholinergic but does have significant antisecretory action. In gastric ulcer disease, it stops gastric acid secretion.

### Acute therapy for hemorrhage

Hemorrhage, the most critical complication, requires vigorous emergency care. In addition to the obvious risks of shock and exsanguination, GI hemorrhage can cause airway obstruction from aspiration of vomited blood or its accumulation in the oropharynx. Emergency care to control such bleeding requires gastric intubation and suctioning and drug therapy to promote clotting.

*Tamponade* with a Sengstaken-Blakemore (S-B) tube is used for emergency control of hemorrhage from esophageal and gastric varices (but only for 48 hours because of the danger of tissue necrosis from balloon pressure). A Minnesota tube, similar to the S-B tube, may also be used. Complications of such intubation may include aspiration of oral secretions or refluxed blood, airway obstruction from balloon displacement, esophageal rupture, and cardiac dysrhythmia from a distended esophagus.

*Nasogastric suctioning* with a double-lumen (Salem sump) or a single-lumen (Levin) large-gauge tube is also performed to control gastric hemorrhage. Some doctors prefer a wide-bore tube, such as an Ewald tube, for clot irrigation. Gastric contents are aspirated, and irrigation is commonly done with iced normal saline solution, but some institutions now recommend saline solution at room temperature instead of ice lavage for upper GI bleeding. This change in procedure is based on the theory that ice causes vagal stimulation as it moves down the esophagus, which, in turn, stimulates gastric secretion of hydrochloric acid and increases motility and thus can aggravate bleeding. Ice may also decrease clotting ability. Saline solution may be contraindicated for lavage in patients with sodium restrictions. For example, water lavage may be preferred in patients with congestive heart failure, kidney impairment, and cirrhosis. Gastric lavage must remove clots before endoscopy can be performed to visualize the bleeding site.

Nasogastric suctioning is also performed in partial or complete gastric obstruction to control gastric fluid accumulation, which can initiate nausea and vomiting, gastric dilatation, or perforation. For such use, an NG tube is connected to intermittent or continuous suction.

*Vitamin K* promotes prothrombin synthesis and increases blood clotting power. In patients with hemorrhage, 10 mg of vitamin K is usually given intramuscularly or subcutaneously. But in severe emergencies, it may be given slowly and cautiously by intravenous route. Blood transfusions may be ordered to replace blood volume in massive bleeding. Fresh frozen plasma may also be given to replace blood-clotting products.

*Vasopressin,* the posterior pituitary diuretic hormone, lowers portal pressure, which may stop active bleeding of esophageal varices by allowing hemostasis and clotting. Its use requires continued monitoring in an intensive care unit. An initial dose of 20 units of vasopressin I.V. may be given diluted in 100 to 200 ml dextrose 5% in water over 10 to 20 minutes. Vasopressin may be given directly into the superior mesenteric artery at a rate of 0.1 to 0.4 unit/minute. This route of administration requires skilled personnel and angiography. Vasopressin lowers splanchnic blood flow and portal pressure by producing mesenteric vasoconstriction and thus may cause abdominal cramping, involuntary bowel evacuation, facial pallor, and, possibly, bowel infarction due to splanchnic vascular constriction. Other hazards with this drug include liver infarcts, cardiac ischemia, and water intoxication. Vasopressin is contraindicated in patients with coronary artery disease.

*Sclerotherapy* may be used for patients with uncontrollable hemorrhage and for poor surgical risks. Sclerosing solutions such as ethanolamine oleate are injected via catheters passed into portal circulation to create variceal thrombosis. Sclerosing solutions may also be given to bleeding varices via rigid endoscopy along the esophageal wall. Acute sclerotherapy has been particularly effective, but long-term sclerotherapy has not stopped rebleeding. Despite the most vigorous treatment, bleeding esophageal varices have a high mortality.

## Special procedures

*Bougienage* dilates the esophagus in an attempt to maintain an adequate lumen and to decrease the LES tone, thus relieving dysphagia in such motor and structural disorders as achalasia and stricture. It stretches and even tears some of the sphincter muscle fibers and leaves the sphincter partially open and weakened so that food and fluids enter the stomach by gravity. So, this treatment may cause subsequent reflux, and only temporary benefit.

Bougienage needs preliminary fasting for 6 to 8 hours, esophageal lavage for patients with achalasia, a topical anesthetic applied to the throat, and sometimes sedation. This procedure risks esophageal perforation and hemorrhage, which usually occur at the cricopharyngeal muscle level. Pain, aggravated by swallowing, and crepitation in the neck and substernal area accompany esophageal perforation. Thoracic esophageal perforation causes dyspnea, pneumothorax, and mediastinal emphysema. Gastric perforation causes abdominal pain radiating to the back, pleural effusion, and cyanosis. Hematemesis may accompany perforation at any level.

A prosthetic plastic or rubber (Celestin) tube may be inserted into the esophagus to maintain the lumen against esophageal carcinoma. This may be only palliative when the prognosis is poor; however, the prosthetic tube allows the patient to eat and swallow.

*Esophageal endoscopy* with a rigid hollow esophagoscope is preferred to remove foreign bodies in the esophagus. Before endoscopy, an anticholinergic drug may be given to inhibit secretions, unless contraindicated. The pharynx is anesthetized with a topical spray such as lidocaine. Then, the instrument is passed as the patient swallows while remaining perfectly still. Care must be taken in dislodging an object with sharp edges.

## Surgical intervention varies

In upper GI disorders, surgery may be necessary to manage an emergency or to provide palliation for incurable disease.

In *esophagomyotomy,* the esophageal muscle wall is cut. A long myotomy may be done for diffuse esophageal spasm. A *cardiomyotomy* (Heller's operation) for achalasia may be performed through the thoracic or abdominal approach. The esophagus' lower end and the cardia are slit to expose but not penetrate the mucosa. Prognosis is generally good, though reflux esophagitis is a complication.

# Surgery for esophageal disorders

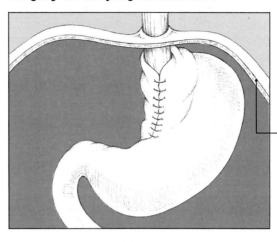

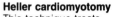

**Nissen fundoplication**
This technique treats hiatal hernia by reducing the hernia and wrapping the fundus around the abdominal esophagus for support.

— Diaphragm

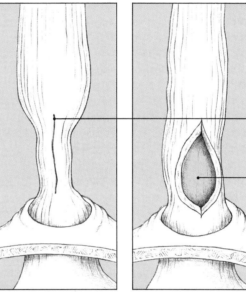

**Heller cardiomyotomy**
This technique treats achalasia by cutting the muscle of the constricted area and allowing the esophageal lumen to expand.

— Incision through constricted area of muscle

— Esophageal mucosa pouching through incision in muscular wall

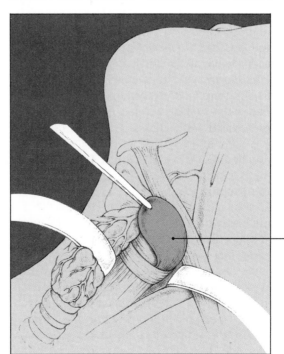

**Cricopharyngeal myotomy**
This technique treats Zenker's diverticulum by removal.

— Diverticulum

## Bougienage to relieve dysphagia

In spasm, stricture, and achalasia, bougienage—forced dilation of the lower esophagus and sphincter—can help relieve dysphagia. An inflatable balloon, guided by fluoroscopy, is inserted and inflated when it reaches the sphincter. Though balloon pressure is monitored, pressure may cause temporary chest discomfort.

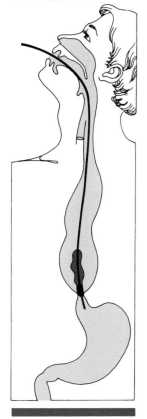

*Polypectomy* (removal of polyps) may be accomplished with a cautery snare by endoscopy or surgical excision. Possibly malignant polyps may be removed by partial gastric resection. Thoracotomy, a surgical incision into the chest wall, is used to approach structures within the chest cavity, for example, to repair esophageal perforation or gastric rupture. Escaped contents such as blood, secretions, and gastric contents are then evacuated from the abdominal or thoracic cavity, and the perforated tissue is repaired and closed.

*Hemigastrectomy* (removal of half of the stomach) may be done for bleeding ulcer disease. *Antrectomy* (partial gastric resection) or *vagotomy* may be done to decrease gastric secretion and to prevent bleeding and perforation in gastric ulcer disease. *Total gastrectomy* may be done in gastric carcinoma, but prognosis is poor. Tumor resection is also possible.

*Resection* (removal of part of a body structure) is done to remove tumors, malignant lesions, and diverticula. Surgery is most successful for lower-third esophageal lesions, although removing obstructions by this treatment is only palliative. A transabdominal approach, which has less surgical risk than thoracotomy, may be possible for certain procedures.

*Esophagogastrectomy* (bringing the stomach up into the chest for anastomosis to the resected esophagus) or replacement of the resected esophagus with a loop of the small intestine generally proves unsatisfactory.

*Fundoplication* (wrapping the fundus around the lower esophagus and suturing the fundus to itself) is used to treat hiatal hernia by compressing the esophagus and aiding LES competence as the stomach distends. This procedure is used only when reflux esophagitis, stricture, and hemorrhage have developed. The Hill procedure narrows the lower esophageal orifice and creates a gastroesophageal flap. The Belsey procedure creates a gastroesophageal angle that enhances LES function. All of these procedures allow an abdominal approach.

### Chemotherapy and radiation

In upper GI tract cancer, chemotherapy tends to be only palliative, offering pain relief. Stomach carcinoma is usually treated with 5-fluorouracil, mitomycin, and other combinations. Remember that antineoplastic agents also damage cells in normal growth, including the gastrointestinal mucous lining, hair follicles, and bone marrow. Therefore, side effects

of anorexia, nausea and vomiting, bleeding gums, stomatitis, and poor wound healing must be weighed against possible benefits.

Radiation treatment may be curative, adjunctive to other therapy such as surgery or chemotherapy, or—for inoperable upper GI cancer—merely palliative (dose of 4,500 to 6,000 rads). It is most useful in carcinoma of the upper third of the esophagus and of some use in carcinoma of the middle third. It gives palliative relief from dysphagia in about one half of squamous carcinoma patients. Radiation therapy may also be used to treat gastric carcinoma. Side effects include nausea and diarrhea. Large radiation doses to the chest may cause tracheal esophageal fistula, which mandates discontinuation of the therapy.

### NURSING MANAGEMENT

Managing the patient with upper GI disorders challenges all your skills, including the ability to give dietary instructions, to give acute care during bleeding crises, and to give psychosocial support during prolonged terminal illness. These varied responsibilities all rest on accurate assessment, the first and always vital element of effective nursing care.

### Accurate assessment vital

Begin by having the patient tell what most concerns him about his condition. Then, carefully ask him about frequency and duration of signs or symptoms and about factors that aggravate or relieve them. Ask specifically about pain or discomfort, dysphagia, vomiting, weight loss, anorexia, respiratory symptoms, and emotional upset.

**Pain or discomfort.** Most esophageal disorders cause discomfort on swallowing, which varies in severity with the disease and its stage. Sharp, stabbing, or burning pain with swallowing or after eating accompanies esophagitis from gastroesophageal reflux, hiatal hernia, esophageal cancer, and ingestion of corrosives. Such pain is aggravated by lying down, bending over, or straining. The patient may describe discomfort as heartburn and may give a history of relief with antacids. He may complain of constricting substernal or back pain with esophageal spasm. Ask specifically about indigestion if you suspect gastric ulcer, bleeding, or carcinoma. The pain will be sharp and unbearable, spreading over the abdomen or chest if gastric or esophageal perforation has occurred.

**Dysphagia.** Ask the patient if he needs to wash down his meals with liquids. Note

## Special uses for wide-bore gastric tubes

Use one of the three wide-bore tubes shown when you need an alternative to the Levin or Salem sump tube. Wide-bore tubes let large volumes of fluid pass through faster, so they're useful when lavaging the stomach of a patient with profuse gastric bleeding or after ingestion of poison. These tubes can't remain in the patient as long as a Levin tube because they're usually passed orally. (If necessary, they can be inserted nasally.) Insert them only long enough to complete lavage and to evacuate stomach contents.

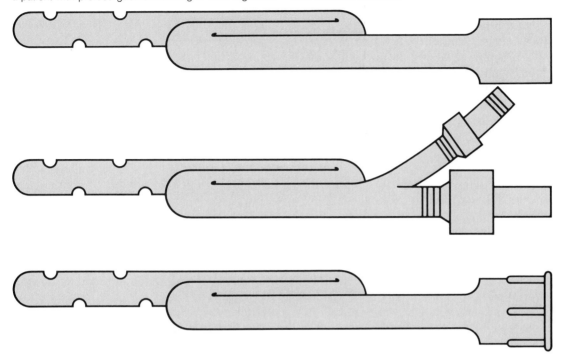

**Ewald tube**
This single-lumen tube, with several openings at the distal end, can be used to aspirate large amounts of gastric contents quickly.

**Levacuator tube**
With this double-lumen tube, the larger lumen is used for evacuation of gastric contents; the smaller, for instillation of an irrigant.

**Edlich tube**
This single-lumen tube has four openings near the closed distal tip. A funnel or syringe may be connected at the proximal end. Like the Ewald tube, the Edlich tube can be used to aspirate large amounts of gastric contents quickly.

whether he has difficulty swallowing solids, liquids, or both to indicate the severity of obstruction. The time of onset of discomfort after swallowing helps localize the obstruction. Discomfort within 5 seconds of swallowing indicates obstruction of the thoracic esophagus, as with Zenker's diverticulum, stricture, or spasm. Discomfort in 5 to 15 seconds indicates carcinoma, a foreign body, or stricture of the lower third of the esophagus. Continuously worsening dysphagia indicates a progressive condition such as cancer; intermittent dysphagia indicates a motor disorder.

**Weight loss.** In many upper GI disorders, weight loss results from the disease itself (cancer), from vomiting, or from fear of eating because of dysphagia and pain. Anorexia is common in cancer.

**Vomiting.** The patient may describe vomitus that looks bloody or resembles coffee grounds if upper GI bleeding has been caused by esophagitis, cancer, or varices. Ask about regurgitation of undigested, foul-smelling food (Zenker's diverticulum) or vomiting of chyme and gastric juice (gastric disorders and those which cause an incompetent LES). Vomiting large amounts of food and secretions indicates complete or almost complete obstruction.

**Respiratory symptoms.** Ask about accompanying shortness of breath and coughing, especially during the night, which may indicate aspiration of refluxed, regurgitated, or retained food from the esophagus into the trachea.

**Emotional upset and other symptoms.** Ask about emotional upsets that worsen symptoms, as in esophageal motor disorders, and onset of GI bleeding. Ask about other symptoms that accompany the chief complaint, such as eructation, halitosis, full feeling in the neck, foul taste in the mouth, gastric fullness, weakness, fatigue, or hoarseness.

### Review the history

Carefully review the patient's personal and family medical history, with special emphasis on drugs, diet, and psychosocial factors.

**Medical history.** Ask about a history of cancer, treated or untreated. Ask if the patient has had any thoracic or abdominal trauma or surgery that may have affected upper GI organs. Traction diverticula often stem from previous thoracic surgery and adhesions; strictures, from trauma to the esophageal mucosa or long-term intubation; and hiatal hernia, from abdominal trauma. Does the patient have a history of diabetes mellitus, which may impair esophageal motility; pernicious anemia, which often predisposes to gastric cancer; or severe congestive heart failure or liver disease, which may cause bleeding varices? Does he have a history of neurologic, neuromuscular, or connective tissue disease, which may cause an esophageal motility disorder?

**Family history.** Remember that gastric carcinoma, ulcers, and other disorders demonstrate a familial tendency. Realizing that blood relatives have had similar problems may hasten diagnosis. Ask about the patient's nearest relatives' ages, their present states of health, and the causes of illness or death of parents, grandparents, brothers, sisters, aunts, and uncles.

**Drug history.** Many patients treat themselves with drugs that can cause relaxed muscles, lowered or increased esophageal sphincter pressure, increased or decreased upper GI tract peristalsis, gastric irritation, and bleeding tendencies. Ask specifically about the use of cholinergics, anticholinergics, aspirin, or other anti-inflammatory agents.

**Psychosocial history.** Obtain a data base of the patient's age, sex, and ethnic origin. These may be diagnostically significant and may help identify contributing dietary patterns. Carefully assess the patient's life-style and occupation. Exposure to air pollutants promotes susceptibility to esophageal cancer. Heavy lifting may precipitate tears, rupture, and reflux. Home- or job-related stress precipitates or worsens many conditions. Check on smoking and use of alcohol because these have also been implicated in esophageal tears and rupture, esophageal varices, carcinoma, and ulcers. Record the specific types and amounts of such substances used. Record the use of coffee and caffeine-containing beverages and the types and amounts of foods consumed. Dietary habits may be related to gastric carcinoma and ulcers and may aggravate hiatal hernia.

Assess the patient's emotional state. Emotions can alter motility, gastric secretions, and blood flow to initiate or worsen upper GI conditions. They may also provoke anorexia, nausea and vomiting, difficulty in swallowing, and dyspepsia, which may have no clear physiologic basis in some patients. Assess the patient's coping style and reliance on support systems. Have these been effective in the past, or are new mechanisms needed? Assess the patient's educational level and intellectual and emotional capacity to understand and deal with his illness and needed self-care. Establish rapport for later interventions.

## Physical examination next
Every patient with a suspected upper GI disorder should have a complete, thorough physical examination.

*Inspect* for emaciation, muscle wasting, and signs of malnutrition. Check for poor skin turgor from dehydration and for pallor from anemia. Be alert for signs of discomfort in the patient's affect—clenched fists and abdominal guarding. Check for the foul-smelling breath of esophageal cancer or diverticula and for the hiccups of late esophageal cancer with metastasis to the phrenic nerve. Watch the patient's vomitus and stools for signs of bleeding. Upper GI bleeding causes frank blood in vomitus but melanotic stools. Abdominal distention may mean stomach perforation.

*Palpate* for tenderness and masses along the inner aspects of the neck and over the stomach area. Local masses causing dysphagia may be seen in the hypopharyngeal area. Tumors within or around the upper GI tract are difficult to palpate unless they are large and advanced. Note if the abdomen is soft and relaxed or rigid and boardlike.

*Percuss* the stomach for characteristic tympany to identify a gastric air bubble. Its absence may indicate achalasia. If percussion reveals a tympanic abdomen, gastric rupture may have occurred.

*Auscultate* to assess swallowing. Normally, a food bolus takes about 6 to 15 seconds to pass through the esophagus into the stomach. Place the stethoscope bell over the xiphoid process while the patient swallows water. When the trickle reaches the LES, you should hear it squirting into the stomach. Swallowing sounds are absent in total esophageal obstruction. A slight delay may mean partial obstruction or a motor disorder such as achalasia.

## Plan appropriate care
Integrating data from the history and physical exam, you now have enough material to form nursing diagnoses and plan interventions.

**Alteration in comfort related to pathology or surgical intervention.** Be alert to changes in the patient's affect and to signs of tachycardia, dyspnea, pyrosis, or discomfort that mean the patient is in pain. Give prescribed narcotics or other analgesic drugs *before* the pain reaches full intensity to provide better relief and to reassure the patient that his pain will not get out of control and that someone cares. Tell the patient when to expect relief to ease his anxiety and enhance relief.

## Fluid and electrolyte imbalances

Without proper intervention, prolonged vomiting and gastric suction can cause serious fluid and electrolyte imbalances. Sodium, potassium, fluid, and hydrochloric acid are lost with gastric secretion. Be alert for the following signs and symptoms of hyponatremia, hypovolemia, hypokalemia, and metabolic alkalosis.

| Hyponatremia | Hypovolemia | Hypokalemia | Metabolic alkalosis |
|---|---|---|---|
| Lethargy | Lassitude | Malaise | Increased muscle tone |
| Headache | Poor skin turgor | Weakness | Irritability |
| Weakness | Dry skin and mucous membranes | Diminished reflexes | Twitching and tremors |
| Confusion | Thirst | Muscle cramps | Tetany |
| Anorexia | Oliguria | Postural hypotension | Tachycardia |
| Abdominal cramping | Weight loss | Paralytic ileus (anorexia, decreased bowel sounds, constipation, nausea, and vomiting) | Depressed respiration |
| Nausea and vomiting | Hypotension | | Nausea and vomiting |
| Diarrhea, convulsions, and coma (These symptoms accompany severe and rapid onset.) | Rapid pulse | Dysrhythmia | Diarrhea |
| | | Weak, irregular pulse | |

To help control pain, control the environment. A noisy environment is tiring and taxing and makes the patient tense. Limit visitors because adequate rest helps the patient obtain full benefit from the analgesics. Relaxation and pleasant surroundings also help relieve pain and tension. Motion usually increases pain, so schedule postoperative turning, coughing, deep breathing, and ambulation to coincide with the onset of benefit from analgesics. But remember, oversedation may make turning, coughing, and deep breathing labored. Help the sedated patient with ambulation.

Keep the patient informed to ease his anxiety, and give him the chance to express his anxiety. Stay with him until he relaxes and his pain subsides. For many patients, reassurance alone is helpful.

Position the patient to promote comfort in upper GI disorders. Elevate the head of the bed, and have him sit in a chair for meals and for 1 hour afterward to prevent discomfort from hiatal hernia or gastroesophageal reflux. Put the patient who has had abdominal surgery in low or semi-Fowler's position to prevent tension on the diaphragm and incision while promoting lung expansion. Have pillows handy for splinting the incision during movement and coughing. Consider your interventions effective if the patient reports relief of pain, sleeps most of the night, and alternates intervals of rest and activity during the day.

**Fluid volume deficit related to vomiting, gastric drainage, and possible upper GI hemorrhage.** Note the quantity and characteristics of emesis. Administer antiemetics as ordered, and provide a quiet, calm environment because stimulation may provoke vomiting, especially in an anxious patient. Clear emesis from the patient's mouth, and change linen promptly.

Nasogastric suctioning may be ordered to relieve obstruction and distention causing vomiting. Monitor the tube's patency, and record the amount and characteristics of gastric drainage. If the patient vomits around the NG tube, irrigate to ensure its patency. Sedation may be necessary. Use normal saline solution, unless contraindicated, rather than water (because of the potential for sodium depletion through the gastric mucosa) for irrigations to assure patency. Give parenteral fluids as ordered to maintain fluid and electrolyte balance while the patient is receiving nothing by mouth and is losing fluid and electrolytes through suctioning. Be alert for dehydration, overhydration, and electrolyte imbalance. Carefully monitor vital signs and record all intake and output. Notify the doctor of any change in vital signs or urine output below 30 ml/hour for 2 consecutive hours. Observe emesis or NG drainage for bright red or coffee-ground appearance. Bleeding into the thoracic or abdominal cavity from erosion or perforation or after surgical intervention may cause abdominal tenderness; rigidity; difficult breathing; bloody chest-tube drainage; signs of shock such as hypotension; rapid, thready pulse; deep, rapid respirations; cold, clammy skin; pallor; apprehension; and restlessness.

Measure, report, and record all bleeding

## How to use a Sengstaken-Blakemore tube

For emergency control of hemorrhage from esophageal varices, the Sengstaken-Blakemore (S-B) tube is used by exerting pressure on esophageal varices. Its triple lumen provides inflation of the esophageal balloon, placement of the gastric balloon, and suction of gastric contents. To use this tube:
• Inflate the gastric balloon to about 250 cc of air and the esophageal balloon to a pressure of 20 to 40 mm Hg (usually 35 mm Hg).
• Anchor the S-B tube securely with slight traction. Tape the tube to a sponge block or a football helmet.
• Inflate the esophageal balloon with a Y connector attached to the appropriate lumen and a mercury manometer and its inflation bulb.
• Double-clamp the gastric balloon port and the esophageal balloon port.
• Irrigate hourly to evaluate gastric bleeding or esophageal blood leaking into the stomach. If needed and ordered, put a second nasogastric tube *above* the esophageal balloon to help detect blood leakage and, along with suctioning, to prevent aspiration.

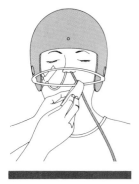

from emesis, suction or chest drainage, or the surgical site. But bleeding may not be evident initially. Test for occult blood in the stools and tube aspirate by the guaiac or hematest method. A patient who has lost considerable blood has a low hemoglobin level and tires easily from inadequate oxygenation to all tissues and, therefore, requires extra rest.

Bleeding in esophageal varices is not associated with pain and epigastric tenderness as is gastric ulcer bleeding. Bleeding in esophageal varices is usually bright red and profuse. Report such bleeding to the doctor immediately. If an I.V. infusion is not already running and the doctor is not immediately available, start an infusion of dextrose 5% in water or normal saline solution to prevent further deterioration and circulatory collapse. Use an 18G needle or cannula if a good vein is available to allow later blood transfusions, if needed. If not, use any available vein, preferably in the upper extremities, to replace fluid and prevent hypovolemic shock.

The doctor may apply tamponade with an esophageal tube such as an S-B tube for emergency control of hemorrhage from esophageal varices. Manometers are attached to the esophageal tube for pressure readings. Your main responsibility during such treatment is to maintain the tube's position and the prescribed pressure. Irrigate the gastric lumen often to see if bleeding diminishes. The initial lavage may be with iced water; however, continued irrigations may be with iced normal saline solution. Iced solutions help control bleeding by constricting blood vessels. (Iced water lavage may not be policy in some hospitals.)

The inflated esophageal balloon suppresses swallowing, so frequent oral suctioning may be necessary to prevent aspiration of accumulated saliva. The doctor may order an NG tube inserted in the other nostril to be connected to intermittent suction. This is not needed with a Minnesota esophagogastric tamponade tube or a Linton tube because they have an extra port for esophageal suction. If you do use a supplemental tube, measure the approximate distance carefully, so this tube doesn't touch or interfere with the esophageal balloon. Maintain the patient in semi-Fowler's position to facilitate breathing and prevent aspiration. Evaluate vital signs frequently, and record intake and output. The patient tends to mouth-breathe because of the large nasal tube, so conscientious oral hygiene is essential to prevent mucous mem-

brane encrustation, drying, and cracking.

Stay with the patient throughout such treatment. This frightening experience requires the assurance of close observation and the knowledge that someone is there to prevent aspiration and choking.

The tube may be left in place for gastric aspiration after the balloons have been deflated. This makes hasty reinflation possible if bleeding recurs. The doctor may order periodic deflation of the esophageal balloon to reduce the risk of necrosis.

You may need to give blood transfusions. If so, follow hospital protocol; double-check for the right blood for the right patient. Watch the patient for untoward reactions, such as itching, rash, fever, chills, back pain, dyspnea, and chest pain. Oxygen is usually administered to enhance hemoglobin saturation for increased availability to tissues.

Nasogastric suctioning without tamponade is also done for gastric hemorrhage. Gastric contents are aspirated, and irrigation is done with iced normal saline solution. A large-bore tube such as an Ewald is used to remove clots and allow rapid fluid exchange. Irrigation may be continuous for profuse bleeding, but associated suctioning must be done gently to prevent further tissue damage. Iced water may be used for some irrigations in patients, such as those with congestive heart failure, who require sodium restriction.

Monitor vital signs often; maintain body temperature, which may be greatly lowered from blood loss or iced irrigations. Give extra blankets if needed, but don't apply too much external warmth because, in the hypovolemic patient, blood should stay in vital organs and not be drawn to the skin by external heating.

Administer drugs as ordered. Vitamin K is usually given during the emergency stage and later when clotting studies are checked. Vasopressin administration requires special surveillance. Because of its effect on blood pressure and its antidiuretic effect, monitor blood pressure and intake and output carefully. After hemorrhage stops, dosage is gradually discontinued after 48 hours.

Consider your interventions effective if vomiting has ceased, tube aspirate and stools are free of blood, and the patient shows no signs of dehydration or electrolyte depletion.

**Alteration in nutrition related to decreased food intake.** Your goals for patients with this diagnosis are to maintain adequate body weight and to prevent upper GI distress.

After treatment with decompression and

suctioning, clamp the NG tube used for compression, and give small amounts of water to assess the patient's tolerance. Note his complaints of nausea, fullness, or pain while the tubing is clamped. Gradually increase fluid after the tube has been removed. Progress from clear liquids to small, bland, easily tolerated feedings. Administer antacids before, with, or after meals as ordered. Watch for incomplete gastric emptying with distention developing over a few days. Encourage the patient to slowly take as much food as possible without experiencing discomfort. Make sure the diet contains protein and vitamin C for tissue repair. High-calorie and liquid nutrient supplements may also help the patient with long-term obstruction. Provide a peaceful environment for eating to enhance swallowing in the patient with a motor disorder.

A patient who retains food in the esophagus may complain of a bad taste in the mouth with accompanying nausea and vomiting. Good oral hygiene is essential; lavage may be necessary. Pressing over the area of Zenker's diverticulum may help express the retained food. Give a drink of water after meals to rinse esophageal contents and to exert pressure on the gastroesophageal sphincter to relax it and permit passage of food.

A patient with carcinoma within or near the upper GI tract may experience anorexia, weight loss, poor nutrition, and nausea and vomiting not only from the malignancy but also from chemotherapy or radiation. Give mouth care every 2 hours with antiseptic mouthwash, diluted hydrogen peroxide, or nystatin solution to prevent stomatitis, which may occur in immunosuppressed patients. Avoid giving extremely hot or cold fluids to prevent further oral and esophageal irritation in a patient with cancer or esophagitis. Note the amounts and kinds of all fluid and food intake. If needed, consult a dietitian for a 24-hour calorie count and nutrient evaluation. Weigh the patient at least weekly, always before breakfast and in the same amount of clothing.

Consider your interventions successful if the patient maintains his weight and tolerates progression of diet without nausea, vomiting, or pain.

**Knowledge deficit related to self-care after discharge.** Your goals are to help the patient understand needed changes in diet, activity, and life-style; to ensure that he learns the dosage and schedule of drug therapy; and to help him accept the need for follow-up visits.

Gear your teaching to the patient's intellectual and emotional capabilities, basing your teaching plan on his current knowledge. Provide literature if available. Ask the patient to express his understanding of his disorder. Schedule teaching sessions when family members can be present.

Be sure the patient understands the effects on his disorder of alcohol, smoking, bending, straining, coughing, caffeine-containing beverages, and highly seasoned foods. He should understand his need for a high-calorie, high-protein diet with vitamin C to promote energy and tissue repair. Teach the patient to avoid tight, constricting clothing (especially girdles on women). Teach him to eat slowly to avoid overdistention and to chew food thoroughly. To prevent reflux, advise him to sleep with three pillows or to raise the head of his bed on blocks.

With the doctor, provide weight counseling for obese or emaciated patients and seek referral for the alcoholic patient. Encourage the patient to discuss his problem and his feelings about alcohol. Teach him about prescribed drugs and their side effects; provide a dosage schedule in writing if appropriate. Tell the patient to avoid over-the-counter drugs that contain aspirin or caffeine or that effervesce. Warn the patient with gastric ulcers, a history of upper GI bleeding, or a tendency to reflux to check with his doctor or pharmacist about antacids and over-the-counter preparations. Give the patient your unit's phone number at discharge, and encourage him to call with further questions or just for support. Review all instructions, and make sure he has an appointment card with his doctor's phone number for follow-up visits.

Consider your interventions effective if the patient can correctly plan a sample day's menu and can list foods he must avoid, if he can express necessary changes, if he makes a commitment to avoid smoking and alcohol, and if he knows his drug dosage and schedule.

### Overall evaluation
Whether your interventions are curative or palliative, your main goals are to make the patient comfortable and to help him keep himself comfortable. You have achieved these goals if you have been able to maintain the patient's fluid and electrolyte balance, have prevented vomiting and bleeding, have maintained his nutrition, and have taught the patient how to care for himself and how to cope with his disorder.

**Points to remember**

• Dysphagia is the most common complaint of patients with esophageal disorders due to mechanical or structural obstruction.
• A Zenker's diverticulum may be unnoticed until food and secretions are retained for several days, enlarging the pouch and raising the risk of pulmonary aspiration or complete esophageal obstruction.
• Esophageal rupture is usually related to alcohol intoxication and often follows vomiting.
• Hiatal hernia is common in the general population; however, it may be ignored as simple indigestion after a heavy meal or confused with more serious heart disease.
• Gastric and esophageal bleeding are life-threatening complications of other GI disorders that may require emergency management with balloon tamponade, irrigation, various medications, and supportive care.

# 9 RECOGNIZING LOWER G.I. OBSTRUCTIONS

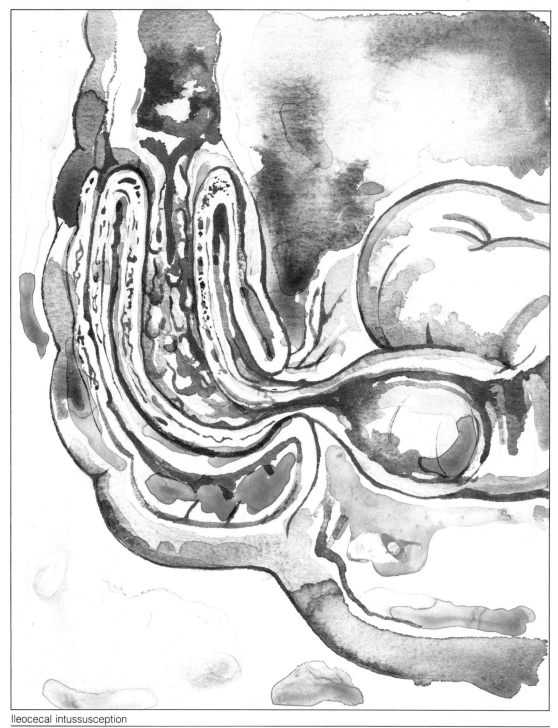

Ileocecal intussusception

ntestinal obstructions occur in all age-groups and are responsible for approximately 20% of the patients treated for acute abdominal pain. Intestinal obstructions are also dangerous and, unless they are correctly and promptly treated, can become life-threatening within hours.

Unfortunately, delayed treatment is not uncommon because the initial signs and symptoms of an obstruction can be so subtle that they are easily overlooked, or because the signs and symptoms obscure the diagnosis. For example, colonic obstruction in an adult may not cause severe symptoms for several days; by then, the patient's distended colon is progressively more vulnerable to perforation. Early symptoms of small-intestine obstruction—abdominal pain, nausea, and hyperactive peristalsis—may lead to a diagnosis of transient viral disease. In the meantime, continuous accumulation of fluids in the intestine creates the risk of hypovolemia and shock.

Partly because intestinal obstructions can be so difficult to identify promptly, they carry a mortality ranging from 10% for simple obstructions to 50% for strangulated obstructions. Obviously, then, the key to caring for a patient with intestinal obstruction is to recognize and treat it quickly before it causes irreversible damage. To do so, you must understand its causes, complications, and presenting symptoms.

## What causes intestinal obstruction?

An intestinal obstruction results from narrowing of the intestinal lumen or inhibited motility of its contents. The majority of obstructions have mechanical causes (see *Mechanical obstructions predominate,* pages 138 and 139). Blockage may be extrinsic, from pressure outside of the lumen, as with a hernia or adhesions; or intrinsic, from narrowing at the lumen itself, as with tumor growth or congenital malformations.

Although the majority of patients you'll see will have mechanical obstructions, many patients will have obstructions from neurogenic causes that result in decreased or absent peristalsis. Like mechanical obstructions, neurogenic obstructions can be either congenital or acquired.

## Congenital intestinal obstructions

Congenital malformations cause most intestinal obstructions in infants. In fact, congenital obstructions—and their sequelae—are so common that they account for one third of all hospitalizations of infants and children. The most common congenital obstructions are mechanical: atresias (complete absence or closure of the intestinal lumen) and stenoses (narrowing of the intestinal lumen). Less common mechanical obstructions include hernias, malrotation, and meconium ileus; a less common neurogenic obstruction is aganglionic megacolon (Hirschsprung's disease).

*Atresias* and *stenoses* usually occur in the small intestine, but a stenosis which is an exception is imperforate anus. In this congenital defect, a membrane partially or completely closes the anus. About 80% of infants born with this defect have a congenitally absent anus (anal agenesis). Their intestines end in blind pouches inside the perineum. This defect results from an abnormal division of the fetal hindgut into the urogenital region and the rectum during the 7th week of gestation. It's frequently accompanied by rectobladder fistulas and other severe congenital anomalies.

*Congenital hernias*—a source of obstruction most common in male infants—develop during the 7th month of gestation. At that time, the testicle descends into the scrotum, preceded by the peritoneal sac. If the sac closes incompletely, it leaves an opening through which a loop of the intestine can protrude. The ring of muscle around the loop squeezes it closed, blocking off the portion of the intestine distal to the hernia.

*Malrotation,* a less common cause of obstruction, occurs during the 10th week of gestation. If the intestine fails to rotate normally during that week, it remains twisted, causing total obstruction.

In *meconium ileus,* excessive secretion of thick, sticky mucus reduces motility in the intestine. In this condition, which is found in children with mucoviscidosis (also called cystic fibrosis), feces combine with thick mucus to cause the obstruction.

In *Hirschsprung's disease,* a segment of colon lacks the ganglion cells responsible for intestinal motility. Absence of these cells causes abnormal peristalsis, constipation, and finally, obstruction.

## Acquired intestinal obstructions

Obstructions also develop from acquired disorders. Like the congenital disorders, they're categorized as mechanical or neurogenic, but about 90% of them are mechanical. Most obstructions of the small intestine result from adhesions or hernias, whereas most obstruc-

## Mechanical obstructions predominate

Most intestinal obstructions result from intrinsic or extrinsic structures that narrow or close the intestinal lumen. These mechanical obstructions can be congenital or acquired.

**Congenital**
Atresia
Imperforate anus
Hernia
Malrotation

**Acquired**
Adhesion
Inflammatory stricture
Hernia
Tumor
Intussusception
Volvulus
Foreign object
Fecal impaction
Endometriosis
Extraintestinal mass
Emboli
Telangiectasia
Impaired peristalsis

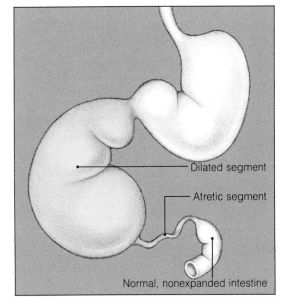

In *atresia*, the most common cause of intestinal obstruction in newborns, anomalous development of part of the intestinal wall causes complete occlusion of the lumen.

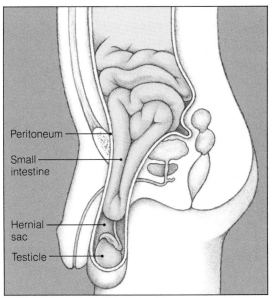

In *inguinal hernia*, a weakening of the abdominal wall permits a loop of intestine to descend into the scrotum. Constriction by the muscle in the abdominal wall obstructs and strangulates the loop.

tions of the large intestine result from malignant tumors in the colon.

*Adhesions* are the bands of granulation and scar tissue that develop in some patients after a surgical incision. Adhesions encircle the intestine and obstruct the flow of intestinal fluids by constricting the lumen. Bowel obstruction can also result from edema or stricture at a surgical site when a bowel resection and reanastomosis is performed. Subsequent edema from manipulation or stricture from a too-tight suture line will narrow the lumen and cause obstruction. This is especially true in the ileum because it is the narrowest part of the intestine.

*Inflammatory strictures* obstruct the intestine from within. They are caused by abdominal trauma; chronic inflammatory diseases, such as Crohn's disease; acute infections; or radiation therapy to the abdominal area. In each of these cases, inflammation of the intestinal wall causes edema, which narrows the lumen. Many strictures are temporary, resolving in 7 to 10 days, when the edema disappears. But some strictures become permanent because scars formed during healing narrow the lumen.

Acquired *hernias* cause most obstructions to the small intestine in adults. The hernias result from a weakened area of abdominal wall (usually the inguinal area) and increased intraabdominal pressure. This increased pressure can result from obesity, pregnancy, heavy lifting, or strenuous coughing. The pressure

forces a loop of intestine through the weakened section of abdominal wall; then the ring of muscles around the protruding intestine constricts it, causing the obstruction.

More than 50% of the obstructions in the large intestine result from *malignant tumors,* and approximately 60% to 70% of these occur in the sigmoid colon or rectal area. (See *Common sites of colorectal cancer,* page 144.) Adenocarcinoma, the most common of these tumors, obstructs the intestine with polypoid lesions that project into the lumen of the rectosigmoid area or with annular lesions that encircle the intestine.

Benign *polyps,* which occur in 10% to 12% of American adults, also can cause colonic obstructions. Colonic polyps, arising from the mucosa and extending into the lumen, may be pedunculated or sessile. (See *Colonic polyps,* page 145.) These polyps seem to increase the likelihood of cancer. Their potential for malignancy is greatest if polyps are multiple, if any polyp is greater than 2 cm in diameter or is of the villous type, or if there is a family history of colon cancer.

In familial polyposis, a genetic disorder characterized by hundreds of polyps, polyps are both pedunculated and sessile and develop within the entire large intestine. Polyps usually develop first at puberty and increase the likelihood of cancer to almost 100% by age 40.

Another acquired obstruction, intussusception, is most commonly seen in infant boys

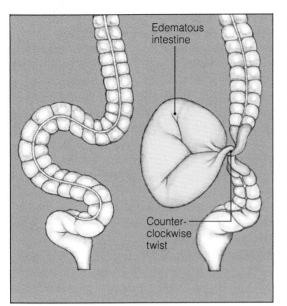

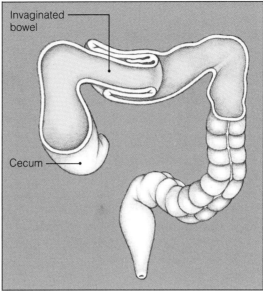

In *volvulus,* the intestine twists at least 180°, causing obstructions both proximal and distal to the loop, obstructing intestinal flow, and causing ischemia. Necrosis rapidly occurs.

In *intussusception,* most common in infants, a portion of the bowel telescopes or invaginates into an adjacent bowel portion. Peristalsis then propels the portion further along the bowel, pulling more bowel along with it.

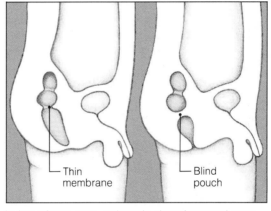

In *imperforate anus,* embryonic cloacal or rectal membranes obstruct the anus. The obstruction can range from mild, such as a thin membrane between the anus and rectum (see illustration at left), to severe, such as anal agenesis, in which the rectum ends in a blind pouch in the abdomen (see illustration at right).

up to age 18 months. Its cause is unknown. In such obstruction, one part of the bowel telescopes into another. (In most cases, the ileum telescopes into the cecum at the ileocecal valve.) In adults, the condition usually follows repeated bouts of bowel obstruction or benign or malignant tumors.

Another mechanical obstruction with an unknown cause is *volvulus.* In this condition, the intestine develops a 180° twist, strangulating the twisted loop. This usually occurs in the sigmoid colon. It is most prevalent in elderly, institutionalized men with chronic constipation.

*Foreign objects* can also block the intestine, especially the lumen, the narrowest section. Pins, bones, or small toys are the most common foreign objects. But gallstones, particles of food, mucus, or drugs can also obstruct the intestine. In a severely dehydrated patient, such objects can create a calcified mass, called a *bezoar.* In a patient with chronic renal failure, for example, a bezoar may develop from large doses of aluminum hydroxide gel and dehydration.

In *endometriosis,* another disorder that narrows the intestinal lumen, endometrial tissue is found in tissue other than the uterus, typically (in 12% to 34% of patients) in the bowel segments near the uterus, usually in the colon or rectum. The endometrial tissue causes fibrosis, inflammation, and necrosis within the bowel lumen.

Dehydration may also lead to intestinal

obstruction by *fecal impaction.* More often, impaction occurs in patients with chronic constipation or inhibited intestinal motility, in patients who chronically fail to respond to the defecation stimulus, in aged or immobilized patients with decreased peristalsis, and in patients who abuse laxatives.

*Masses outside the intestine* can also cause intestinal narrowing. For example, abscess or tumor development in an adjacent organ or pregnant uterus can put pressure on the intestine and cause it to become smaller.

Finally, mechanical obstructions can result from vascular causes, such as *emboli* or *atherosclerotic narrowing* of a mesenteric vessel.

## Atherosclerotic vessel changes

Like coronary and cerebral arteries, visceral arteries are prone to vascular disease. Atherosclerosis deposits plaques of lipids and cholesterol, which narrow the arterial lumen (see middle drawing) and reduce the elasticity of the vessel wall (see bottom drawing). The sluggish blood flow that results may cause thrombi, which, in turn, may lead to ischemia and intestinal infarction resulting in bowel obstruction.

**Normal artery**

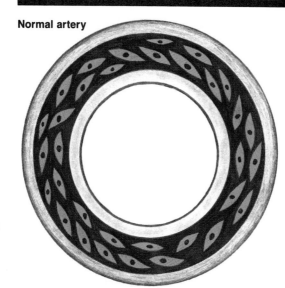

**Early**

Reduced elasticity —

Lipid and cholesterol deposits —

**Late**

Narrowed arterial lumen —

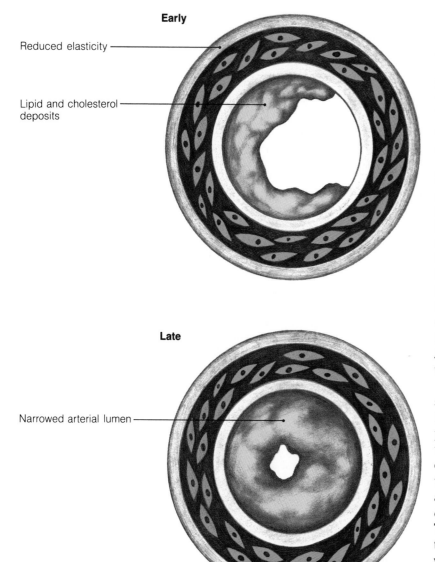

(See *Atherosclerotic vessel changes.*) These obstructions can become life-threatening quickly—resulting in irreversible intestinal ischemia within 40 minutes. Another vascular condition, *telangiectasia,* obstructs the GI tract by dilating the capillaries and venules of the mucous membranes throughout the entire GI tract. Telangiectasia is an autosomal dominant variant of vascular purpura. Lesions are commonly seen in the buccal mucosa, tongue, nose, and lips and extend throughout the entire GI tract.

Acquired obstructions may also result from neurologic impairment of peristalsis (paralytic ileus). Such obstruction in adults most commonly results from surgery. It occurs to some extent in every patient who has abdominal surgery, probably because of an overactive sympathetic nervous system response to the stress of surgery. But it may also result from exposure of the intestine to the atmosphere, surgical manipulation, and anesthesia. Most often, paralytic ileus resolves spontaneously in 2 to 3 days. This type of impairment can also result from blunt abdominal trauma, chemical irritants, electrolyte disturbances, and vascular insufficiency. In infants, acquired paralytic ileus is most often associated with pneumonia.

### PATHOPHYSIOLOGY

Any obstruction can have grave consequences on body homeostasis if it's serious enough to interfere with the intestine's normal digestion and absorption of over 8 liters of nutrients, fluid, and digestive juices each day. (See *Fluid handling by the GI tract.*) The small intestine digests or absorbs the majority of nutrients, trace metals, and fluids, sending these vital elements into the systemic circulation. The large intestine absorbs more salt and water. And the colon stores the dehydrated feces until they can be eliminated.

These functions are so crucial that an obstruction to the flow of food and fluid at any level can quickly lead to life-threatening complications. Whatever the cause, the obstruction creates two major pathophysiologic events: distention of the intestine proximal to the obstruction and systemic dehydration and electrolyte imbalance. (See *Complications of intestinal obstruction,* pages 142 and 143.) The speed with which these events occur and the complications that follow depend on whether the obstruction is partial or complete and whether it's in the small or large intestine. Of course, the severity of complications also depends on the timeliness of treatment. Without treatment, severe obstruction can cause irreversible damage within a few hours and death within 12 to 24 hours. The damage starts with distention.

## Complications of intestinal distention

Distention occurs in the section of the intestine proximal to the obstruction for several of the following reasons: the patient continues to swallow air, he may continue to ingest food and fluids, and his GI tract continues to secrete gastric juices and to acquire other gastric fluids from the liver and pancreas. Unable to bypass the obstruction, the fluids accumulate in the section of the intestine proximal to the obstruction, distending the intestinal walls.

As distention progresses, the unremitting pressure on the intestinal mucosa causes it to become necrotic and gangrenous. This is called strangulation. In strangulation, circulation is compromised, making the distended area ischemic. If ischemia persists longer than a few hours, the affected portion may suffer irreversible damage and gangrene. Damage to the wall of the intestine changes its permeability. The result: Toxins from the intestine leak into the peritoneum, causing bacterial peritonitis and ultimately septic shock. In addition, increased intraluminal pressure impairs venous return by the inferior vena cava. This may lead to thrombosis and formation of emboli, which further compromise the circulatory system. Hemorrhage into the lumen and weeping of plasma add to systemic hypovolemia.

Within 12 to 24 hours, the accumulation of gases and fluids proximal to a severe obstruction exceeds the intestine's ability to distend. Finally, the pressure perforates the distended portion of the bowel, spewing fecal material into the peritoneum, producing chemical peritonitis. In the meantime, the patient's condition has already been compromised by increasingly severe dehydration.

## Complications of reduced absorption

Dehydration is just one of the severe systemic problems that result from accumulation of fluids, nutrients, and electrolytes. The more severe the obstruction, the more fluid is sequestered in the intestine proximal to the obstruction. And more fluid sequestered there means less fluid available to the systemic circulation. How much fluid is involved? In 6 to 12 hours, nearly half the body's plasma

## Fluid handling by the GI tract

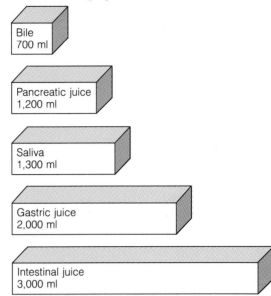

In addition to the 2,000 ml of fluid an average person ingests each day, the GI tract secretes, digests, and absorbs over 8,000 ml of digestive juices in the proportions shown above.

volume may be sequestered in the intestine proximal to a complete obstruction. The result is severe dehydration and electrolyte imbalance. In time, hyponatremia, hypochloremia, acidosis, metabolic acidosis, and hypovolemic shock develop.

In a severe obstruction, each complication tends to create another, so that each problem reinforces another. One complication of distention, for example, is ischemia. Ischemia may cause thrombosis, and thrombosis may send emboli into the systemic circulation, where they'll block off other vessels. This will cause further pooling of blood and additional complications, depending on the organs involved. Of course, the pooling of blood also intensifies hypovolemic shock, vomiting contributes to dehydration and metabolic acidosis, and so on.

## Symptoms of obstruction

The three main symptoms of obstruction are pain, vomiting, and constipation. These symptoms vary in severity and onset according to the location of the obstruction.

*Pain* results from distention and also from peristalsis, which becomes increasingly strong as the intestine tries to force its contents past the obstruction.

*Vomiting* occurs as the body tries to relieve the distention. It occurs early in high small-intestinal obstructions and late, or not at all, (*continued on page 144*)

# Complications of intestinal obstruction

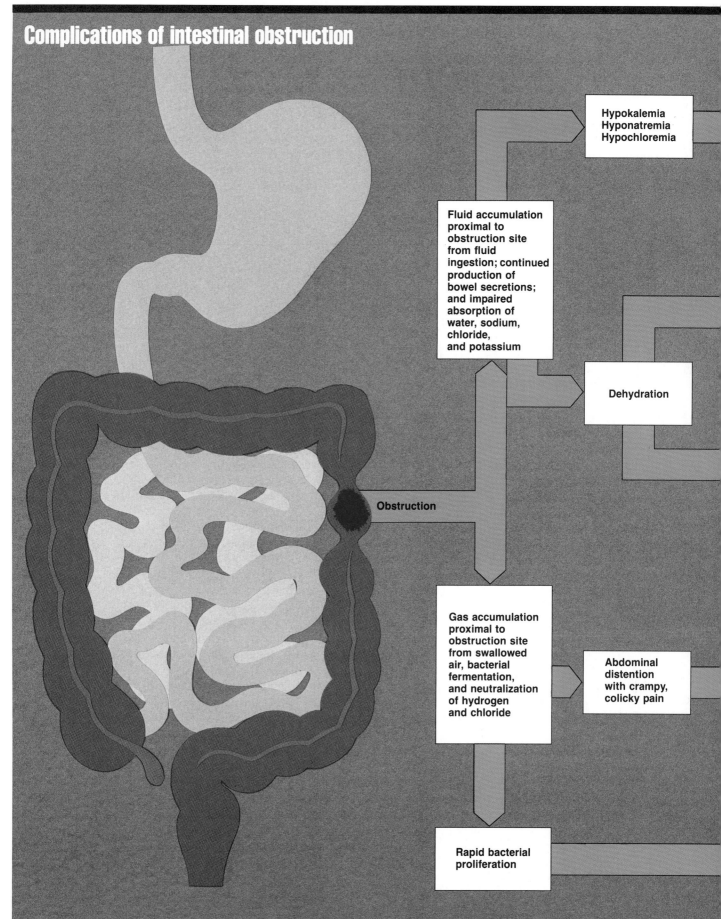

Hypokalemia
Hyponatremia
Hypochloremia

Fluid accumulation proximal to obstruction site from fluid ingestion; continued production of bowel secretions; and impaired absorption of water, sodium, chloride, and potassium

Dehydration

Obstruction

Gas accumulation proximal to obstruction site from swallowed air, bacterial fermentation, and neutralization of hydrogen and chloride

Abdominal distention with crampy, colicky pain

Rapid bacterial proliferation

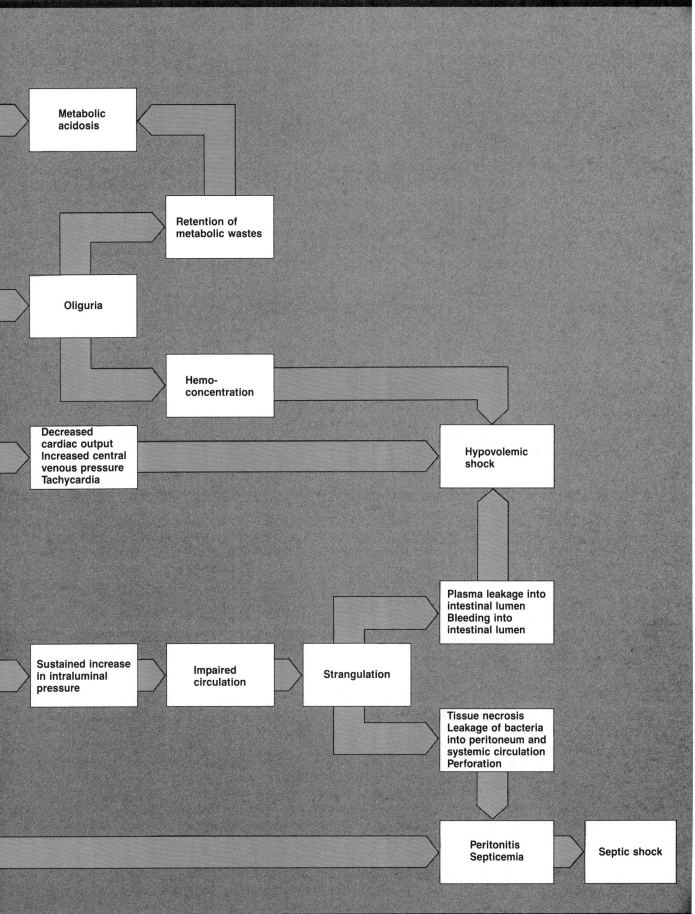

in lower intestinal and colonic obstruction. Obviously, in the latter case, distention is more marked.

*Constipation* also varies according to the level of obstruction. In small-intestinal involvement, bowel movements may continue if there are fecal contents distal to the obstruction. Constipation usually occurs early and is absolute in large-intestinal obstructions. Also, liquid stool may leak around a partial obstruction.

## MEDICAL MANAGEMENT
Diagnosis of an intestinal obstruction depends primarily on the history and physical examination, but diagnostic tests help make the differential diagnosis and monitor the effectiveness of medical treatment.

### X-rays localize the obstruction
Abdominal X-rays are the most useful diagnostic tests. Upright and lateral abdominal X-rays usually show air and fluid in the intestines when an obstruction's present. The X-ray shows air and fluid throughout the upper and lower GI tract in paralytic ileus. In a mechanical obstruction, it shows a localized collection

of air and fluid—and localized distention.

Besides the plain abdominal X-rays, barium enemas help localize suspected colonic obstructions. Barium swallow isn't safe to use in a possible intestinal obstruction because the barium itself might add to the obstruction—it is more difficult to remove barium instilled via this route.

### Endoscopy permits direct visualization
Proctoscopy, sigmoidoscopy, and colonoscopy permit direct visualization of the lower rectum, anal canal, distal sigmoid colon, and large intestine. They permit the diagnosis of most colonic obstructions and, when a simple polyp is involved, provide a channel for its excision.

The first examination is proctosigmoidoscopy—digital examination, followed by sigmoidoscopy, then proctoscopy. After dilating the anal sphincters during digital examination, the doctor inserts a sigmoidoscope into the anus. He slowly advances the sigmoidoscope through the anal canal, into the rectum, past the rectosigmoid junction, into the distal sigmoid colon. While he slowly withdraws the 10″ to 12″ (25- to 30-cm) sigmoidoscope, he

## Common sites of colorectal cancer
After lung cancer, colorectal cancer is the most common malignancy affecting American adults. It occurs primarily in the rectum and sigmoid colon, progresses slowly, and remains localized for a prolonged period.

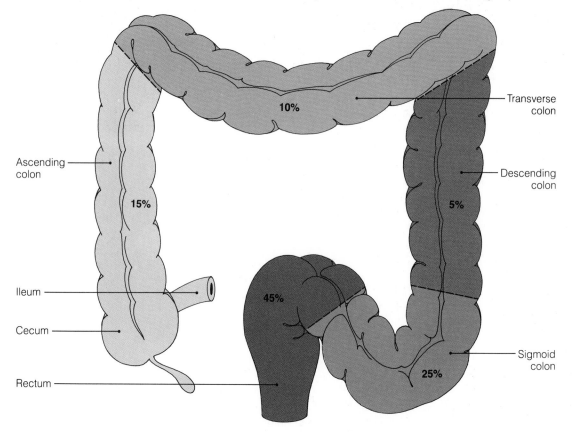

Transverse colon

Ascending colon

Descending colon

10%

15%

5%

Ileum

Cecum

45%

Rectum

Sigmoid colon

25%

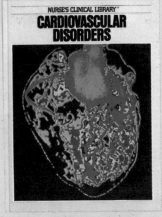
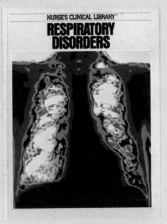
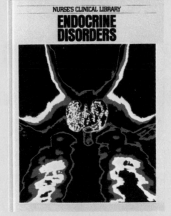
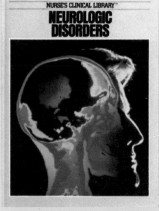
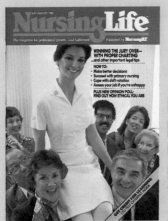

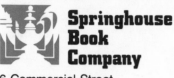
# Introduce yourself to the new NURSE'S CLINICAL LIBRARY™ series.

A comprehensive book for each specific body system disorder. That's what makes this set of books so valuable to nurses. No longer will you have to go to one book for drug information, then another for pathophysiology, and still another for diagnostics. Each book in the NURSE'S CLINICAL LIBRARY is a complete source for each body system disorder. And as a subscriber to the series, you save $3.00 off the single-copy price of each book. Act now. Send the postage-paid card above today!

© 1984 Springhouse Corporation

## Mail the card at left to get your trial copy of NursingLife.

Send no money now. Just mail the card at left and we'll send you a trial copy of NursingLife, the fastest growing nursing journal in the world. You'll discover how to avoid malpractice suits, answer touchy ethical questions, get along better with doctors and other nurses, work better under pressure, and much more. Send for yours today!

opens the bowel lumen with freqent jets of air. At any time, he can pass an electrocautery snare through the sigmoidoscope to remove obstructing polyps or pass a biopsy forceps or culture swab through the sigmoidoscope to collect specimens of suspicious areas of intestinal mucosa. After withdrawing the sigmoidoscope, he inserts a 2¾" (7-cm) proctoscope into the rectum. Again, he inspects the mucosa as he withdraws the instrument. Before obtaining specimens from the anal canal, he injects a local anesthetic since this area of the intestinal lumen is pain-sensitive.

If proctosigmoidoscopy fails to reveal the obstruction, the doctor may perform colonoscopy. In this examination, he passes a 42" to 72" (107- to 183-cm) flexible tube into the ascending colon and cecum, using abdominal palpation or fluoroscopy to guide the colonoscope through the large intestine. He can remove polyps with an electrocautery snare and obtain biopsy specimens during the examination.

### Laboratory tests monitor treatment

Laboratory tests can't confirm or rule out an obstruction, but they provide essential information on the patient's fluid and electrolyte status before and during treatment.

*Blood studies.* Serum chloride and potassium levels drop soon after the intestine becomes obstructed; later, plasma bicarbonate, pH, and blood urea nitrogen levels rise, and in response to continuing dehydration, the hematocrit level increases. An elevated white blood cell (WBC) count, with fever and other signs of peritonitis, warns of perforation or strangulation. Repeated blood studies during treatment indicate the patient's response to fluid and electrolyte replacement.

*Stool tests.* Stool tests for occult blood are usually positive in partial obstruction of the large intestine because passage of feces past the obstruction irritates the intestinal mucosa. Gross bleeding indicates impending necrosis and dictates emergency surgery.

*Urinary output.* Urinary output decreases, and specific gravity increases in the patient with an obstruction. During fluid replacement, central venous pressure monitoring helps prevent fluid overload, but urinary output remains the most important indication of adequate blood volume.

### Treatment: Three main goals

Medical treatment has three goals: to decompress the intestine by removing gas and fluid,

## Colonic polyps

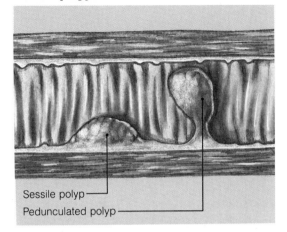

Sessile polyp
Pedunculated polyp

*Pedunculated* polyps are attached to the intestinal wall by a thin stem. In contrast, broad-based *sessile* polyps are attached directly to the intestinal wall.

to maintain fluid and electrolyte balance until intestinal function resumes, and to remove the obstruction or to provide a bypass around it to restore the flow of intestinal contents. Postsurgical and traumatic paralytic ileus usually resolve spontaneously and require no treatment.

**Suctioning decompresses the intestine.** In mild paralytic ileus, nasogastric suctioning or a rectal tube may be adequate. In severe ileus or mechanical obstruction, however, intestinal suctioning is usually necessary. Either a single-lumen Cantor tube or a double-lumen Miller-Abbott tube is effective. After the tube's passed through the nose into the stomach, peristalsis carries it through the pylorus into the duodenum. (Aspirate will be alkaline—turning litmus paper blue—when the tube reaches the duodenum.) Failure of the tube to advance may indicate the location of an obstruction in the small intestine. Then, a series of X-rays can localize the site of obstruction. If the obstruction results from an adhesion, gently forcing the tube through the adhesion may relieve it.

**Intravenous fluids restore balance.** The second goal, fluid and electrolyte balance, requires I.V. infusions. Isotonic sodium chloride and glucose solutions are the mainstays, with frequent adjustments in composition and infusion rate based on changes in serum potassium and chloride levels, hematocrit level, and urine output. (See *Guidelines for fluid replacement,* page 148.) The higher the obstruction, the greater the electrolyte imbalance. The reason: When fluids are sequestered high in the small intestine, electrolytes normally absorbed by the small intestine and

# Understanding ostomies

**M**alignant tumors cause most obstructions in the large intestine. Removal of these tumors frequently requires removal of large sections of the intestine, including the rectum and anus. Ostomy, the most common surgery for these tumors, involves creation of an opening—a stoma—in the abdominal wall for elimination of body wastes. Types of ostomies include:

• *Colostomy.* This is a stoma formed from the colon or large intestine. It's referred to as an ascending, transverse, descending, or sigmoid colostomy, depending on the site of surgery.

Cancer of the rectum requires a procedure called abdominal-perineal resection. In this two-step procedure, a colostomy is formed through an abdominal incision. After the abdominal incision is closed, the colon, anus, and rectum are removed through a perineal incision.

• *Double-barrel colostomy.* This is the creation of a proximal and distal stoma, which may be adjacent or several inches apart. It's usually temporary.

• *Loop colostomy.* In this temporary procedure, proximal and distal openings are created in a loop of bowel brought through the abdominal wall and supported by a plastic rod.

• *Ileostomy.* This stoma in the distal portion of the ileum usually accompanies total removal of the colon and rectum.

**Colostomy**

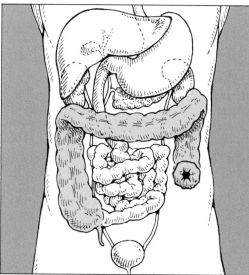

**Double-barrel colostomy**

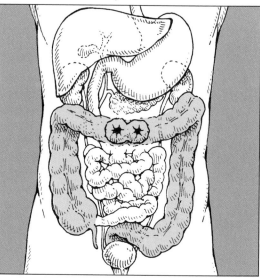

**Loop colostomy**

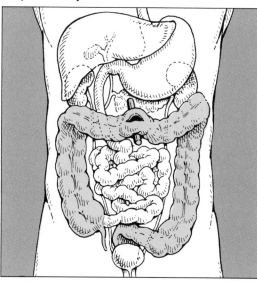

**Ileostomy**

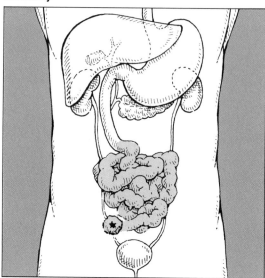

carried into the systemic circulation are sequestered, too.

Blood transfusions are started, and I.V. antibiotics such as clindamycin (Cleocin) are added at the first sign of strangulation.

**Obstructions should be removed.** A third medical goal is to remove the obstruction or make a bypass around it. Intussusception usually responds to hydrostatic pressure given by a barium enema. Meconium ileus resolves after an enema with a hypertonic solution called Gastrografin. And fecal impaction usually resolves after enemas and manual disimpaction. But, most obstructions need surgery.

The surgery may be fairly simple. Such obstructions as adhesions, hernias, polyps, and most cases of volvulus require only a simple laparotomy and repair. But large tumors and necrotic tissue require more extensive surgery. If the tumor or necrosis doesn't involve the colon or rectum, the doctor may remove the obstructed portion of the intestine, then anastomose healthy tissue on either side of the resection with an end-to-end or end-to-side anastomosis. Larger tumors or obstructions will require a partial or total colectomy and the creation of a colostomy or ileostomy. (See *Understanding ostomies.*) In creating an ostomy, the surgeon creates a stoma from healthy tissue proximal to the obstruction by suturing the open end of the intestine to the skin.

The surgeon may create a temporary colostomy if a damaged segment of the intestine seems likely to heal after a rest. In this procedure, a stoma is formed in a loop of intestine brought outside the abdominal wall. The stoma diverts intestinal flow from the damaged area, allowing it to heal. After 6 to 8 weeks, a second procedure restores normal bowel function. This is common in the treatment of Hirschsprung's disease and mesenteric artery thrombosis.

## NURSING MANAGEMENT
In intestinal obstruction, nursing management requires an individualized plan of care and repeated assessments to detect possibly life-threatening changes in your patient's condition. Formulate your care plans after a careful patient history and physical examination.

### Take a detailed patient history
In your initial interview, ask the patient to describe his symptoms, including his chief complaint. Your patient's symptoms are likely to include abdominal pain, vomiting, changes in bowel habits, and abdominal distention. If your patient describes these symptoms, be sure to include these questions.

• Ask about the location, character, intensity, associated events, duration, and frequency of his pain. Pain from an intestinal obstruction is usually generalized because the viscera contain relatively few pain fibers, and most are shared by several organs. Even so, pain from an obstruction in the small intestine is likely to be periumbilical—from the terminal ileum or colon, near the colonic segment. The pain is crampy, intermittent, and more severe in small-intestinal obstructions and milder and more consistent in colonic obstructions. There is little or no pain in paralytic ileus because of decreased or absent peristalsis. And pain from all obstructions is likely to be aggravated by eating.

Observe your patient during the history. The patient with intestinal pain is likely to writhe and shift position constantly, seeking a comfortable position. The patient with inflammation of the peritoneum is likely to lie quite still because any movement worsens the pain.

Be prepared to interrupt your history taking and call the doctor if your questioning reveals possible perforation or strangulation. Severe pain in the lower abdomen after several days of constipation or watery diarrhea may signal imminent perforation of the colon. Severe pain that's lasted several days requires immediate attention, particularly if accompanied by distention, because perforation or strangulation may be imminent. And an abrupt change from intermittent pain to constant pain may also indicate perforation or strangulation.

• Ask about the color, consistency, odor, amount, onset, and duration of any vomiting. Profuse, forceful, bilious vomiting after a feeling of fullness is common with a small-intestinal obstruction. Vomiting with a fecal odor may occur with lower small-intestinal obstruction. The absence of vomiting usually indicates a large-intestinal obstruction.

• Ask about the patient's normal bowel habits: the frequency, color, shape, and consistency of the stool; frequency of constipation or diarrhea; gas pain or flatus; and use of laxatives or enemas. These questions are important because "normal" bowel habits vary greatly. For one patient, two bowel movements a day may be normal; for another, two bowel movements a week.

After finding out what your patient considers normal, you're better able to evaluate the sig-

## Guidelines for fluid replacement

The accumulation of fluid proximal to an intestinal obstruction soon leads to dehydration and electrolyte imbalance. To correct this imbalance, start one or two I.V. lines, using large-bore cannulas to permit rapid infusion.
• Start with an isotonic solution such as Ringer's lactate, adjusting the flow appropriately for the estimated volume loss, as ordered.
• Alternate a 5% glucose solution with the isotonic solution, as ordered, unless renal function is impaired.
• Replace potassium as ordered, not exceeding 40 mEq/hour.
• If strangulation occurs, infuse whole blood or packed cells, as ordered.

nificance of any alterations in bowel habits associated with the current illness. Watery diarrhea stools are common in a partial obstruction. Currant jelly stools are associated with intussusception in infants. Total constipation with no passage of gas is usual in complete obstruction. But don't rule out an obstruction in a patient who reports normal bowel habits despite other signs and symptoms you usually associate with an obstruction. Normal stools may continue for 2 or 3 days after complete obstruction in the small intestine because of fecal material already in the large intestine and colon at the time the obstruction formed.
• Ask the patient whether his abdomen seems swollen and, if so, when the swelling occurred. (If he doesn't know, ask him whether his waistbands have seemed tight recently.) Extreme distention is more likely with a colonic obstruction than with a small-intestinal obstruction because of vomiting.
• Ask about any other recent health problems. About 20% of patients with intestinal obstructions report recent weight loss, anorexia, changes in food tolerance, and increased fatigability. In children, fever frequently accompanies constipation lasting more than 2 days.
• Ask the patient to describe a typical day's menu. If your patient's obstruction is caused by chronic constipation, changing his nutritional habits may be the most important aspect of patient teaching. Find out how much liquid he usually drinks each day and how much whole-grain and high-fiber food he eats. With some patients, prevention of future obstructions is a matter of adding fluid and bulk to the diet.
• Ask whether the patient swallowed a foreign object recently. An obstruction may develop 2 or 3 days after a child swallows a toy or an adult swallows a bone. Without your specific questioning, the family may forget it occurred.
• Finally, get a complete health history: Has your patient had similar symptoms before? If so, what caused them and what relieved them? What about other past or chronic illnesses? A patient with chronic ulcerative colitis is 10 times more likely than other patients to get colonic cancer—the leading cause of obstructions of the large intestine. A patient with atherosclerosis is more likely to develop an obstruction caused by thrombosis and emboli. A patient with chronic renal failure may be taking large doses of aluminum hydroxide gel, a common cause of bezoars.
• Ask about previous abdominal surgery.

Adhesions may cause intestinal obstructions many years after the surgery was performed.
• Get a family health history. Colon cancer or polyposis is more likely if someone else in the family has it.
• Assess the patient's and family's understanding and attitudes toward the illness, and use this assessment as a basis for emotional support and teaching.

### Conduct a physical examination

Before you examine the patient, assess his overall appearance. Look for pallor and lack of facial expression, indicating possible anemia from chronic intestinal bleeding. Note dry, grayish skin and sunken eyes; jerky physical movement; and irritation, which may indicate dehydration and electrolyte imbalance. Record the patient's vital signs, and use these values as baseline data for later vital sign checks. A rapid pulse may indicate dehydration; a rapid pulse accompanied by low blood pressure may indicate severe hypovolemia; fever may accompany prolonged constipation, especially in children; rapid, shallow respirations may indicate that the distended intestine is pressing against the diaphragm.

During your physical examination of the abdomen, note your findings after inspection, auscultation, percussion, palpation, and digital rectal examination.

Inspect the abdomen for distention, scars, and involuntary motility.
• If your patient's a child, be sure to distinguish between distention and a normally protuberant abdomen. In adults and children, marked distention is more likely in paralytic colonic obstruction than in small-bowel obstruction.
• Ask about any scars from surgery not described during the history. The more surgery the patient has undergone, the more likely he is to have obstructing adhesions.
• Inspect the abdomen for visible arterial pulsations and peristaltic movement. Visible peristaltic movement indicates intestinal irritation in most adults and children. (Be sure to distinguish it from abdominal breathing, which is normal in young children.)

Auscultate the four quadrants of the abdomen, starting with those farthest from the pain. (With a child, auscultate the abdomen immediately after the heart and lungs—while the child's used to the stethoscope.) Note any changes from the irregular bubbling or gurgling noises of normal peristalsis. Diminished or absent sounds in all four quadrants

## Assessing fluid and electrolyte balance

| Body system | Fluid excess | Fluid loss/electrolyte imbalance |
| --- | --- | --- |
| Cardiovascular | Bounding pulse, hypertension | Elevated temperature; rapid, weak pulse; extremities cold to touch; hypotension |
| Gastrointestinal | Anorexia, nausea and vomiting, acute weight gain (greater than 5%), increased abdominal girth | Anorexia, nausea and vomiting, thirst, acute weight loss (greater than 5%), constipation, abdominal cramps, longitudinal wrinkles on tongue |
| Integumentary | Pitting edema, pallor, facial edema | Poor skin turgor, dry mucous membranes, drawn facial expression |
| Musculoskeletal | Muscle hypertonicity | Muscle weakness |
| Neurologic | Confusion, apathy | Lethargy, indifference, confusion, coma |
| Ophthalmic | Pitting edema | Sunken eyes |
| Renal | Polyuria (if kidneys are healthy) | Oliguria, anuria |
| Respiratory | Shortness of breath, hoarseness, productive cough, moist rales, dyspnea | Shortness of breath; deep, rapid breathing |

are common in paralytic ileus or peritonitis. Rapid, high-pitched, tinkling sounds or loud, gurgling sounds occur early in an obstruction of the small intestine.

Percuss all four quadrants. As with auscultation, examine the painful quadrant last so that muscle guarding won't disguise any abnormalities. Note the degree of tympany in each quadrant, indicating the amount of distention from air. Tympany without visible distention is common in obstructions of the small intestine.

Palpate all four quadrants for masses, tender areas, and guarding. If you detect any tender areas, check for rebound tenderness by slowly pushing your fingertips into the tender area, then quickly releasing them. A sharp pain at the time of release is common in peritoneal inflammation and may indicate that the bowel has perforated.

Palpate the rectum for nodules, irregularities, tenderness, or fecal impaction.

### Formulate your nursing diagnoses

You'll formulate your nursing diagnoses on the basis of the history, physical examination, diagnostic test results, and medical orders. For a typical patient with obstruction, your diagnoses may include:

**Fluid volume deficit related to vomiting, bleeding, and third-space losses.** Keep a running total of your patient's intake and output. In the intake column, be sure to include small sips of water, ice cubes, and any liquid medications as well as I.V. fluids. Besides urinary

output, include fluid losses from diarrhea, emesis, and tube drainage.

Give I.V. and oral fluids, as ordered. Check balances every 2 to 4 hours—more often in an unstable patient or a small child. Watch values, such as the hematocrit level, for fluid status changes. And note any physical changes that might mean an imbalance (see *Assessing fluid and electrolyte balance*). Report any significant imbalances immediately.

Consider your interventions effective if the patient's intake and output balance within 200 ml; and his skin turgor, orientation, vital signs, and laboratory values are normal.

**Alteration in comfort related to obstruction.** Reduce your patient's anxiety by demonstrating your concern and your confidence that you can help him. Encourage him to report pain immediately for optimal relief. Ask the patient to describe his pain each time you give him an analgesic. Note any changes in the quantity, quality, or location of the pain. Report any significant increase in pain or a change from intermittent, colicky pain to severe, constant pain. Either change may indicate that necrosis or perforation is imminent; and emergency surgery may be necessary to prevent irreversible damage. Monitor the effectiveness of each dose of analgesic, and notify the doctor if it doesn't effectively relieve the pain.

To augment analgesics (or to help relieve the patient's pain if you must withhold analgesics until the diagnosis is made), find out what pain relief techniques your patient uses

## How to irrigate a colostomy

Colostomy irrigation is basically an enema given through a stoma. Before irrigation, explain the procedure and equipment to the patient. Perform the irrigation at the same time each day, allowing an hour for the procedure. To perform the irrigation:
• Fill a container with 1 qt of lukewarm tap water, and run some water through the tubing to remove air.
• Have the patient sit on the toilet or a chair across from the toilet.
• Hang the container at the level of the patient's shoulder.
• Take the protective covering off the stoma, and attach the irrigating sleeve and belt, centering the stoma in the opening.
• Lubricate a cone or catheter, and gently insert it 3″ (7.6 cm) or less into the stoma. Hold the cone or shield firmly against the stoma to prevent retrograde water flow.
• Open the adjustable clamp, and let water flow for 15 minutes. If the patient develops cramps, shut off the water and hold the cone or shield in place until cramping ceases. Then begin again.
• Keep the cone or shield in place for 10 seconds after instilling all the water. Then, gently remove the cone or shield.
• Allow 15 to 20 minutes for drainage. Then dry the bottom of the sleeve and attach it to the top.
• Keep the sleeve in place for about 45 to 60 minutes. Meanwhile, the patient can perform light activities, such as walking or reading.
• Take off the sleeve, clean the stoma, dry the surrounding skin, and attach a protective coating.

at home. Help him use these methods and add other comfort measures, such as back rubs, changes in positioning or ambulation, distraction, and imagery.

The obstruction itself or the nasogastric or intestinal tube inserted to relieve it may cause discomfort from nausea. Give antiemetics as ordered, and help your patient relieve his nausea with slow, deep breaths. Remove vomitus promptly; air the room; and change your patient's gown and linen, as needed. Offer oral hygiene two or three times per shift. Check the tube frequently for position and patency, and irrigate it with small amounts of normal saline solution, as necessary. (Document the type and amount of drainage every 8 hours or as ordered.)

Consider your interventions successful if the patient remains free from pain, nausea, and vomiting.

**Constipation related to trauma, decreased activity, low fluid intake, or disease.** In the patient whose obstruction results from chronic constipation and fecal impaction, relieve the impaction manually and with enemas to stimulate defecation and add volume to the stool.
• If your patient has a fecal impaction, the doctor may order an oil retention enema to soften fecal material before evacuation. Warm the solution to 105° F. (40.6° C.) before administering it. Pinch or clamp the tube momentarily if your patient develops cramps or an urge to defecate, and ask him to breathe deeply. Encourage him to retain the enema for 20 to 30 minutes.
• If your patient's scheduled for intestinal surgery, the doctor may order a medicated enema to reduce intestinal bacteria. Follow the steps for administering an oil retention enema.
• If your patient is constipated, the doctor will probably order a cleansing enema. Use warm saline solution for the enema rather than soap, which irritates the bowel mucosa, or tap water, which is hypotonic and causes fluid shifts. Warm the solution, and instill as much solution as the patient can retain, clamping the tube to stop the flow temporarily if he develops cramps or the urge to defecate. Encourage him to retain the enema for at least 10 minutes.
• If the doctor orders suppositories to soften fecal material and to stimulate defecation, place them so that they touch the rectal mucosa—not the center of the fecal mass.

Encourage the patient to achieve natural bowel regulation by drinking 8 to 10 glasses of liquid a day; eating fibrous foods, such as

raw fruit, vegetables, and whole-grain cereals; eating natural laxatives, such as prunes and raisins; and exercising. If the patient's chronically constipated or laxative-dependent, show him that natural regulation is possible by encouraging liquids, fibrous foods, and ambulation and leg-raising exercises. Help him achieve normal bowel habits by assuring him privacy and ample time for defecation at the same time each day. If possible, choose a time that will prove convenient when the patient returns home.

If your patient has a colostomy, introduce new foods one at a time, and help him determine which cause constipation, diarrhea, or gas. Your patient is most likely to have trouble with gas-producing foods, such as cabbage and broccoli, and difficult-to-digest foods, such as nuts and corn. If he prefers or requires irrigation to regulate his stools, schedule the irrigations in the hospital to fit the patient's at-home schedule. Use 500 to 1,000 ml of warm tap water (see *How to irrigate a colostomy*), and perform the irrigations daily or less often, as needed. Clean the stoma thoroughly after irrigation.

Your interventions are effective if the patient develops normal bowel habits without dependence on laxatives or enemas and if your colostomy patient passes stools with minimal odor at predictable intervals.

**Infection related to interrupted skin integrity from trauma or immobility.** In the postoperative patient, the surgeon will change the initial dressing. After that, clean the wound and change the dressing at least daily.

In an infant with anal repair, dressings are of little use. Keep the wound open to air, and clean the perineum after bowel movements and urination. Position the infant to keep pressure off the wound.

In an adult with a perineal wound, position the patient to keep pressure off the wound; irrigate regularly with 200 to 500 ml of warmed saline, diluted peroxide, or antibiotic solution; and use a heat lamp to facilitate healing. After the patient's ambulatory, keep the wound clean with frequent sitz baths or a hand-held shower. Tell your patient that the wound may take 6 to 8 months to heal, although most wounds heal within 3 months.

In colostomy patients, apply a commercial skin preparation to the intact skin before attaching the drainage bag. If the skin becomes irritated from drainage, apply aluminum gel or a commercial product before attaching the bag. Follow these additional mea-

sures to maintain skin integrity around the stoma.
• Empty the ostomy bag whenever it's one-third to one-half full. Letting it fill increases the weight and may loosen the seal.
• When you change the ostomy bag, wash the area around the stoma with warm water and a mild, nonperfumed soap.
• After irrigation, wash the stoma thoroughly with soap and water.

In all patients, give routine skin care, schedule regular position changes, and massage pressure points regularly. Watch particularly for skin breakdown in a malnourished or elderly patient.

Your interventions are successful if wounds heal with good skin approximation, if skin around the stoma is intact, and the patient's temperature and WBC count are normal.

**Knowledge deficit related to anxiety and unfamiliarity.** Develop your patient's trust and confidence from the beginning by orienting him to the unit, his room, and hospital procedures. Throughout his care, explain each procedure or treatment, repeating the explanation as necessary to be sure the patient understands. If pain medication must be withheld because it's masking symptoms, explain the reason to the patient and family to reduce their anxiety.

Begin discharge teaching as soon as possible, explaining the disease to the patient and his family at their level of understanding and formulating realistic teaching objectives. A plan for the patient with a lower GI disorder will include preventive steps, such as better nutrition, exercise, and medication, and knowledge of the signs and symptoms of recurrence.

If your patient's had surgery, include wound care in your teaching. If he has an ostomy, teach him and his family to care for the ostomy, starting with simple things and adding a step each time. Supplement your explanations with models and with pamphlets the patient can take home.

Your interventions are successful when your patient can describe and perform the basics of follow-up and preventive care.

**Disturbed body image related to nonintegration of change.** Give your colostomy patient time to look at his stoma and decide how much involvement he wants his family to have in its care. Talk over his feelings and decisions with him to help him feel more comfortable discussing the stoma. Encourage questions, and answer them completely and

honestly. If you can't answer them, be sure to find out the answers. Next—beginning with simple tasks such as clamping the bag—get your patient involved in stoma care, and include the family if he desires. Keep adding tasks until the patient can perform colostomy care independently. But don't limit your interventions to physical care of the ostomy. Talk to him about his plans for returning to work, continuing hobbies, traveling, and so forth. Give him a list of contacts if he needs help or supplies after discharge.

Your interventions have succeeded when the patient can freely discuss his colostomy and care for it.

**Alteration in parenting related to interrupted bonding and knowledge deficit.** If your patient is an infant with a congenital obstruction, evaluate the parents' needs before and after surgery. Follow their cues in deciding when they need someone to talk to and when they need to be alone. Avoid prolonged separations of the infant and his parents, which inhibit bonding. Encourage the parents to hold their infant as much as possible.

Continue to offer emotional support despite the fact that the parents may make you the target for their angry and guilty feelings. Assure parents that they can form a close bond with their infant despite hospitalization, and supply them with up-to-date information on their infant's condition in language they can understand and in a way that assures them they aren't to blame for their infant's disorder.

Include the parents in planning and giving their child's care as much as possible. Make sure they feel comfortable giving any special nutritional, wound, or colostomy care before their child is discharged.

You can't assess the parents' emotional adjustment because it's likely to take months: some parents remain depressed by a congenital defect for years after their child's birth. Consider your interventions a success if the parents seem more comfortable talking about their infant's condition and can demonstrate their ability to care for him.

### The nursing challenge
Signs and symptoms of intestinal obstructions come in a baffling variety. But after you understand their causes and underlying pathophysiology, you're ready to put your assessment skills to work. Using these skills to help you formulate nursing diagnoses and an individualized care plan, you're able to give your patient prompt, effective care.

**Points to remember**

• Lower GI obstructions result from many congenital and acquired disorders and occur in people of every age.
• Most obstructions result from mechanical blockage, but some result from impaired peristalsis or vascular insufficiency.
• Medical treatment has three goals: to reduce distention, to restore fluid and electrolyte balance, and to restore intestinal flow.
• Your challenge is to recognize signs of obstruction promptly, to detect complications before they become life-threatening, and to devise a care plan to meet varied patient needs.

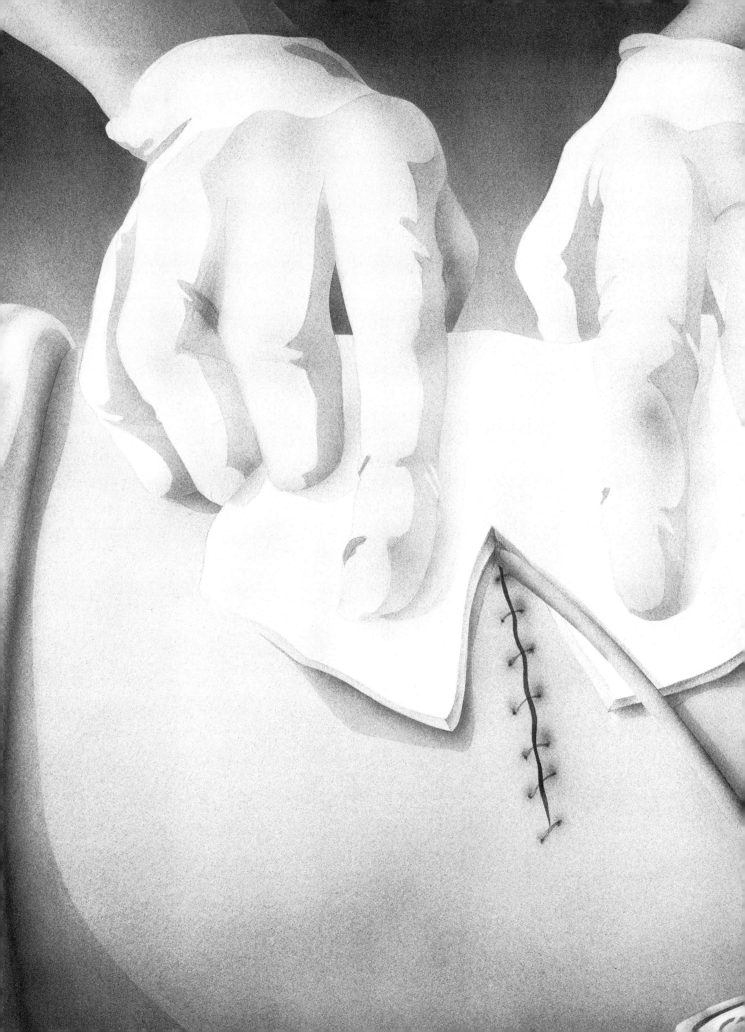

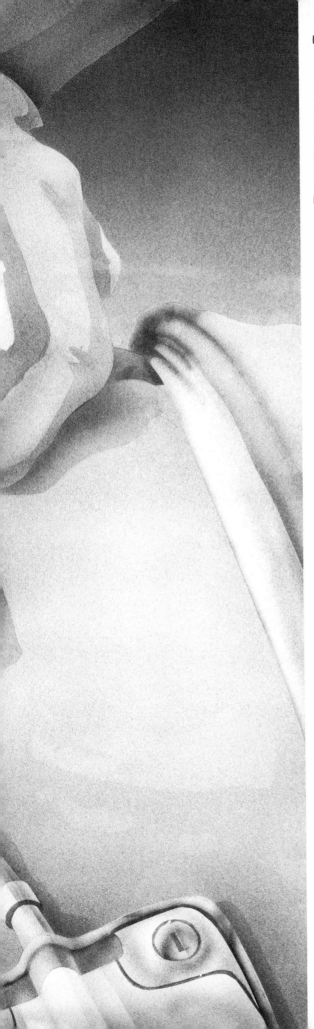

# ACCESSORY ORGAN DISORDERS

# 10 TREATING LIVER DISORDERS

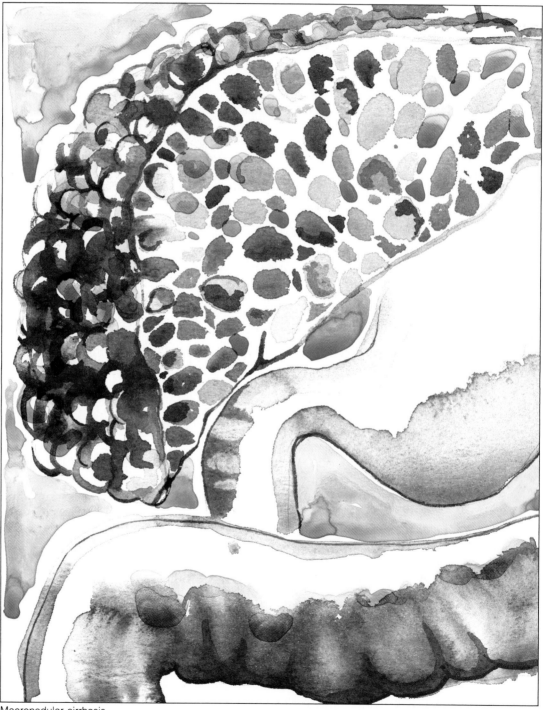

Macronodular cirrhosis

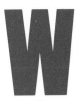ith some dramatic exceptions, liver disease usually develops insidiously. In fact, its characteristic signs, jaundice and ascites, often signal advanced disease. What's worse, overt liver disease may rapidly progress to the life-threatening complications of bleeding varices and hepatic encephalopathy.

How to improve this grim prognosis? First, by recognizing predisposing factors—most notably, alcoholism—you can promote prompt diagnosis by uncovering subtle, early signs of disease in the high-risk patient. Second, by learning how to prevent or manage complications—as described in this chapter—you can help curb progression of disease and minimize residual liver dysfunction.

### Identifying risk factors
In the United States, liver disease strikes more men than women and more nonwhites than whites. Alcoholics are at high risk, especially for fatty liver and cirrhosis. Hemodialysis patients, homosexuals, intravenous drug abusers, and hospital staff are particularly susceptible to viral hepatitis. Chronic liver disease may, in turn, predispose the patient to portal hypertension, hepatic encephalopathy, and, rarely, primary liver tumors.

### PATHOPHYSIOLOGY
A review of pathophysiology shows that disease can alter liver structure and compromise essential functions. Hepatic necrosis leads to fibrotic regeneration of cells, yet this process typically fails to restore function. As a result, liver disease impairs protein, fat, and carbohydrate metabolism; fluid and electrolyte balance; lymphatic drainage; coagulation; and detoxification.

### Fatty liver
As the term implies, "fatty liver" (steatosis) refers to excessive accumulation of fat within hepatic cells. It most often results from chronic alcoholism, with severity of liver disease directly related to alcohol consumption. Other causes include diabetes mellitus, obesity, Cushing's syndrome, prolonged protein deprivation and starvation, Reye's syndrome, and pregnancy. Intravenous tetracycline therapy, prolonged intravenous hyperalimentation, and intestinal bypass surgery can also lead to fatty liver.

Normally, hepatic cells hydrolyze serum triglycerides into glycerol and free fatty acids for use by the body. However, triglycerides—and trace amounts of cholesterol and phospholipids—may accumulate within hepatic cells owing to increased mobilization of fat stores or to increased synthesis or decreased hydrolysis of triglycerides in the liver. In fatty liver associated with alcoholism, triglyceride-laden hepatic cells may enlarge, merge with other cells, and form fatty cysts. In fatty liver associated with other causes, fat remains in small droplets. Excessive fat accumulation may cause inflammation and necrosis, resulting in cirrhosis. Although fatty liver is usually reversible, it may lead to recurrent infection or sudden death from fat emboli to the lungs.

### Hepatitis
An acute inflammation of the liver, hepatitis occurs in viral and nonviral forms.

**Viral hepatitis.** This form of hepatitis includes types A, B, and non-A, non-B. Highly contagious type A hepatitis, the most common viral type, is transmitted via fecal-oral and parenteral routes. It typically spreads through ingestion of contaminated food or water, often in outbreaks that can be traced to ingestion of raw shellfish from polluted waters. Despite such epidemics, mortality associated with type A hepatitis is low.

Transmitted parenterally, type B hepatitis typically spreads through contaminated blood, needles, or medical or dental instruments or through contact with contaminated semen or saliva. Epidemics are rare, but this form of hepatitis produces a higher mortality, which increases with age.

Type non-A, non-B hepatitis is transmitted parenterally by blood transfusions and hemodialysis and has the mildest clinical course.

In viral hepatitis, mononuclear leukocytes and a virus infiltrate the parenchyma and portal tracts, causing swelling, cellular degeneration, and autolysis. Irregular, patchy necrosis appears with autolysis. Although necrosis and cellular regeneration occur simultaneously, liver function remains compromised. Necrosis of bile-secreting cells causes cholestasis. Severe, widespread necrosis may cause degeneration of the underlying reticulin framework. Fibrosis and nodular regeneration eventually progress to chronic active hepatitis or postnecrotic cirrhosis. Fulminant hepatitis denotes massive necrosis and fibrosis.

**Nonviral hepatitis.** This form of hepatitis follows exposure to hepatotoxins, most commonly, carbon tetrachloride, alcohol, isoniazid, thiazide diuretics, and acetaminophen. It's

## Esophageal varices: Common and often deadly

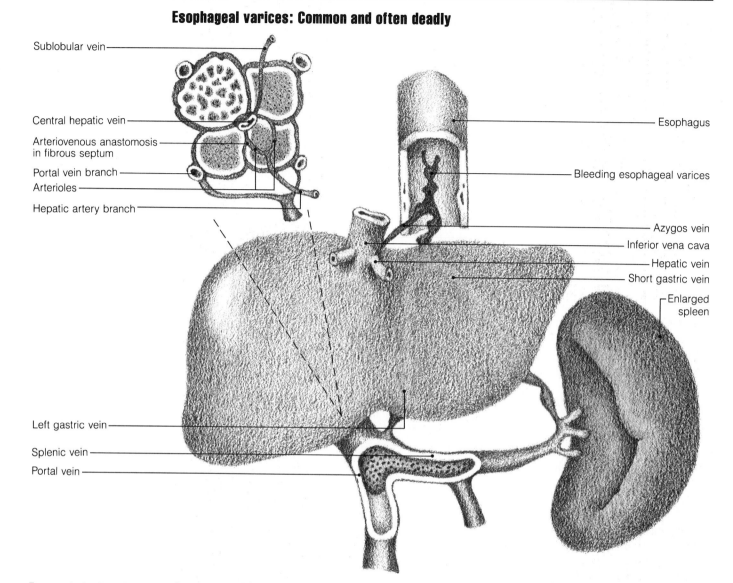

Sublobular vein

Central hepatic vein

Arteriovenous anastomosis
in fibrous septum

Portal vein branch

Arterioles

Hepatic artery branch

Esophagus

Bleeding esophageal varices

Azygos vein

Inferior vena cava

Hepatic vein

Short gastric vein

Enlarged
spleen

Left gastric vein

Splenic vein

Portal vein

Frequently the first sign of portal hypertension, esophageal varices may complicate liver disease. They develop when hepatic fibrosis compresses hepatic veins, impeding outflow through the vena cava and increasing portal pressure. Arteriovenous shunting further compromises blood supply. Eventually, rising portal pressure causes blood to back up in the spleen and establishes collateral circulation between the portal and caval systems via the left gastric and short gastric esophageal veins. But these thin-walled vessels accommodate portal circulation poorly; they become dilated and are often the source of massive hematemesis.

characterized by diffuse fatty infiltration, inflammation, and necrosis. Inflammation occurs rapidly, and necrosis follows within 24 to 48 hours.

### Cirrhosis
Characterized by diffuse necrosis followed by fibrotic regeneration of hepatic cells, cirrhosis has various causes and exists in several clinically distinct forms. *Laennec's cirrhosis,* the most common, is typically associated with alcoholism and related malnutrition. Biliary cirrhosis results from bile duct diseases, which impede bile flow. *Postnecrotic cirrhosis* follows various types of hepatitis. *Pigment cirrhosis* stems from disorders such as hemochromatosis. *Cardiac cirrhosis,* a rare type, results from right ventricular failure. *Idiopathic cirrhosis* has no known cause.

In early types of cirrhosis, the liver is enlarged and fatty. In advanced stages, it be-

comes shrunken and nodular as fibrous bands dissect the liver into small, irregular clumps of nonfunctional tissue. Fibrotic regeneration unites portal tracts yet compresses portal circulation. Narrowing of portal venules reduces outflow, enhancing necrosis. Increased vascular resistance eventually causes abnormal shunting between arterioles and venules, producing ischemia in central lobule areas and increasing portal pressure.

### Tumors
Primary liver tumors are usually associated with cirrhosis but can be linked to other predisposing factors, including fungal infection *(Aspergillus flavus),* viral hepatitis, excessive use of anabolic steroids, trauma, nutritional deficiencies, and exposure to hepatotoxins. Such tumors are most prevalent in Asia and Africa, possibly because of related protein and vitamin deficiencies.

Primary liver tumors may involve the parenchymal cells (hepatomas), the bile duct cells (cholangiomas), or both. Typically, these tumors arise in areas of necrosis or fibrotic regeneration. Tumor growth may erode adjacent blood vessels, causing intraperitoneal bleeding. Metastatic tumors occur 20 times more often than primary liver tumors. In fact, the liver is one of the most common sites of metastasis from other primary cancers, particularly those of the colon, rectum, stomach, pancreas, esophagus, lung, or breast, and melanoma.

## Complications of liver disease

*Portal hypertension,* the most common complication of liver disease, usually results from cirrhosis, but it may also stem from portal vein thrombosis, hepatic vein obstruction caused by tumor or thrombosis (Budd-Chiari syndrome), or, rarely, pancreatitis that has affected the splenic vein.

In portal hypertension, impaired blood flow from the portal system to the vena cava promotes formation of collateral vessels that shunt blood from the high-pressure portal system into lower-pressure veins. As a result, varices that may be life-threatening commonly develop in the esophagus, stomach, and rectum. (See *Esophageal varices: Common and often deadly.*) Variceal rupture may cause fatal exsanguination.

*Hepatic encephalopathy,* a neurologic syndrome, may also complicate chronic liver disease. Typically, it results from elevated serum ammonia levels caused by gastrointestinal bleeding. Metabolic alkalosis, ingestion of hepatotoxic drugs, an alcoholic spree, shock, and hypoxia may also provoke or deepen hepatic encephalopathy.

Normally, ammonia produced by protein breakdown in the bowel is converted to urea in the liver. However, impaired hepatocellular function and portal circulation shunting cause ammonia to bypass the liver and spill into the blood. Elevated levels of serum ammonia act as a direct toxin to brain cells, inhibiting neurotransmission and cerebral metabolism and ultimately producing coma.

## Metabolic effects of liver disease

Liver disease can significantly impair metabolism of bilirubin, carbohydrates, proteins, and hormones.

**Bilirubin metabolism.** Normally, free bilirubin is absorbed into hepatic cells, conjugated into a water-soluble form, channeled through bile ducts, and excreted with bile into the duodenum. However, hepatocellular damage or bile duct obstruction increases free bilirubin levels, causing jaundice, hyperbilirubinemia, light-colored stools, and dark, amber-colored urine. Concomitantly decreased bile salt levels impair absorption of fat-soluble vitamins. Vitamin K deficiency interferes with hepatic synthesis of prothrombin, compounding the risk of bleeding that arises from deficiency of plasma proteins.

**Carbohydrate metabolism.** Occurring in the liver, glycogenesis, glycogenolysis, and gluconeogenesis operate in carbohydrate metabolism. Severe liver disease impairs these processes, causing hypoglycemia marked by fatigue, lethargy, and weight loss.

**Protein metabolism.** Also based in the liver, protein metabolism involves deamination of amino acids, conversion of ammonia to urea, and formation of plasma proteins. Deamination transforms amino acids for energy use or storage; impaired deamination causes fatigue. Conversion of ammonia to urea prevents buildup of toxic serum ammonia levels; impaired conversion causes hepatic encephalopathy marked initially by slight personality changes, then by asterixis, confusion, lethargy, stupor, and eventually coma.

Formation of plasma proteins supports tissue building, coagulation, and adequate intravascular volume; impaired formation causes poor healing, ecchymoses, bleeding tendencies, and intravascular fluid transudation. This fluid shift results in peripheral edema, compromised renal blood flow, and ascites (see *How ascites develops in portal hypertension,* pages 158 and 159). Eventually, generalized massive edema (anasarca) may develop with pleural effusion, pericardial effusion, and congestive heart failure. Hepatorenal syndrome may follow, marked by azotemia, hyperkalemia, and oliguria or anuria. Urine sodium levels may decrease, while protein levels increase.

**Hormone metabolism.** Liver disease also upsets hormone metabolism. Impaired catabolism and biliary excretion of estrogens cause spider nevi; palmar erythema; menstrual irregularities; and gynecomastia, testicular atrophy, impotence, and loss of body hair in males. Impaired catabolism of aldosterone results in high serum and urinary levels, which contribute to ascites. Testosterone and progesterone metabolism may also be impaired.

*(continued on page 160)*

## How ascites develops in portal hypertension

Ascites, an accumulation of serous fluid in the abdominal cavity, may develop in portal hypertension as a result of a combination of factors, including disrupted hepatic blood flow, altered protein metabolism, and altered hormone catabolism. Its development produces a grossly swollen abdomen, which raises the diaphragm, making respiration more difficult. As a result, ascites may also compromise mobility.

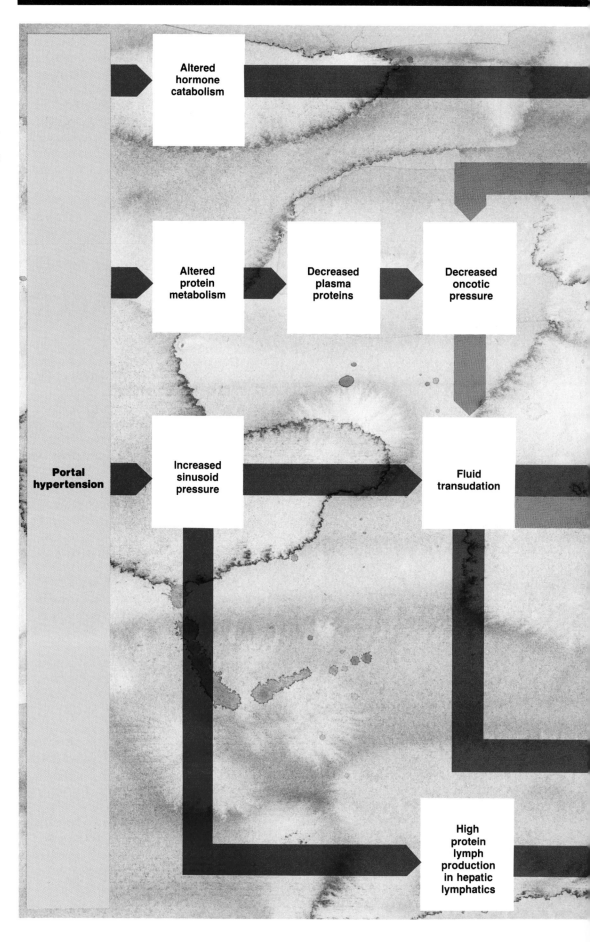

Portal hypertension

Altered hormone catabolism

Altered protein metabolism → Decreased plasma proteins → Decreased oncotic pressure

Increased sinusoid pressure → Fluid transudation

High protein lymph production in hepatic lymphatics

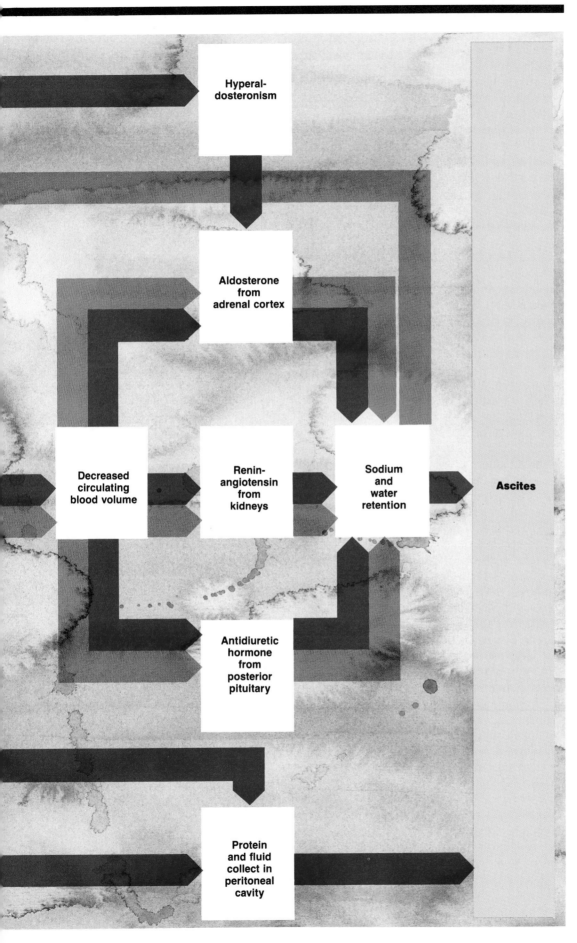

## MEDICAL MANAGEMENT

Because liver disease typically presents few telltale signs in its early, most treatable stage, a thorough history and physical examination are vital to detect predisposing factors. Laboratory tests of blood, urine, and stool measure altered enzyme and hormone levels and blood components; sophisticated radiologic studies reveal abnormal structural changes and help define the severity of disease.

### Confirming diagnostic tests

The following tests help confirm diagnosis of liver disease:

**Blood tests.** Enzymes, proteins and protein metabolites, lipids, carbohydrates, and hematologic factors may be altered in liver disease. *Enzyme tests.* Elevated liver enzyme levels occur with hepatocellular or biliary tissue necrosis. Serum glutamic-oxaloacetic transaminase and serum glutamic-pyruvic transaminase levels rise in hepatitis, cirrhosis, and liver tumors. Alkaline phosphatase levels rise in biliary tract obstruction. Lactic dehydrogenase levels rise in obstructive jaundice, hepatic metastasis, and hepatitis.
*Protein and protein metabolite tests.* Decreased serum albumin and total protein levels reflect impaired hepatic synthesis of protein. A reversed albumin:globulin ratio may occur with increased gamma globulin production in hepatitis, cirrhosis, hepatic malignancy, and obstructive jaundice.
*Lipid and carbohydrate tests.* Decreased serum cholesterol levels reflect impaired hepatic synthesis. Decreased serum glucose levels accompany malnutrition—common in alcohol-related liver disease—and impaired gluconeogenesis. Elevated serum ammonia levels indicate impaired hepatic synthesis of urea and typically occur in advanced disease or after surgical shunting procedures. The total level of bilirubin increases in liver disease, although its conjugated fraction decreases. The level of alpha-fetoprotein, a globulin, is usually elevated in liver tumors.
*Hematologic tests.* These tests include the complete blood count (CBC), prothrombin time, and an antigen test. Decreased red blood cells (RBCs) and hematocrit or hemoglobin levels reflect the liver's inability to store hematopoietic factors (iron, folic acid, and vitamin $B_{12}$), which results in anemia. Decreased white blood cells and thrombocyte levels appear with splenomegaly in cirrhosis. Lymphocyte and monocyte levels may increase in hepatitis. Increased prothrombin time accompanies decreased synthesis of prothrombin, impaired vitamin K absorption, or both. Hepatitis-associated antigen (HAA) appears in early type B hepatitis.

**Urine and stool tests.** Increased urine urobilinogen and reduced fecal urobilinogen levels accompany hepatocellular jaundice due to cirrhosis or hepatitis. Diminishing urine sodium levels may accompany rising aldosterone levels in liver disease. A positive fecal occult blood test may indicate GI bleeding from varices in portal hypertension.

**Radiologic studies.** Abdominal X-rays may show an elevated diaphragm, liver enlargement, and organ displacement in hepatitis, cirrhosis, and advanced tumors. Angiography may diagnose portal hypertension and tumor invasion. Superior mesenteric arteriography visualizes the hepatic vasculature to evaluate cirrhosis and portal hypertension. Splenoportography, used to evaluate portal hypertension and to stage cirrhosis, generally defines the venous system more clearly than superior mesenteric arteriography; however, it fails to outline the portal vein and, often, the splenic vein in portal hypertension associated with reverse venous blood flow. The liver scan detects abnormal hepatic structure, tumors, and cysts and also evaluates liver disease.

**Other tests.** Liver biopsy reveals tissue changes characteristic of hepatitis, cirrhosis, fatty liver, hemochromatosis, and malignancies. Endoscopy helps locate GI bleeding.

### Supportive therapy

Treatment of liver disease is essentially supportive and aims to preserve optimal liver function. Supportive measures include bed rest, dietary restrictions, and drug therapy. Bed rest reduces metabolic requirements and promotes cellular regeneration.

**Diet.** A high-carbohydrate diet prevents hypoglycemia and breakdown of energy reserves. However, fats should be avoided because they're usually poorly tolerated, especially in jaundice. Abstinence from alcohol is also mandatory. A high-protein diet aids cellular regeneration in hepatitis, but it is contraindicated in encephalopathy or ascites.

**Drug therapy.** Although controversial, steroids may be given in hepatitis and cirrhosis to reduce inflammation, to enhance appetite, and to inhibit fibrosis. Typically, they're given with antacids to reduce the risk of GI bleeding. Long-term use of corticosteroids is contraindicated in liver disease. Antiemetics may be given to relieve nausea, but phenothiazines are contraindicated because of their chole-static effect. Sedatives, barbiturates, and hepa-totoxic narcotics to relieve pain or prevent insomnia must be administered cautiously be-cause of impaired metabolism.

Administration of immune serum globulin within a week after exposure to type A hepa-titis provides protection for up to 6 months. Prophylactic administration of hepatitis B im-mune globulin may confer immunity to type B hepatitis. A high-titer hepatitis B immune globulin is approximately 70% effective in preventing type B hepatitis.

Although prognosis is poor for patients with liver cancer, their tumors may be treated with chemotherapy through either regional perfusion directly into the hepatic artery or systemic intravenous perfusion.

### Managing complications essential

Despite supportive therapy, the patient may develop potentially life-threatening complica-tions—ascites, bleeding varices, hepatic en-cephalopathy, and hepatorenal syndrome—all of which demand prompt intervention.

**Ascites.** Restriction of sodium, protein, and fluids helps reduce fluid retention in ascites. Diuretics promote fluid excretion. Spironolac-tone blocks the action of aldosterone, which causes sodium and chloride retention. How-ever, diuresis may cause hypokalemia and hy-ponatremia, which may precipitate or aggra-vate hepatic coma. Infusion of salt-poor albumin increases osmotic pressure, resulting in reabsorption of ascitic fluid and enhanced renal perfusion. Paracentesis—the aspiration of ascitic fluid from the peritoneal cavity—may relieve dyspnea associated with ascites. However, routine paracentesis is no longer recommended because ascites tends to recur rapidly and protein depletion follows each procedure.

**Bleeding varices.** Gastric lavage with iced saline solution—or iced water in ascites—helps constrict bleeding vessels. Continuous infusion of vasopressin (at a rate of 0.4 unit/ minute) reduces portal blood pressure. Esophagogastric tamponade with a Seng-staken-Blakemore triple-lumen tube applies pressure to the bleeding site. Sclerotherapy hardens bleeding vessels, promoting thrombo-sis. Vitamin K administered I.M. enhances clotting. Occasionally, massive blood transfu-sions may be necessary to raise hematocrit levels. Close monitoring of serum calcium and ammonia levels is mandatory with transfu-sions of stored blood. Stored blood contains

# Morphologic classification of cirrhosis

When the cause of cirrhosis is unclear or when overlap-ping causes appear, morphologic markers can charac-terize cirrhosis more precisely. These markers—*micronodular, macronodular,* and *mixed*—assess cirrho-sis according to size and distribution of nodules and histopathologic changes.

**Micronodular**

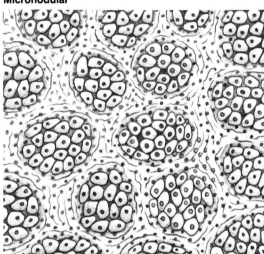

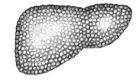

Regenerative nodules (under 3 mm in diameter) of uniform size involve all lobules. Connective tis-sue is thick and regular.

**Macronodular**

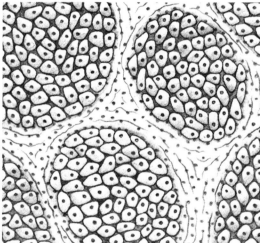

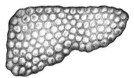

Regenerative nodules (over 3 mm in diameter) vary in size and appear throughout all lobules. Connective tissue is slen-der and distorted.

**Mixed**

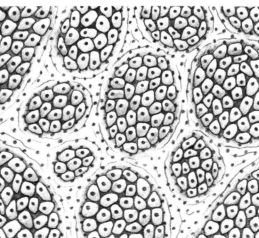

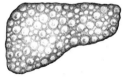

Macronodules and micronodules appear in approximately equal portions.

# Surgical shunts for portal hypertension

Shunting procedures aim to reduce portal pressure and control bleeding esophageal varices by diverting blood from the portal venous system collateral vessels. However, these procedures carry significant risks, among them, hepatic encephalopathy, hemorrhage, and liver failure.

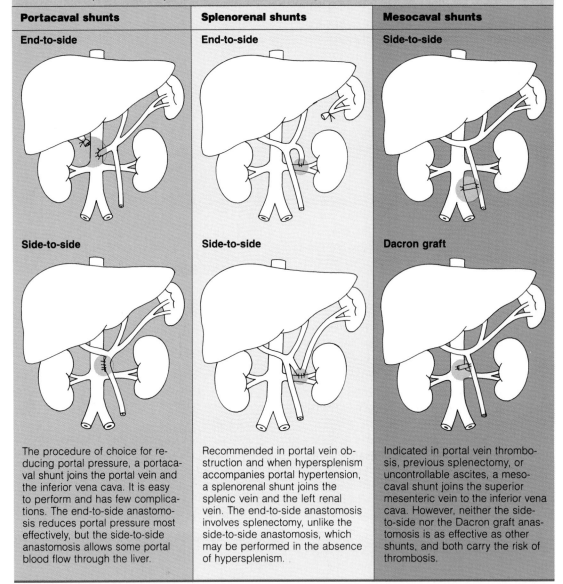

| Portacaval shunts | Splenorenal shunts | Mesocaval shunts |
|---|---|---|
| **End-to-side** | **End-to-side** | **Side-to-side** |
| **Side-to-side** | **Side-to-side** | **Dacron graft** |

The procedure of choice for reducing portal pressure, a portacaval shunt joins the portal vein and the inferior vena cava. It is easy to perform and has few complications. The end-to-side anastomosis reduces portal pressure most effectively, but the side-to-side anastomosis allows some portal blood flow through the liver.

Recommended in portal vein obstruction and when hypersplenism accompanies portal hypertension, a splenorenal shunt joins the splenic vein and the left renal vein. The end-to-side anastomosis involves splenectomy, unlike the side-to-side anastomosis, which may be performed in the absence of hypersplenism.

Indicated in portal vein thrombosis, previous splenectomy, or uncontrollable ascites, a mesocaval shunt joins the superior mesenteric vein to the inferior vena cava. However, neither the side-to-side nor the Dacron graft anastomosis is as effective as other shunts, and both carry the risk of thrombosis.

citrate, which binds with calcium and can dramatically reduce serum ionized calcium. Citrate intoxication may also follow impaired hepatic metabolism. Because stored blood also contains high levels of ammonia, transfusion also compounds the risk of hepatic encephalopathy.

**Hepatic encephalopathy.** Treatment involves decreased dietary intake of protein to eliminate ammonigenic material from the GI tract (because normal bacterial degradation of amino acids in the gut produces ammonia); catharsis to produce osmotic diarrhea and to prevent accumulation of ammonigenic blood proteins and nitrogenous body wastes; neomycin and kanamycin to suppress bacterial flora, preventing them from converting amino acids into ammonia; and lactulose to increase colonic acidity, to prevent bacterial growth, and to promote excretion of ammonia. Occasionally, hemodialysis can temporarily clear some toxins from the blood. Similarly, exchange transfusions may provide dramatic but temporary relief.

**Hepatorenal syndrome.** A possible outcome of hypovolemia in liver disease, hepatorenal syndrome may respond to restricted sodium and fluid intake. If azotemia is severe, hemodialysis, though only minimally effective, may be performed.

### Surgery: Shunting or resection
Typically, surgery for liver disease is performed only when conservative measures prove ineffective. Portacaval shunting, the most common procedure, diverts blood from the portal venous system to the inferior vena cava and aims to prevent or control bleeding varices. However, this surgery carries significant risks. Infusion of blood into the inferior vena cava may cause acute pulmonary edema and ventricular overload in the postoperative period. And because shunting prohibits conversion of ammonia to urea, chronic hepatic encephalopathy may result. (See *Surgical shunts for portal hypertension*.)

Peritoneovenous shunting, using the LeVeen shunt, helps control intractable ascites. Triggered open by inspiration, a one-way pressure-sensitive valve within the shunt drains ascitic fluid from the abdominal cavity into the superior vena cava.

Surgical resection may help improve prognosis in liver malignancy confined to a specific lobe or segment. Lobectomy is the treatment of choice in primary liver tumors, but wedge resection may be effective for small tumors. Total liver resection has not proven successful.

### NURSING MANAGEMENT
Detecting early signs of liver disease and preventing complications are your major nursing goals. To achieve these goals, you'll need to rely on a firm data base from the history and physical examination.

### Comprehensive history essential
Begin the history by having the patient describe his chief complaint. Ask about precipitating factors, such as diet or activity. If the patient reports more than one complaint, determine their relationship. Typically, the patient with early liver disease reports vague symptoms, such as malaise, anorexia, indigestion, flatulence, nausea and vomiting, weight loss, and abdominal pain. The patient with hepatitis may also report arthritis-like joint pain.

Next, ask the patient about his medical history, including previous hospitalizations and surgery. Cardiac disease often accompanies liver disease and worsens portal hypertension and ascites. Advanced biliary tract disease may cause hepatocellular jaundice. Chronic liver disease, infectious diseases such as Reye's syndrome, and any benign or malignant tumors may predispose to liver dysfunction.

Explore the family history. A few rare liver diseases, such as hemochromatosis (excessive iron absorption) and Wilson's disease (excessive copper retention), are hereditary.

Ask the patient to describe his home and work environment. Chronic exposure to insecticides, carbon tetrachloride, paraquat, nitrosamines, hydrocarbons, and metals may cause hepatotoxicity.

Determine if the patient consumes alcohol. If so, how much? Because the alcoholic often deliberately underestimates how much he drinks, confirm alcohol consumption with family members.

Ask about drug history. Intravenous tetracycline therapy may cause fatty liver; steroids and oral contraceptives may cause cholestasis or liver tumors. Some common nonprescription drugs, notably acetaminophen, may have hepatotoxic effects.

Obtain a diet history. Ask about recent changes in appetite and about food intolerances, especially to fatty foods.

Review the patient's psychosocial history. Focus on his concerns about hospitalization and recovery. Does he have a strong support network? Is he independent and coping effectively? If necessary, has he sought counseling for alcohol dependence?

After you complete the history, have the patient write his name and address for baseline data on handwriting, a skill that may deteriorate with hepatic encephalopathy.

### Physical examination for telltale signs
Begin the physical examination by noting the patient's general appearance. Liver disease usually causes jaundice, which produces icteric skin, sclera, and oral mucosa. Spider nevi along the face and upper trunk and palmar erythema may also be apparent. Frailty and muscular atrophy may indicate malnutrition. (See *Signs and symptoms of liver disease,* page 164.) Note the patient's breath odor. A sweet, musty odor (fetor hepaticus) characterizes impaired metabolism of methionine.

**Record vital signs.** Watch for rapid respirations—possibly the result of pulmonary compression due to liver enlargement or ascites. Hypotension and tachycardia may reflect anemia or decreased blood volume in ascites. A slightly elevated temperature may indicate hepatitis.

## Signs and symptoms of liver disease

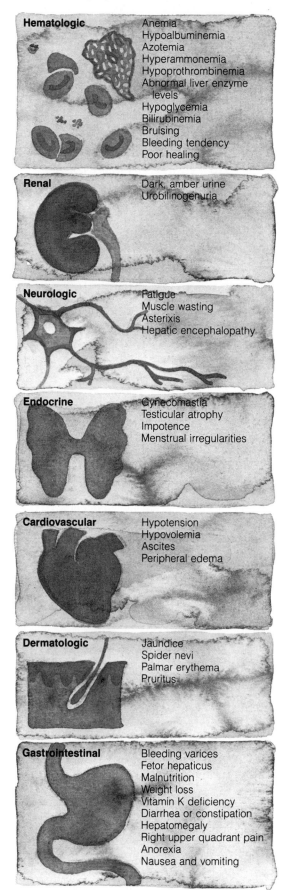

**Hematologic**
Anemia
Hypoalbuminemia
Azotemia
Hyperammonemia
Hypoprothrombinemia
Abnormal liver enzyme
  levels
Hypoglycemia
Bilirubinemia
Bruising
Bleeding tendency
Poor healing

**Renal**
Dark, amber urine
Urobilinogenuria

**Neurologic**
Fatigue
Muscle wasting
Asterixis
Hepatic encephalopathy

**Endocrine**
Gynecomastia
Testicular atrophy
Impotence
Menstrual irregularities

**Cardiovascular**
Hypotension
Hypovolemia
Ascites
Peripheral edema

**Dermatologic**
Jaundice
Spider nevi
Palmar erythema
Pruritus

**Gastrointestinal**
Bleeding varices
Fetor hepaticus
Malnutrition
Weight loss
Vitamin K deficiency
Diarrhea or constipation
Hepatomegaly
Right upper quadrant pain
Anorexia
Nausea and vomiting

**Observe the skin.** Inspect the skin for dryness, ecchymoses, poor wound healing, and loss of pubic and axillary hair in males. Then palpate for poor skin turgor and peripheral edema. These signs may reflect hypoproteinemia, hypovolemia, coagulopathy, or endocrine imbalance. Also check for clubbing of the fingers and cyanosis caused by hypoxia due to arteriovenous shunting.

**Assess the abdomen.** Check for abdominal distention and caput medusae (dilated, superficial abdominal blood vessels), which may accompany portal hypertension. Auscultate for abnormal bowel sounds, associated with diarrhea or constipation, which often occur in liver disease. If you note a vascular hum over the right quadrant, suspect hemangioma. Palpate for right upper quadrant tenderness, hepatomegaly, an irregular and nodular liver surface, and splenomegaly. Test for a fluid wave, indicating ascites. Percuss the abdomen for shifting dullness, which also occurs in ascites. If liver height is above 4¾" (12 cm), percussion also reveals hepatomegaly.

**Evaluate neurologic status.** Watch for disorientation and deterioration of mental capacity, which may signal onset of life-threatening hepatic failure. Monitor the patient's ability to solve addition and subtraction problems, his handwriting, and his responses to simple oral commands. Note slowed speech patterns, drowsiness, and restlessness. Ask family members to help you evaluate personality changes, an early sign of hepatic encephalopathy. Watch for asterixis (liver flap or flapping tremor), a sign of neurologic irritation. Typically, asterixis is induced by extending the arm and dorsiflexing the wrist.

As part of continuing assessment, be alert for hematemesis and melena, which may indicate bleeding varices. If the patient is not jaundiced at admission, watch for its initial signs, such as yellow sweat, dark urine, and light-colored stools. Monitor urine output for oliguria, which may signal hepatorenal syndrome.

### Formulate nursing diagnoses

After you've gathered comprehensive assessment data, formulate nursing diagnoses with appropriate goals and interventions. Expect to include the following nursing diagnoses in your care plan for the patient with liver disease.

**Actual fluid volume deficit related to upper GI bleeding.** To promote fluid balance, you'll need to control bleeding varices and to maintain cardiovascular stability. Infuse dextrose 5% in water or normal saline solution to maintain systolic blood pressure above 90 mm Hg or in the patient's low-normal range. However, avoid infusing high-volume saline solution in patients with ascites. If ordered, transfuse with whole blood or blood components (packed RBCs, fresh frozen plasma). Monitor vital signs, urine output, and central venous pressure (CVP) at least hourly. Notify the doctor if blood pressure drops, CVP falls below 5 cmH$_2$O, or urine output falls below 30 ml/hour. Check for orthostatic hypotension by taking serial blood pressure measurements with the patient supine, in semi-Fowler's position, and sitting in bed with his legs supported. Decreasing serial pressures signal inadequate blood volume. Check heart rate and rhythm on a cardiac monitor.

Also monitor inflation pressure of the Sengstaken-Blakemore tube, if inserted. Perform gastric lavage until returns are clear. Monitor vasopressin infusion; use an infusion device to ensure controlled flow.

Obtain CBC data, including hemoglobin and hematocrit levels, every 4 hours. Check stools and gastric aspirate for blood.

Assess ascites and edema daily. Measure abdominal girth at the same time every day. Administer salt-poor albumin I.V., as ordered. Give 25 to 100 g of 25% albumin daily at a rate no faster than 3 ml/minute. Following administration, watch for signs of circulatory overload (dyspnea, tachycardia, and chest pain). Notify the doctor promptly if you detect a third heart sound or crackles in the lung field on auscultation.

If necessary, prepare the patient for insertion of a LeVeen shunt. (See *Managing ascites: The LeVeen shunt,* page 166.) Restrict sodium intake and I.V. infusions of saline solution. Administer diuretics as ordered, noting their effect. Because fluid and electrolyte imbalance may precipitate coma, monitor serum electrolyte levels closely and administer potassium replacements as needed. To detect hepatorenal syndrome early, monitor serum creatinine and blood urea nitrogen levels daily, and record hourly urine output. Notify the doctor if oliguria or azotemia develops or if urine specific gravity exceeds 1.015. If necessary, prepare for emergency dialysis.

Consider your interventions effective if upper GI bleeding is controlled; vital signs are adequate; and hemoglobin, hematocrit, and serum electrolyte levels are within normal limits.

**Alteration in comfort related to right upper quadrant tenderness and jaundice.** Your goals are to maintain activities of daily living, to promote rest, and to relieve pain. Maintain bed rest (with bathroom privileges for the ambulatory patient). To promote circulation and relieve muscle tension, administer back rubs before daytime naps and before bedtime. Schedule treatments to allow periodic rest. Provide at least 90-minute intervals of uninterrupted sleep at night to ensure rapid-eye-movement-stage sleep. Administer drugs to relieve pain and to enhance rest, as ordered. Because liver disease impairs metabolism, morphine sulfate and barbiturates are generally contraindicated in liver disease. Other narcotic analgesics and sedatives should be used cautiously, in reduced doses.

Ensure good hygiene and provide comfort. Change the patient's position frequently to avoid decubiti. Administer perineal care and keep buttocks clean and dry, especially for the patient with diarrhea. Avoid using soap and starched linen if the patient has jaundice. To relieve pruritus and prevent skin breakdown, administer cholestyramine or antihistamines, apply oil-based lotions, or give cool baking-soda baths. Provide frequent oral care, especially if the patient has a nasogastric and/or Sengstaken-Blakemore tube. If the patient's anorectic, provide oral care immediately before meals to enhance intake.

If the patient's not in danger of hepatic encephalopathy, encourage a high-protein, high-calorie diet to promote hepatocellular regeneration. Administer corticosteroids to increase appetite, if ordered. To improve well-being, encourage family members and friends to visit, as allowed by hospital policy. Identify and encourage interests and hobbies the patient can pursue in the hospital or at home during recovery. Encourage the patient to express fears and anxieties that may intensify discomfort.

Consider your interventions effective if the patient obtains restful sleep and relief from discomfort.

**Ineffective breathing pattern related to ascites and painful postoperative incision.** Your goals are to promote easy, unlabored respirations and to prevent postoperative respiratory complications. Begin by placing the patient in high-Fowler's position to promote optimal chest expansion. Advise the patient with ascites to avoid wearing constrictive undergarments or clothing that compresses the abdomen, pushing the diaphragm upward.

# Managing ascites: The LeVeen shunt

A welcome alternative to traditional medical and surgical treatments, the LeVeen shunt drains ascitic fluid into the superior vena cava. Inserted under sedation and local anesthesia, the shunt consists of a peritoneal tube, a venous tube, and a one-way valve controlling fluid flow. The valve opens when intraperitoneal pressure exceeds superior vena caval pressure by at least 3 cmH$_2$O—which occurs on inspiration. Use of an abdominal binder and inspiration against resistance via a blow bottle enhance fluid drainage. The one-way valve prevents backflow of blood into the tubing, thus eliminating the risk of clotting and shunt occlusion.

### Nursing care

Your daily postoperative care includes the following:
• Teach the patient to take deep breaths against resistance for 15 minutes, four times daily.
• Check incision wounds (one on the right side of the abdomen and one in the right subclavian area) for bleeding, redness, swelling, drainage, and hematoma formation.
• Apply dry, sterile dressings.
• Monitor vital signs frequently, and watch for signs of hypovolemia or hypervolemia.
• Measure abdominal girth, and weigh the patient daily.
• Apply a firm abdominal binder 24 hours after surgery to enhance drainage.
• Record intake and output.
• Monitor complete blood count and serum electrolyte, blood urea nitrogen, creatinine, and albumin levels daily.
• Administer antibiotics, diuretics, and potassium replacements, as ordered.
• Watch for complications, such as leakage of ascitic fluid from incisions, subcutaneous bleeding, disseminated intravascular coagulation, wound infection, septicemia, shunt occlusion, and cardiac overload.

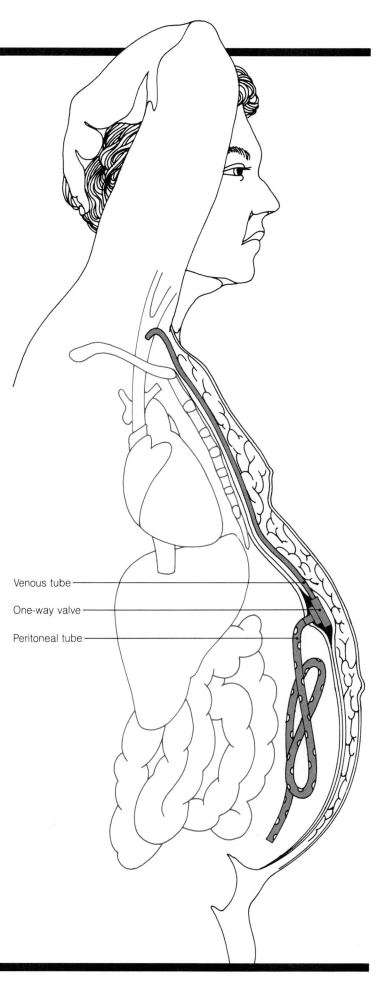

Venous tube

One-way valve

Peritoneal tube

Monitor respirations closely, including their rate, depth, pattern, and sound. Describe abnormal breath sounds. Note whether the patient uses abdominal or thoracic muscles for breathing. Also check for symmetrical respiratory expansion. Administer humidified oxygen as needed. Monitor blood gases to assess respiratory sufficiency.

After surgery, encourage deep breathing 6 to 10 times hourly to prevent atelectasis. Assist the patient with intermittent positive pressure treatments or incentive spirometry, if necessary. Also help the patient change position and cough hourly to prevent pooling of secretions and pneumonia. Splint the incision to ease tension and discomfort during coughing. Auscultate breath sounds every 4 hours. Notify the doctor about adventitious sounds or purulent, foul-smelling sputum.

Assist with paracentesis if necessary. Have the patient empty his bladder, then help him sit upright in a chair or in bed with his feet firmly supported at the bedside. As the doctor performs the procedure, monitor cardiovascular and respiratory status. After the catheter is removed, apply a sterile dressing. Document the color and amount of aspirated fluid—usually several liters—on the intake and output record. Take the patient's vital signs every 15 minutes for the first hour and frequently thereafter for 24 hours after the procedure. Observe for shock caused by fluid shift from intravascular to interstitial space.

Consider your interventions effective if the patient's respirations are even, unlabored, and of normal rate (between 12 and 20) and if signs of respiratory infection are absent.

**Alteration in thought processes related to elevated serum ammonia levels.** Your goals are to preserve neurologic status and to control serum ammonia levels. Monitor neurologic status every 4 hours, including level of consciousness; orientation to person, place, and time; handwriting skills; and ability to solve addition and subtraction problems, to follow simple and complex commands, and to interpret common proverbs. Also check for asterixis. Notify the doctor of neurologic deterioration.

To control serum ammonia levels, administer high colonic or Fleet enemas, as ordered—usually every 4 to 6 hours. Administer neomycin P.O. or by enema, as ordered. Administer lactulose P.O. or by a nasogastric tube hourly or as ordered. Maintain a low-protein, low-sodium diet, but encourage high-calorie feedings. If GI bleeding develops, perform vigorous gastric lavage to decrease intestinal protein load. Monitor serum ammonia levels at least every 8 hours in progressive hepatic encephalopathy. If coma develops, monitor neurologic status every 2 hours. Assess level of consciousness, pupillary activity, muscle strength and tone, reflexes, and posture.

Consider your interventions effective if the patient remains alert and oriented and his serum ammonia level decreases.

**Disturbance in self-concept related to chronic alcoholism or serious illness.** Your goals are to encourage the patient to express his concerns, to help him acknowledge and cope with his illness, and to promote independence and self-care. To achieve these goals, first establish a trusting relationship with the patient by maintaining continuity of care. Always address him by name, and take time to get to know him and his family. Explain care procedures, and allow the patient to participate whenever possible. Encourage him to express his concerns. Try to spend time each day talking with him about his illness. Urge the alcoholic patient to stop drinking. Arrange to have an Alcoholics Anonymous volunteer talk with him. Watch for manipulative behavior as the patient struggles to cope with his illness.

Support a positive self-concept by promoting self-care and encouraging socialization at mealtimes. Assure the patient that jaundice and ascites are usually temporary. If the patient has terminal liver disease, protect his dignity by encouraging independence and providing comfort. Recognize the stages of death and dying elaborated by Dr. Elisabeth Kübler-Ross, including shock and denial, anger, bargaining, depression, and acceptance. Support the patient and his loved ones during each stage.

Consider your interventions effective if the patient expresses his feelings and concerns about his illness, acknowledges his alcoholism and actively seeks help, and performs self-care whenever possible.

### Many roles in one
When caring for the patient with liver disease, you'll undoubtedly need to fill several roles, among them, teacher, friend, and care provider. For example, dietary instruction helps promote recovery in fatty liver, while skillful acute care helps forestall liver failure in hepatic encephalopathy. Knowing what to expect in the patient with liver disease will help you fill your many roles effectively.

## Points to remember

• Most commonly associated with chronic alcoholism, fatty liver involves excessive accumulation of fat within hepatic cells, resulting in inflammation and necrosis.
• Hepatitis, an acute inflammation of the liver, occurs in viral and nonviral forms; viral hepatitis includes type A, type B, and type non-A, non-B. Highly contagious type A hepatitis occurs most frequently.
• Cirrhosis is characterized by diffuse necrosis followed by fibrotic regeneration of hepatic cells. Although its etiology is diverse, it most commonly results from alcoholism.
• Primary liver tumors are rare, but the liver is one of the most common sites of metastasis from other primary tumors.
• A life-threatening complication of liver disease, hepatic encephalopathy results from toxic effects of elevated serum ammonia levels.
• Liver disease may produce widespread metabolic effects, including impaired metabolism of bilirubin, carbohydrates, protein, and hormones.
• Nursing management focuses on early detection of liver disease and preventing or treating its complications, including ascites, bleeding varices, hepatic encephalopathy, and hepatorenal syndrome.

# 11 CORRECTING GALLBLADDER DISORDERS

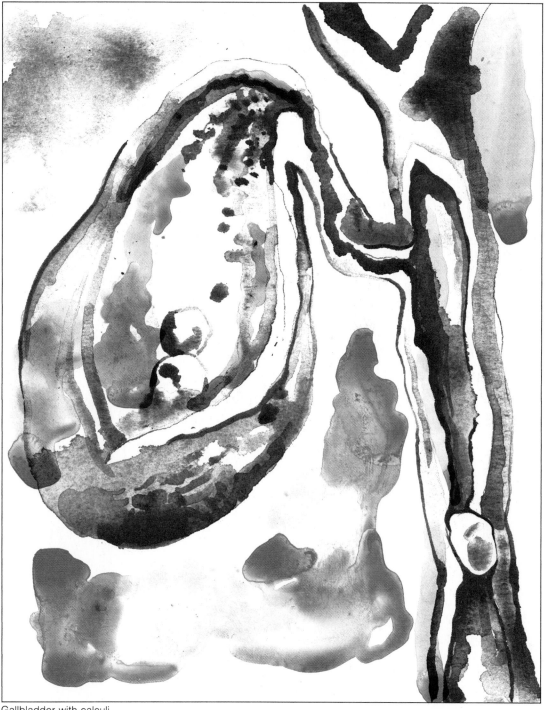

Gallbladder with calculi

Cholelithiasis, the leading biliary tract disease, affects over 20 million Americans and accounts for the third most common surgical procedure performed in the United States—cholecystectomy. Considering these statistics, you're sure to care for patients with this disease often. You may even regard it—and the patients who have it—as routine. But such patients require more than routine nursing care. Cholelithiasis typically follows an unpredictable course. It may cause debilitating pain; it often requires surgery to relieve biliary obstruction, and such surgery may lead to acute complications. These potential problems have important implications for nursing care. With effective preoperative teaching, you can help prevent infection, pulmonary embolism, and other complications that prolong recovery. Equally important, your discharge teaching helps the patient comply with dietary restrictions and, in some cases, to confidently perform T-tube care. This chapter will help you provide such information to the patient with this common, but challenging, disease.

## Who gets biliary tract disease?
Caucasians and native Americans of the Navajo and Pima tribes have the highest incidence of biliary tract disease. Women ages 20 to 50 are affected almost three times more frequently than men, but after age 50, both sexes are affected equally.

## Puzzling etiology
No one knows exactly how gallstones form, but abnormal metabolism of cholesterol and bile salts is a likely cause. Diet, altered hormone levels, and certain drugs and disorders may be at work. A high-calorie, high-cholesterol diet, often associated with obesity, causes increased synthesis and biliary secretion of cholesterol. Elevated estrogen levels (the result of postmenopausal therapy, oral contraceptives, pregnancy, or multiparity), and the antilipemic clofibrate also increase cholesterol secretion. Diabetes mellitus, ileal disease, hemolytic disorders, liver disease, and gallbladder inflammation also contribute to gallstone formation.

## PATHOPHYSIOLOGY
Gallstones are generally classified as cholesterol stones or pigment stones. Cholesterol stones—large, pale yellow, and occurring singly or in groups—form secondary to metabolism of cholesterol and bile salts. Most cholesterol stones are not pure cholesterol but a mixture of cholesterol, calcium salts, bile acids, fatty acids, protein, and phospholipids, with some fraction of bile pigment at their center. Pigment stones—small, black or dark brown, and usually found in groups—form secondary to metabolism of unconjugated bile pigments. They contain bile salts, bilirubin, proteins, and calcium. Both types of stone may be present simultaneously.

## How cholesterol stones form
Cholesterol, a lipid, isn't soluble in an aqueous solution such as bile without the presence of bile salts and lecithin, a phospholipid. These substances form clusters, called *micelles*, within which cholesterol dissolves. During fasting the level of cholesterol exceeds the levels of bile salts and lecithin, producing small amounts of cholesterol-saturated bile. However, this bile is readily diluted by normal bile within the gallbladder, yielding a predominantly unsaturated bile. A marked imbalance between levels of cholesterol and of bile salts and lecithin causes supersaturated bile, the first phase of cholesterol stone formation.

Generally, stone formation occurs in three phases: chemical imbalance, crystallization, and precipitation. (See *Pathogenesis of gallstones,* pages 170 and 171.)

**First phase, imbalance.** In the first phase, a defect in the hepatic metabolism of biliary lipids—which increases cholesterol secretion and decreases levels of bile salts and lecithin—usually accounts for supersaturated bile. A reduced bile salt pool, biliary stasis, and gallbladder inflammation may also cause or contribute to supersaturated bile. Normally, when the amount of bile salts available for cholesterol metabolism decreases, new bile salts form. However, excessive excretion of bile salts, as in ileal disease, or a defective bile feedback mechanism may decrease the bile salt pool. Failure of the gallbladder to empty completely or to concentrate bile normally may cause biliary stasis. Pregnancy, diabetes mellitus, or prolonged sitting may interfere with normal emptying of the gallbladder. Gallbladder inflammation, as in acute cholecystitis, promotes breakdown of lecithin (which normally holds cholesterol in solution), produces debris that helps crystallize stones, and interrupts normal absorption of bile salts.

**Second, crystallization.** Next, cholesterol undergoes two transformations. In nucleation—a process that's not fully under-

## Pathogenesis of gallstones

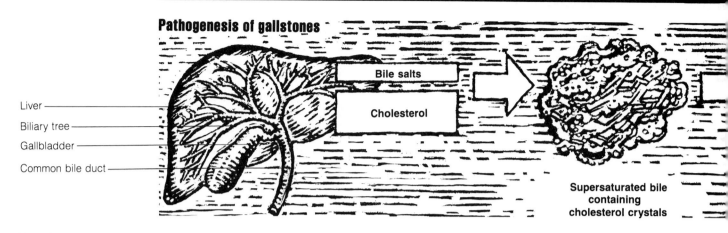

Liver
Biliary tree
Gallbladder
Common bile duct

Bile salts

Cholesterol

**Supersaturated bile containing cholesterol crystals**

Normally, a balance of bile salts, lecithin, and cholesterol maintains cholesterol's solubility in bile. Increased cholesterol, decreased bile salts, or both upset this balance, producing supersaturated bile, the first—or chemical imbalance—phase of gallstone formation. Nucleation—the formation of cholesterol crystals—and flocculation—the aggregation of such crystals—occur in the second phase. In the third phase, these macrocrystals precipitate out of bile.

stood—cholesterol crystallizes in the supersaturated bile. Then, in flocculation—the aggregation of crystals—such substances as bacteria, bilirubin, and epithelial cells act as seeding agents to attract cholesterol crystals. As flocculation continues, these microcrystals become macrocrystals.

**Third, precipitation.** These macrocrystals grow large enough to precipitate out of solution, thus completing cholesterol stone formation. Cholesterol stones may remain "silent" or may dislodge into the gallbladder neck, cystic duct, or common bile duct, triggering symptoms. Generally, gallstones produce overt symptoms within 10 years of formation.

### How pigment stones form
Enzyme imbalance, increased bilirubin secretion, and biliary stasis probably contribute to pigment stone formation. These stones develop when deconjugated bilirubin combines with calcium to form calcium bilirubinate. Normally, bile inhibits formation of this compound; it contains enough glucaric acid to inhibit the enzyme beta-glucuronidase, which deconjugates bilirubin. Infection upsets this balance, allowing rapid deconjugation of bilirubin. Hemolysis and chronic liver disease increase bilirubin secretion, causing a similar imbalance. Similarly, obstruction or anomalies of the bile ducts may promote biliary stasis, enhancing precipitation of stones.

### Acute cholecystitis
Whether gallstones are classified as pigment or cholesterol stones, their development sets the stage for acute cholecystitis, among other disorders. Acute cholecystitis develops when gallstones lodge near or within the cystic duct, causing acute gallbladder inflammation. Obstruction interrupts the normal flow of bile, causing increased intraluminal pressure decreased venous return, and vascular conges-

tion. The edematous, distended gallbladder eventually becomes ischemic, resulting in tissue sloughing and gangrene. Vasodilation may precipitate interstitial hemorrhage and thrombus formation. Bacterial infection is common, producing a fibrinopurulent exudate over the gallbladder's surface.

Acute cholecystitis produces various GI signs and symptoms, such as nausea, anorexia, and vomiting. Severe pain in the right upper quadrant and epigastrium that worsens on inspiration and with movement is common. Jaundice occurs infrequently. Symptoms often disappear within 72 hours, when the stone falls back into the gallbladder or passes through the duct.

### Chronic cholecystitis
Gallstones may also cause chronic cholecystitis, persistent gallbladder inflammation, which follows repeated attacks of acute cholecystitis or develops insidiously. In chronic cholecystitis, the gallbladder shrinks, becomes fibrotic, and may adhere to neighboring organs. Biliary stasis and increased intraluminal pressure are also characteristic.

Chronic cholecystitis produces only vague symptoms unless a stone causes obstruction or spasms of Oddi's sphincter. Obstruction of the cystic or common duct causes biliary colic—steady, intense pain—in the right upper quadrant that often radiates to the shoulder blades (due to splanchnic fibers synapsing with phrenic nerve fibers) and persists for 3 to 4 hours. Persistent obstruction may precipitate attacks of acute cholecystitis. Other signs and symptoms include nausea from intolerance of fatty foods, abdominal fullness, heartburn, excessive belching, constipation, and diarrhea. Various disorders may complicate chronic cholecystitis. Repeated attacks of acute cholecystitis cause porcelain gallbladder—asymptomatic calcification of the gall-

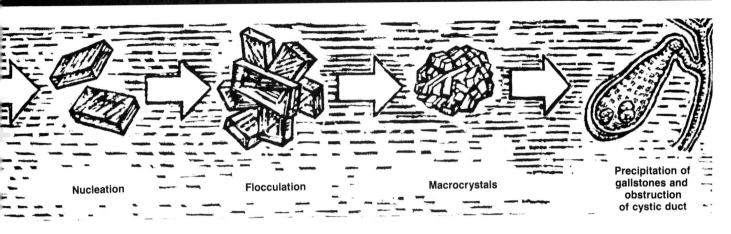

Nucleation — Flocculation — Macrocrystals — Precipitation of gallstones and obstruction of cystic duct

bladder characterized by a translucent, greyish-white appearance and loss of function. Prolonged cystic duct obstruction may cause empyema—intraluminal abscess—or hydrops—distention of the gallbladder with clear, sterile mucus. Chronic erosion of the gallbladder wall may produce fistulas.

### Choledocholithiasis
Gallstones frequently migrate to the common bile duct via the cystic duct, then travel through the ampulla of Vater into the duodenum, where they're eliminated. However, in choledocholithiasis, these stones lodge at the lower end of the common duct near the ampulla, causing partial or complete biliary obstruction. Although choledocholithiasis may produce no symptoms, it can cause jaundice, biliary colic, ascending cholangitis, or pancreatitis. (See *Obstructive jaundice: How its signs and symptoms develop,* page 172.)

### Cholangitis
Often associated with choledocholithiasis, cholangitis involves infection of the bile ducts. It commonly follows bacterial or metabolic alteration of bile salts. Charcot's triad—spiking temperatures and shaking chills coinciding with biliary colic and obstructive jaundice—is its chief symptom. Ascending cholangitis, inflammation of the biliary tree, occurs when intestinal bacteria invade the ductal system. Acute suppurative cholangitis results when pus forms in the ducts, leading to hepatic abscess, septicemia, and shock. Prolonged obstruction associated with hepatocellular dysfunction—sclerosing cholangitis—leads to biliary cirrhosis. This, in turn, can cause hepatic failure, portal hypertension, and death.

### Gallstone ileus
As the term implies, gallstone ileus involves small-bowel obstruction by a gallstone. Typically, the gallstone travels through a fistula between the gallbladder and small bowel and lodges at the ileocecal valve. This obstruction causes pain, distention, and bilious vomiting.

### Gallbladder cancer
Adenocarcinoma and squamous cell carcinoma of the gallbladder typically infiltrate the liver and bile ducts. These rare cancers appear most frequently in patients with preexisting gallstone disease. Characteristic signs and symptoms of gallbladder cancer include anorexia, weight loss, nausea, vomiting, malaise, jaundice, and right upper quadrant pain, which may be acute or dull. However, these signs and symptoms frequently appear late with cystic or common bile duct obstruction.

### MEDICAL MANAGEMENT
Successful medical management of biliary tract disease begins with a thorough history and physical examination to detect predisposing factors and diagnostic tests to evaluate biliary patency and jaundice. Treatment typically includes surgery.

### Tests for biliary patency
*Oral cholecystography,* the procedure of choice in suspected gallstone disease, reliably detects gallstones in nonjaundiced patients. It can also detect abnormal gallbladder size, gallbladder displacement secondary to tumor, and spontaneous passage of stones. However, an elevated serum bilirubin level interferes with proper visualization.

*Cholescintigraphy (HIDA scan),* a safe, simple, nuclear imaging scan, outlines biliary tract patency and is especially reliable for visualizing the cystic duct. Because it permits faster diagnosis than oral cholecystography, cholescintigraphy is indicated in suspected acute cholecystitis and when liver disease elevates serum bilirubin levels.

## Obstructive jaundice: How its signs and symptoms develop

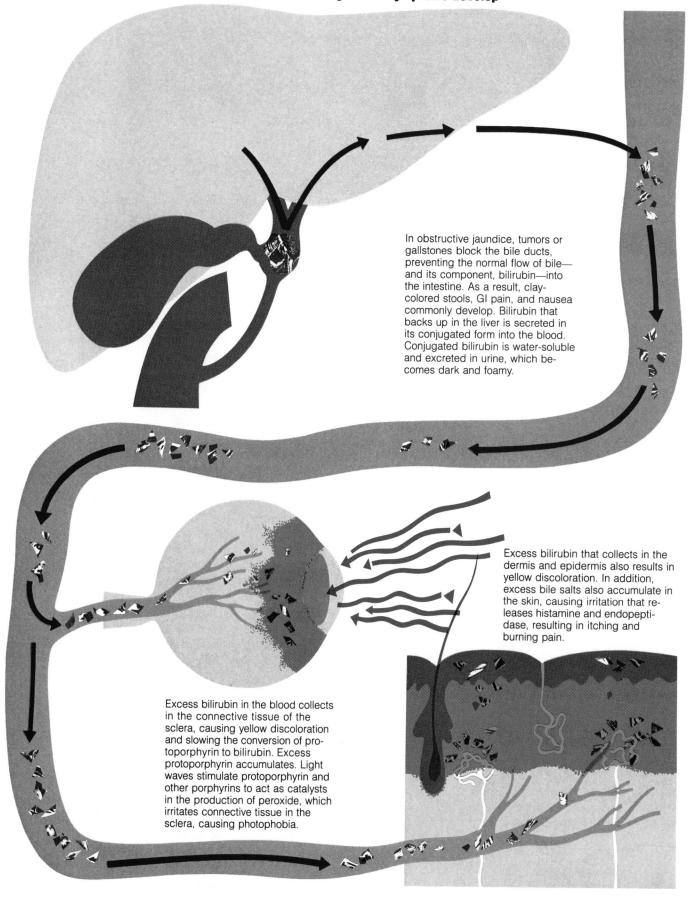

In obstructive jaundice, tumors or gallstones block the bile ducts, preventing the normal flow of bile—and its component, bilirubin—into the intestine. As a result, clay-colored stools, GI pain, and nausea commonly develop. Bilirubin that backs up in the liver is secreted in its conjugated form into the blood. Conjugated bilirubin is water-soluble and excreted in urine, which becomes dark and foamy.

Excess bilirubin that collects in the dermis and epidermis also results in yellow discoloration. In addition, excess bile salts also accumulate in the skin, causing irritation that releases histamine and endopeptidase, resulting in itching and burning pain.

Excess bilirubin in the blood collects in the connective tissue of the sclera, causing yellow discoloration and slowing the conversion of protoporphyrin to bilirubin. Excess protoporphyrin accumulates. Light waves stimulate protoporphyrin and other porphyrins to act as catalysts in the production of peroxide, which irritates connective tissue in the sclera, causing photophobia.

*Gallbladder ultrasonography* helps identify biliary tract obstruction, such as choledocholithiasis and gallbladder carcinoma. It's the procedure of choice in evaluating jaundice and in patients with liver disease or iodine allergy.

When results of ultrasonography or oral cholecystography appear inconclusive, a *computerized tomography (CT) scan* may establish the level and cause of obstruction by showing intrahepatic or extrahepatic bile duct dilatation. But, like ultrasonography, the CT scan usually fails to reveal small stones, tumors, or strictures that cause partial obstruction.

*Cholangiography*—via the intravenous, percutaneous transhepatic, or T-tube route—defines the site and extent of biliary obstruction. Elevated serum bilirubin levels may limit visualization of the biliary tree in intravenous cholangiography. Also, all three routes involve the risk of hypersensitivity reactions to the contrast medium.

*Endoscopic retrograde cholangiopancreatography (ERCP)* aids diagnosis of biliary duct cancer, helps locate calculi and stenosis in the hepatobiliary tree, and evaluates obstructive jaundice.

### Tests for jaundice
Jaundice is categorized as *nonobstructive* (secondary to abnormal function of the cells and ducts within the liver) or *obstructive* (secondary to impaired bile flow out of the gallbladder or along the bile ducts). *Serum bilirubin* reflects increased conjugated and unconjugated bilirubin levels in both types of jaundice. Similarly, *urine bilirubin* reflects increased bilirubin in both types of jaundice. Other tests distinguish between these types.

Elevated *serum cholesterol levels* may indicate obstructive jaundice. Decreased *urine* or *fecal urobilinogen levels* suggest obstructive jaundice.

*Serum enzyme* tests also help to evaluate jaundice. A sharp elevation of *alkaline phosphatase* levels may indicate obstructive jaundice. *Serum glutamic-oxaloacetic transaminase (SGOT)* and *serum glutamic-pyruvic transaminase (SGPT)* reflect the extent of liver damage in jaundice. Markedly increased levels usually occur in nonobstructive jaundice, whereas moderately increased levels occur in obstructive jaundice. A sudden rise in *serum amylase* levels suggests pancreatitis, which is often related to choledocholithiasis.

The *duodenal drainage* test identifies cholesterol and calcium bilirubinate crystals associated with cholelithiasis and jaundice and helps diagnose hepatic and pancreatic disease, parasitic infections, and biliary tract tumors.

### Supportive therapy
In biliary tract disease, supportive therapy aims to relieve abdominal distention, to maintain fluid and electrolyte balance, to manage pain, to prevent or control infection, and to restore normal nutritional status. Nasogastric intubation relieves abdominal distention and nausea. Intravenous therapy helps prevent or correct hypovolemia, dehydration, and electrolyte imbalance—the result of vomiting caused by common bile duct obstruction. Typically, I.V. therapy includes sodium and potassium replacements.

Drug therapy with narcotic analgesics, anticholinergics, and, occasionally, certain vasodilators helps manage pain. Narcotic analgesics, such as morphine sulfate and hydromorphone hydrochloride, tend to induce spasm of Oddi's sphincter and to increase biliary pressure, but meperidine hydrochloride, used judiciously, can be effective. Anticholinergics help prevent biliary contraction, relax smooth muscle, and decrease ductal tone during milder attacks of pain. Nitroglycerin, amyl nitrite, and papaverine also help control smooth muscle spasm.

Drug therapy also helps prevent and control infection. Parenteral administration of antibiotics or aminoglycosides is recommended during acute attacks and for prophylaxis in elderly and diabetic patients.

Vitamin and diet therapy may be necessary to restore normal nutrition. Biliary tract disease often impairs internal synthesis of vitamin K and decreases absorption of the other fat-soluble vitamins, A, D, and E. Vitamin K may be administered I.M. in acute cholecystitis because of poor absorption; the other fat-soluble vitamins are administered orally in chronic cholecystitis. When acute inflammation subsides, the patient is placed on a low-fat diet, excluding red and fatty meats, fried foods, and pastries. This fat-restricted diet inhibits the release of cholecystokinin, the enzyme that stimulates gallbladder contraction and causes inflammatory attacks.

**Surgery: The answer for many.** When supportive therapy fails to control biliary disease, surgery usually brings relief.

*Cholecystectomy,* removal of the gallbladder, is indicated in gallstone disease and carcinoma. Usually performed after acute inflammation subsides, it relieves symptoms in over 95% of patients. Cholecystectomy may also

## Techniques for removing retained gallstones

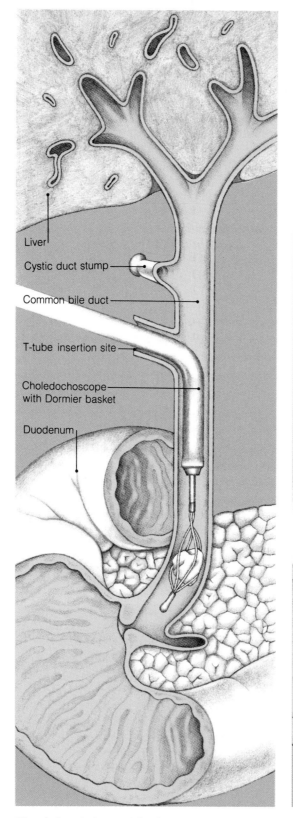

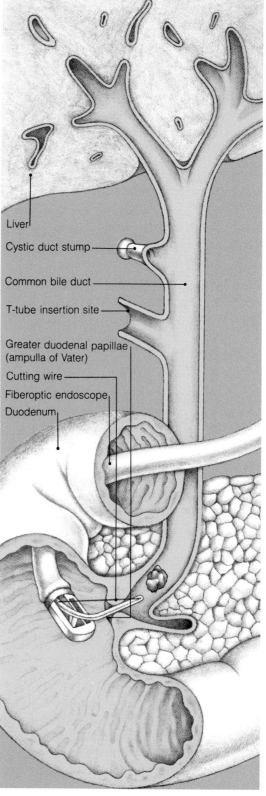

After cholecystectomy, retained stones may cause symptomatic obstruction of the bile ducts. Identified by T-tube cholangiography, these stones can be removed through two relatively safe techniques. In the first technique, a Dormier basket introduced through a choledochoscope or catheter in the T-tube tract snares the retained stone. When this technique fails, endoscopic retrograde papillotomy may be performed. In this technique, a fiberoptic endoscope is introduced into the duodenum to the greater duodenal papillae (ampulla of Vater). An incision at this site then allows the stone to pass into the duodenum.

be recommended for asymptomatic patients, depending on age, weight, and health history. Generally, it's recommended for those under age 50 who are not obese and who have no concurrent health problems, such as angina pectoris or recent myocardial infarction.

*Choledochotomy,* an exploratory procedure involving incision into the common bile duct, allows removal of ductal stones (choledocholithotomy). Temporary insertion of a T tube afterward decompresses the biliary tree, reduces edema, and promotes wound healing.

*Cholecystostomy,* placement of a catheter into the gallbladder, promotes gravity drainage of bile to an external collection system. Often an emergency procedure, it's indicated when bile flow is completely obstructed, empyema or rupture is suspected, or the patient is a poor surgical risk. Performed under local anesthesia, this procedure usually controls pain and fever sufficiently so that a cholecystectomy can be performed.

*Choledochoscopy,* direct visualization of the biliary tract via an endoscope, allows postoperative removal of retained common duct stones. Performed through a T tube or an incision in the common bile duct, it's also useful for evaluating bile duct tumors, filling defects within the biliary tree, and impacted stones. It's contraindicated in biliary sepsis or when the duct is too small to accommodate the choledochoscope.

*ERCP,* commonly used as a diagnostic procedure, allows passage of common duct stones into the duodenum. (See *Techniques for removing retained gallstones.*)

Performed after resection of biliary cancer, *cholecystoduodenostomy* and *cholecystojejunostomy* involve anastomosis of the gallbladder and small intestine to relieve symptoms of obstruction.

## Nonsurgical alternatives
Dissolution of cholesterol stones by *oral administration of bile salts,* such as chenodeoxycholic acid, offers one alternative to surgery. However, such treatment dissolves only small stones, which then tend to recur; it's best suited for elderly patients with mild or asymptomatic gallstone disease and those who are poor surgical risks.

A second treatment, *percutaneous insertion of a transhepatic biliary catheter,* decompresses obstructed extrahepatic bile ducts so that bile can flow freely. It's performed under fluoroscopic guidance and involves percutaneous insertion of a cannula sheath and a guide wire across the liver parenchyma into the common bile duct and duodenum.

## NURSING MANAGEMENT
Because the patient with biliary tract disease has so many diverse needs, he's certain to challenge your nursing skills. When you first meet him, chances are he'll be in acute abdominal distress or dreading surgery, yet only dimly understanding what it involves. He'll need keen assessment from the start to evaluate his condition, to understand his emotional needs, and to monitor his clinical status.

### Begin with the patient history
To obtain a thorough patient history, ask the following types of questions:

**About the chief complaint.** Have the patient describe his chief complaint. Note its frequency, duration, and location. *Pain, GI distress,* and *jaundice* are the most common chief complaints associated with biliary tract disease. *Pain* from acute cholecystitis—occurring a few hours after a heavy meal—begins in the right upper quadrant, radiates to the right scapula or shoulder tip, and worsens on inspiration. Pain from cholelithiasis begins in the midepigastrium, intensifies, and radiates to the back. Attacks of pain from cholecystitis and gallstone obstruction usually last only a few hours, unless pancreatitis has developed. *GI distress,* with nausea and vomiting occurring 3 to 6 hours after a heavy or fatty meal, usually indicates gallbladder disease. Lying down exaggerates this distress. *Jaundice* may present a number of signs, including claycolored stools, bile-stained semen and sweat, dark urine, and discolored skin and sclera.

**About medical history.** Find out when biliary tract disease was first diagnosed and the details of subsequent treatment. Ask about a history of Crohn's disease, ileal resection, and vagotomy, which may precede cholesterol stones, and of liver disease or hemolytic anemia, which may precede pigment stones.

**About dietary habits and drug use.** Does the patient consume high-calorie, fatty foods, such as dairy products, fatty meats, and bakery items? Such a diet promotes excessive cholesterol secretion. Find out the name and dose of any drug the patient's taking. Oral contraceptives, postmenopausal estrogen, and clofibrate may influence gallstone formation. Antipsychotics, such as chlorpromazine hydrochloride, and antiemetics, such as prochlorperazine maleate, may cause cholestasis and dark urine.

**About family history.** Do any of the patient's family members have heart disease, diabetes mellitus, or biliary tract disease? If so, this history may aid differential diagnosis.

**About psychosocial concerns.** Note how the patient copes with his illness. Does he fear surgery or recurring illness? Does he fear extended hospitalization that could impair his ability to meet family or work responsibilities? Does he have financial worries that may interfere with treatment or recovery?

### Physical examination: Focus on the abdomen

Physical assessment of the patient with biliary tract disease demands keen inspection and palpation, particularly of the abdomen. But first, inspect the patient's general appearance, especially his posture, for signs of distress. Guarding of the right side and abdomen, restlessness, and shallow respirations may indicate pain. Next, inspect the skin, scleras, oral mucosa, and inner forearm for evidence of jaundice. Also check for poor skin turgor and dry mucosa, which may indicate dehydration.

Take vital signs. Tachycardia characterizes severe pain and may also occur with fever, hypovolemia, and dehydration. Hypotension may occur with dehydration. Low-grade fever often accompanies cholecystitis and dehydration; fever above 102° F. (38.8° C.) usually signals cholangitis, empyema, pancreatitis, hepatic abscess, or biliary fistulas.

Then, inspect and palpate the abdomen. Note abdominal distention, which may result from perforation, pancreatitis, or peritonitis. Right upper quadrant and right epigastric tenderness usually indicates biliary tract disease; left epigastric tenderness indicates pancreatitis. Abdominal rigidity and right upper quadrant tenderness (usually radiating to the midback) signal peritoneal irritation. Palpation on deep inspiration may elicit increased tenderness and arrested inspiration (Murphy's sign), suggesting cholecystitis. Normally, the gallbladder can't be palpated. However, in acute cholecystitis and porcelain gallbladder, palpation may reveal the gallbladder as a tender mass below the liver.

### Nursing diagnoses guide intervention

To set appropriate goals and plan intervention, begin by formulating nursing diagnoses—precise definitions of the patient's actual or potential problems that you're qualified to treat. Expect to see the following nursing diagnoses in biliary tract disease.

**Alteration in comfort related to gallbladder inflammation and biliary duct spasms.** Your goals are to relieve epigastric distress and to control acute pain. To achieve these goals, administer meperidine hydrochloride, amyl nitrite, and nitroglycerin, as ordered, to help relieve pain and to relax the biliary tract's smooth muscle. Assess drug effectiveness, and note how frequently the patient requires additional doses. Observe for side effects, such as nausea, vomiting, flushing, and hypotension. Effects may occur within minutes of sublingual administration of nitroglycerin or administration of meperidine hydrochloride. To avoid impaired respirations, splint the abdomen with pillows until pain subsides. Watch for compromised respirations, and auscultate the lungs for rales and rhonchi.

Try to promote a quiet, restful environment. Turn the patient every 2 hours to relieve pressure, and provide frequent oral hygiene. Encourage the patient to verbalize fear and anxiety in order to reduce stress and pain.

Consider your nursing interventions successful if the prescribed drugs control pain, the patient's fear and anxiety ease, and he rests comfortably.

**Alteration in fluid and nutritional status related to fatty food intolerance.** When biliary tract disease causes fatty food intolerance, the patient may experience severe vomiting or loss of appetite. Your goals are to maintain fluid and electrolyte balance and to prevent negative nitrogen balance. If ordered, begin I.V. fluid replacement immediately and administer antiemetics, noting their effectiveness. Watch closely for central nervous system depression, especially if phenothiazine antiemetics are administered concomitantly with narcotics, and provide safety measures.

Nasogastric intubation may be necessary to relieve abdominal distention, nausea, and vomiting. If so, maintain intermittent suction. Irrigate the nasogastric tube with normal saline solution (irrigation with water may lead to hyponatremia). Provide frequent oral hygiene and administer ice chips, if allowed.

Monitor serum electrolyte levels, daily weight, and intake and output. Also watch carefully for signs of dehydration, such as poor skin turgor, coated tongue, and oliguria. If the patient is recovering from acute cholecystitis, begin a progressive low-fat diet regimen, including small portions of proteins and carbohydrates. Avoid foods that produce flatulence. Encourage the patient to increase food intake gradually, and provide periodic reas-

# Tips for T-tube care

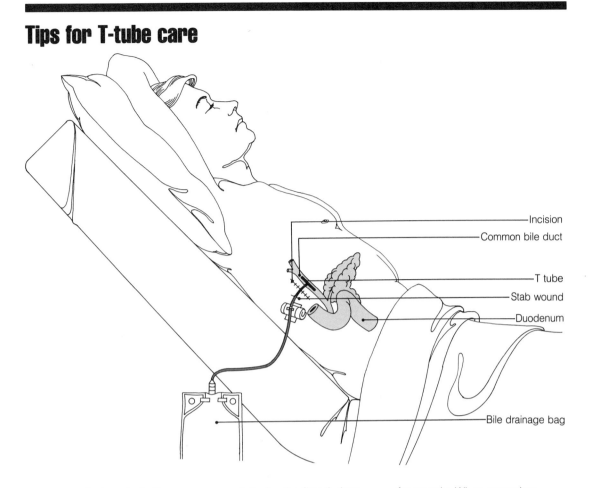

Incision
Common bile duct
T tube
Stab wound
Duodenum
Bile drainage bag

Usually inserted after cholecystectomy and common bile duct exploration, a T tube allows decompression of the biliary tree and postoperative removal of retained stones. Review these tips to ensure proper T-tube care.

• Immediately after surgery, place the patient in a low Fowler's position to maintain T-tube patency and to promote bile drainage. This also relieves pressure on the diaphragm and facilitates breathing.

• Monitor T-tube drainage. During the first few hours after surgery, drainage will appear bloody and then gradually change to a greenish-brown color. Notify the doctor if bile remains bloody longer than 6 hours.

• To prevent undue tension on the tube and to record bile output, empty the drainage bag into a measuring container each shift or when the drainage bag is two-thirds full. Measure and record the amount of drainage. Expect 400 to 1,000 ml of drainage daily for the first 2 days, then a gradual decrease in volume once bile resumes normal flow. Expect stool color to return to normal as drainage decreases.

• Include bile drainage in the patient's intake/output record to ensure accurate fluid and potassium replacement. If drainage exceeds 500 ml/day, bile may be replaced orally or by nasogastric tube. For oral administration, chill the bile and mix it with fruit juice. Bile salts, such as florantyrone, may be given instead of the patient's bile.

• If drainage decreases dramatically and the patient has chills, fever, abdominal pain, and epigastric distress, suspect T-tube or ductal obstruction. If leakage around the T-tube site accompanies these symptoms, suspect bile peritonitis or biliary fistulas. Notify the doctor immediately, and document your observations. T-tube irrigation or further exploration for retained stones may be necessary.

• Change the T-tube dressing frequently. When removing soiled dressings, carefully inspect the incision (and stab wound, if a Penrose drain has been inserted). Note redness, irritation, and drainage. Expect serosanguineous drainage. Notify the doctor if drainage is bloody, purulent, or bile-saturated.

• Using aseptic technique, cleanse the incision with hydrogen peroxide to remove dried drainage. Apply an antiseptic ointment, such as povidone-iodine, if ordered.

• To apply a dressing, slit two gauze pads and fit them around the T tube so the slits overlap.

• Clamp the T tube at intervals, as ordered. Clamping at mealtime evaluates the adequacy of bile flow. Watch for nausea, vomiting, abdominal cramping, and bile leakage around the T tube, indicating impaired bile flow. Unclamp the tube and notify the doctor immediately. If clamping is well tolerated, assist the doctor in T-tube removal, which usually occurs 7 to 10 days postoperatively.

# Caring for the patient with a transhepatic biliary catheter

The transhepatic biliary catheter, an internal bile drain, is commonly inserted when inoperable liver, pancreatic, or bile duct carcinoma obstructs bile flow. It's also used preoperatively in biliary obstruction and in hepatic dysfunction secondary to obstructive jaundice and biliary sepsis. Immediately after insertion, the catheter is connected to a drainage bag to remove blood and debris.

During the first 24 hours after insertion, watch for fever, chills, and hypotension; blood and food particles in the catheter; excessive drainage (over 1,500 ml/day); dislodged sutures around the catheter disk; and external visualization of the catheter's side holes. These findings indicate catheter malfunction, which can cause biliary sepsis or bile peritonitis, both serious complications. To maintain patency, irrigate the catheter daily with no more than 20 ml of sterile saline solution to avoid excessive distention of the biliary tree and abdominal cramping. Next, cleanse the skin around the catheter disk with an antiseptic, and apply sterile dressing. Observe for bile leakage.

If no complications develop within 4 days, the bag is removed and the catheter capped to allow bile drainage into the duodenum. Be alert for complications after the catheter has been capped. Notify the doctor and immediately reconnect the drainage bag to ensure adequate drainage. Prepare the patient for fluoroscopy and, possibly, for catheter replacement.

If the patient is discharged with the catheter in place, you'll need to ensure good home care. Teach him and his family how to irrigate, cleanse, and dress the catheter site. Also instruct them to watch for bile leakage, infection, and other signs of catheter malfunction and to report them promptly.

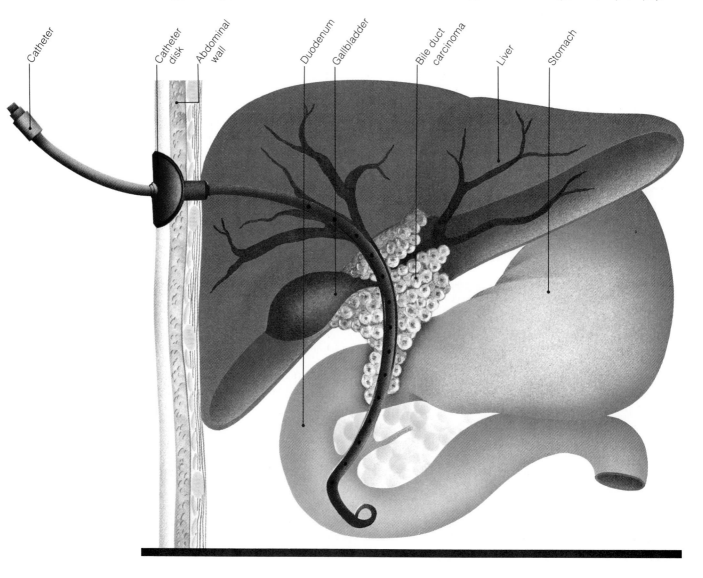

Catheter · Catheter disk · Abdominal wall · Duodenum · Gallbladder · Bile duct carcinoma · Liver · Stomach

surance if his recovery is slow.

Consider your nursing interventions successful if the patient maintains adequate fluid and electrolyte balance, no longer experiences nausea and vomiting, and gradually increases his oral intake.

**Impaired skin integrity related to jaundice.** Your nursing goals are to control pruritus and to prevent skin breakdown. First, be alert for signs of jaundice—brown, frothy urine; clay-colored stools; yellow skin and scleras—and promptly notify the doctor if they develop. To reduce pruritus, use unstarched linen. Give tepid sponge and sodium bicarbonate baths, and apply calamine lotion. If necessary, massage the skin with cocoa butter to stimulate circulation. To prevent decubiti, turn the patient frequently, pad pressure points, and encourage ambulation. If the patient has a T tube, keep the insertion site clean and dry. Change the dressing frequently, using Montgomery straps to secure it in place.

Provide emotional support since jaundice can significantly affect the patient's self-image. If the patient has treatable biliary tract disease, assure him that jaundice is probably temporary. If the patient has inoperable biliary cancer, contact a hospice or the hospital's social services department for assistance.

Consider your nursing interventions successful if pruritus subsides with no skin breakdown and the patient effectively copes with jaundice.

**Potential injury related to postoperative complications.** Your goal is to prevent bleeding, infection, and pulmonary and circulatory complications. Thorough preoperative teaching can do much toward achieving this goal. Stress the importance of coughing and deep breathing, early ambulation, pain control, and adequate nutrition after surgery. Assess the patient's preoperative nutritional status, as well as his fluid and electrolyte balance. Monitor serum protein and prothrombin levels. If ordered, give I.V. albumin to increase serum oncotic pressure and I.M. vitamin K to promote absorption of fat-soluble vitamins and to help correct coagulation problems.

To prevent bleeding, apply pressure to puncture sites, use small-gauge needles for injections, and inspect the skin frequently for bleeding and bruising. Inspect vomitus, nasogastric aspirate, stools, and urine for blood.

To prevent infection, maintain strict asepsis when changing surgical dressings, especially if perforation has occurred (see *Tips for T-tube care,* page 177.) Watch for fever and right upper quadrant pain, which may signal subhepatic abscess.

To prevent pulmonary complications—such as pooling of secretions, atelectasis, and pneumonia—turn the patient frequently. Help him cough and deep breathe every 2 hours. Splint his abdomen with pillows to reduce pain caused by diaphragmatic pressure secondary to abdominal distention. Also auscultate the lungs for rales and rhonchi.

To prevent circulatory complications, apply antiembolism stockings and encourage leg exercises and early ambulation. Remember that obesity increases the risk of pulmonary and circulatory complications.

Consider your nursing interventions successful if the patient has an uneventful recovery from surgery and gradually resumes activities of daily living.

**Knowledge deficit related to biliary tract disease.** Your goals are to teach the patient the signs and symptoms of biliary tract disease and to promote compliance with treatment. Before discharge, instruct the patient and his family to immediately report signs of bile peritonitis, wound infection, and obstructive jaundice. Have the patient avoid strenuous activity; encourage him to resume activity gradually with moderate daily exercise, such as walking. Assess his need for ongoing care, particularly if he's discharged with a T tube in place. Suggest community resources, such as visiting nurses.

Review the prescribed drug regimen with the patient, and stress the importance of compliance. Help him plan dietary changes that limit fat and caloric intake. Tell him to avoid pastries, nuts, avocados, gravies, and fatty, organ, or smoked meats. Instruct him to avoid foods that cause flatulence, and advise against overeating and irregular mealtimes.

Consider your nursing interventions successful if the patient recognizes the signs and symptoms of biliary tract disease; plans sample menus that follow the prescribed diet; knows the name, dose, schedule, and side effects of each prescribed drug; and makes arrangements for follow-up visits.

### A well-earned reward

Caring for the patient with biliary tract disease undoubtedly has its special rewards. A good recovery from surgery—the result of effective pre- and postoperative teaching—is one reward. Discharging the patient confidently—knowing he understands his disease and how to care for himself at home—is another.

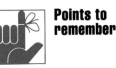

**Points to remember**

• Gallstones occur in 10% to 20% of the general population, with the highest incidence in women, Caucasians, certain native American tribes, and the elderly.

• Midepigastric or right upper quadrant pain radiating to the back or referred to the right scapula or shoulder blade commonly occurs in biliary tract disease.

• Biliary colic, jaundice, and vomiting are characteristic signs of common duct obstruction.

• Diagnostic evaluation of the biliary tract to pinpoint stones may include contrast X-ray studies, ultrasonography, and nuclear imaging scan.

• Primary nursing goals in biliary tract disease are to relieve pain, to ensure adequate nutrition, to prevent postoperative complications, and to provide thorough patient teaching. Such teaching includes instructing the patient about diet, medications, and activity level and encouraging ongoing care.

# APPENDICES

## Mouth disorders

### Salivary gland disease

| Disorder | Causes/predisposing factors | Signs and symptoms | Treatment |
|---|---|---|---|
| **Mumps** (epidemic parotitis) | Exposure to paramyxovirus | Acute bilateral, nonsuppurative swelling, reaching peak in 24 to 48 hours; fever, mild malaise | Analgesics for pain<br>Antipyretics for fever<br>Fluid replacement<br>Respiratory isolation<br>Vaccine for prophylaxis |
| **Staphylococcal parotitis** | Exposure to *Staphylococcus aureus* in debilitated and postoperative patients, typically with ascending infection of Stensen's duct<br>Predisposing factors of poor oral hygiene, dehydration, and decreased saliva production | Sudden onset of severe pain, fever, and swelling of parotid | Antibiotics<br>Good oral hygiene |
| **Sialadenitis** | Usually associated with sialolithiasis (salivary stone) | Pain and swelling at mealtime from obstructed salivary flow | Antibiotics to control infection<br>Stone removal |

### Tongue disease

| Disorder | Causes/predisposing factors | Signs and symptoms | Treatment |
|---|---|---|---|
| **Glossitis** | Exposure to *Streptococcus*, irritation or injury (jagged teeth, ill-fitting dentures, biting during convulsions, alcohol, spicy foods, smoking, sensitivity to toothpaste or mouthwash), vitamin B deficiency, anemia, skin conditions (lichen planus, erythema multiforme, pemphigus vulgaris) | Reddened, ulcerated or swollen tongue, which may obstruct airway; painful chewing and swallowing; speech difficulty | Removal or treatment of underlying cause<br>Topical anesthetic mouthwash or systemic analgesics (aspirin and acetaminophen for painful lesions)<br>Good oral hygiene; vigorous chewing<br>Avoidance of hot, cold, or spicy foods and alcohol |
| **Median rhomboid glossitis** | Cause unknown | Asymptomatic, elevated, rhomboid-shaped reddish lesion on midline of dorsal surface, often causing cancerphobia | No specific treatment needed, although lesion may persist for years |
| **Black hairy tongue** | Cause unknown but *Candida* often present | Usually painless discoloration of the tongue (yellow, brown, or black patches) with hairlike elongation of filiform papillae | Good oral hygiene (including daily tongue brushing) |
| **Fissured tongue** | Cause unknown<br>Sometimes congenital | Deep grooves or furrows in tongue; mild pain after eating acidic or spicy foods | Good oral hygiene<br>Avoidance of acidic or spicy foods |
| **Geographic tongue** (erythema migrans) | Cause unknown | Asymptomatic, variable, maplike configuration of smooth erythematous patches with well-marked borders that may disappear, then reappear | No successful treatment |

## Periodontal disease

| Disorder | Causes/predisposing factors | Signs and symptoms | Treatment |
|---|---|---|---|
| **Acute marginal gingivitis** | Local irritation, such as calcareous deposits on teeth, food impaction, ill-fitting dentures, rough or malaligned surfaces<br>May be aggravated by allergies, pregnancy, mouth breathing | Friable, edematous, reddened, and possibly cyanotic gums that bleed easily and are painful after brushing and eating | Removal of irritant<br>Debridement and curettage of inflamed, ulcerated gingival lining |
| **Acute necrotizing ulcerative gingivitis** (trench mouth) | Exposure to fusiform bacillus or spirochete<br>Predisposing factors of gum flaps, crowded teeth, malocclusion, fatigue, stress, alcohol, smoking, nutritional deficiency | Painful, superficial bleeding ulcers with grayish pseudomembrane (ulcers eventually become punched-out lesions), foul taste, halitosis, fever, malaise, and lymphadenopathy | Antibiotics (penicillin or erythromycin P.O.) for infection<br>Analgesics, as needed<br>Hourly mouth rinses (with equal amounts of hydrogen peroxide and warm water)<br>Soft, nonirritating diet; rest; no alcohol or smoking |
| **Chronic necrotizing gingivitis** | Accumulation of plaque | Usually asymptomatic; gums may bleed after brushing and eating | Good oral hygiene<br>Chemical antiplaque agents, such as 0.2% chlorhexidine gluconate |
| **Periodontitis** | Untreated gingivitis, malocclusion, early sign of hypovitaminosis, diabetes, blood dyscrasias | Suppurative, but usually painless; bleeding, itching, or burning gums; foul taste; vague jaw pain; loosening of teeth and, eventually, tooth loss; temperature sensitivity from root exposure<br>Throbbing pain, swelling, fever, and lymphadenopathy from systemic infection | Scaling, root planing, and curettage to control infection<br>Correction of malocclusion<br>Splinting of mobile teeth<br>Plastic and reconstructive surgery in advanced disease<br>Good oral hygiene |

## Oral mucosal disease

| Disorder | Causes/predisposing factors | Signs and symptoms | Treatment |
|---|---|---|---|
| **Candidiasis** | Exposure to *Candida albicans*<br>Predisposing factors of debilitating disease, such as diabetes, and antibiotic, corticosteroid, and antimetabolite therapy | Pearly white, curdlike lesions surrounded by erythematous mucosa | Nystatin<br>Nonirritating diet |
| **Leukoplakia** | Continuous mechanical or chemical irritation (lip or cheek biting, ill-fitting dentures, smoking) | Painless, white, hyperkeratotic lesions<br>Possible degeneration of chronic inflammation into squamous cell carcinoma | Removal of irritant<br>Topical vitamin A<br>Long-term monitoring, possibly with excisional biopsy |
| **Acute herpetic stomatitis** | Exposure to herpes simplex virus | 1- to 2-day prodrome of sore throat, fever, headache, malaise, nausea, vomiting, and mouth pain followed by eruption of small vesicles or shallow papulovesicular ulcers and swollen bleeding gums | Bland or liquid diet and, in severe cases, I.V. fluids and bed rest<br>Antihistamines in aqueous rinse with cracked ice applied to lips before meals |
| **Allergic or contact stomatitis** | Sensitivity to antibiotics, mouthwashes, topical anesthetics | Generalized inflammation | Removal of irritant<br>Topical steroids for severe inflammation |
| **Aphthous stomatitis** (canker sores) | Predisposing factors of stress, fatigue, anxiety, and menstruation | 2- to 48-hour prodrome; burning sensation; painful, shallow ulcers covered by necrotic slough and surrounded by a bright erythematous zone | Topical anesthetic, such as Orabase<br>Avoidance of irritating foods |

# Gastrointestinal drugs

## Antacids

| Drug, dose, and route | Interactions | Side effects | Special considerations |
|---|---|---|---|
| **Aluminum and magnesium hydroxides**<br>5 to 30 ml of suspension t.i.d. and at bedtime. For peptic ulcer, administer dose more frequently (1 hour before and 3 hours after meals and at bedtime)<br><br>**magaldrate (aluminum-magnesium complex)**<br>Same as for aluminum and magnesium hydroxides | *Amphetamines, ephedrine, pseudoephedrine:* increased pharmacologic effects. Monitor for excessive CNS stimulation.<br>*Iron salts:* decreased therapeutic response to iron. Separate antacid dose by several hours.<br>*Salicylates:* decreased effectiveness. May need to increase salicylate dose.<br>*Sodium polystyrene sulfonate:* risk of metabolic alkalosis. Avoid use, if possible.<br>*Tetracycline:* decreased antibiotic effects from diminished absorption. Separate antacid dose by at least 2 hours. | Constipation, diarrhea, hypermagnesemia | Shake suspension well; give with small amount of water to ensure passage to stomach. When administering drug through nasogastric tube, be sure tube is patent and properly positioned. After instilling drug, flush tube with water to ensure complete dose and to maintain tube patency.<br>    Monitor serum magnesium levels in patients with mild renal impairment. Symptomatic hypermagnesemia usually occurs only in severe renal failure.<br>    Warn patient not to take drug indiscriminately or to change antacids without consulting the doctor.<br>    If patient experiences diarrhea or constipation with one preparation, suggest an alternate one. |

## Anticholinergics

| Drug, dose, and route | Interactions | Side effects | Special considerations |
|---|---|---|---|
| **atropine**<br>0.25 to 0.6 mg P.O. q 4 to 6 hours | *Digoxin:* elevated blood levels due to increased gastrointestinal absorption. Monitor carefully.<br>*Haloperidol, phenothiazines:* decreased antipsychotic effect of atropine. Monitor for lack of drug effect. | Confusion or excitement in elderly patients, palpitations, blurred vision, dry mouth, urinary hesitancy and retention, constipation | Instruct patient to avoid driving and other demanding activities if he's drowsy or dizzy or has blurred vision. Advise him to drink plenty of fluids to help prevent constipation. Offer gum, sugarless hard candy, or pilocarpine syrup to relieve mouth dryness.<br>    Use cautiously in hot or humid environments to prevent drug-induced heatstroke. Administer smaller doses to elderly patients.<br>    Other anticholinergic drugs may increase vagal blockage. |
| **methantheline**<br>50 to 100 mg P.O. q.i.d. (before meals and at bedtime)<br><br>**propantheline**<br>15 mg P.O. t.i.d. before meals and 30 mg at bedtime | *Digoxin:* elevated blood levels due to increased gastrointestinal absorption. Monitor carefully. | Confusion or excitement in elderly patients, palpitations, blurred vision, dry mouth, urinary hesitancy and retention, constipation | Instruct patient to avoid driving and other demanding activities if he's drowsy or dizzy or has blurred vision. Advise him to drink plenty of fluids to help prevent constipation. Offer gum, sugarless hard candy, or pilocarpine syrup to relieve mouth dryness.<br>    Use cautiously in hot or humid environments to prevent drug-induced heatstroke. Administer smaller doses to elderly patients.<br>    Other anticholinergic drugs may increase vagal blockage. |

## Antiemetics

| Drug, dose, and route | Interactions | Side effects | Special considerations |
|---|---|---|---|
| **benzquinamide**<br>50 mg I.M. q 3 to 4 hours p.r.n. | None significant | Drowsiness, hypotension | Give I.M. injection in large muscle mass. Use deltoid area only if it's well developed. Aspirate syringe for I.M. injection to avoid inadvertent I.V. injection.<br>    Reconstituted solution is stable for 14 days at room temperature. Store dry powder and reconstituted solution in light-resistant container. |
| **prochlorperazine**<br>5 to 10 mg P.O., I.M., or rectally t.i.d. or q.i.d. | *Antacids:* inhibited absorption of oral phenothiazines. Separate prochlorperazine dose by at least 2 hours.<br>*Anticholinergics, including antidepressants and antiparkinson agents:* increased anticholinergic activity, aggravated parkinson-like symptoms. Use together cautiously.<br>*Barbiturates:* may decrease phenothiazine effect. Monitor for decreased antiemetic effect. | Extrapyramidal reactions, orthostatic hypotension, ocular changes, blurred vision, dry mouth, constipation, urinary retention, mild photosensitivity | Store drug in light-resistant container. Slight yellowing does not affect potency; however, discard markedly discolored solutions.<br>    To prevent contact dermatitis, avoid spilling concentrate or diluted solution on your hands or clothing.<br>    Dilute oral concentrate with tomato or fruit juice, milk, coffee, carbonated beverage, tea, water, soup, or pudding. |
| **thiethylperazine**<br>10 mg P.O., I.M., or rectally daily, b.i.d. or q.i.d | *Antacids:* inhibited absorption or oral phenothiazines. Separate prochlorperazine dose by at least 2 hours.<br>*Anticholinergics, including antidepressants and antiparkinson agents:* increased anticholinergic activity, aggravated parkinson-like symptoms. Use together cautiously.<br>*Barbiturates:* may decrease phenothiazine effect. Monitor for decreased antiemetic effect. | Extrapyramidal reactions, orthostatic hypotension, ocular changes, blurred vision, dry mouth, constipation, urinary retention, mild photosensitivity | To prevent nausea and vomiting associated with anesthesia and surgery, give deep I.M. injection on or shortly before terminating anesthesia. Never give intravenously.<br>    Warn patient about hypotension. Advise him to stay in bed for 1 hour after receiving drug.<br>    If drug contacts skin, wash immediately to prevent contact dermatitis. |

## Antiemetics (continued)

| Drug, dose, and route | Interactions | Side effects | Special considerations |
|---|---|---|---|
| **trimethobenzamide**<br>250 mg P.O. t.i.d. or q.i.d.;<br>200 mg I.M. or rectally<br>t.i.d. or q.i.d. | None significant | Pain at I.M. injection site, drowsiness, dizziness | Don't use suppositories if patient is hypersensitive to benzocaine hydrochloride or similar local anesthetics. Give deep I.M. injection into upper outer quadrant of gluteal muscle to reduce pain and local irritation.<br>    Warn patient of possible drowsiness and dizziness. Caution him not to drive or perform activities requiring alertness until CNS response to drug is determined. |

## Anti-infectives

| Drug, dose, and route | Interactions | Side effects | Special considerations |
|---|---|---|---|
| **ampicillin**<br>250 mg to 1 g P.O., I.M., or I.V. q 6 hours | *Aminoglycoside antibiotics:* separate ampicillin dose by at least 1 hour. Also, don't mix together in the same I.V. container. | Diarrhea, nausea, vomiting, maculopapular skin rash, hypersensitivity | When giving drug intravenously, mix with dextrose 5% in water ($D_5W$) or saline solution. Don't mix with other drugs or solutions; they might be incompatible.<br>    When giving drug orally, watch for GI disturbances. Food may interfere with absorption, so give drug 1 to 2 hours before meals or 2 to 3 hours after. |
| **cefazolin**<br>500 mg to 1 g I.M. or I.V. q 6 to 8 hours | *Probenecid:* may increase blood levels of cephalosporins. Use together cautiously. | Thrombophlebitis at I.V. injection site, maculopapular skin rash, diarrhea | Use cautiously in patients with impaired renal function and in those with sensitivity to penicillin. Avoid doses greater than 4 g daily in patients with severe renal impairment. Ask patient if he's ever had any reaction to cephalosporins or penicillin before administering cefazolin.<br>    If I.V. therapy lasts longer than 3 days, alternate injection sites. Use small I.V. needles in the larger veins.<br>    About 40% to 75% of patients receiving cephalosporins show a false-positive direct Coombs' test; only a few of these indicate hemolytic anemia. |
| **chloroquine hydrochloride**<br>**chloroquine phosphate**<br>160 mg to 200 mg chloroquine hydrochloride I.M. daily for no more than 11 days; then, 1 g chloroquine phosphate P.O. daily for 2 days followed by 500 mg daily for 2 to 3 weeks | None significant | Visual disturbances (reversible), dose-related retinopathy (may be irreversible), blood dyscrasias, ototoxicity, photosensitivity | Record baseline ophthalmologic status; then monitor status during therapy. Report blurred vision, increased sensitivity to light, or muscle weakness. Also assess hearing before, during, and after therapy, especially with long-term drug use. Take complete blood counts frequently during therapy.<br>    Warn patient that excessive exposure to sun may exacerbate drug-induced dermatoses. |
| **emetine**<br>1 mg/kg S.C. or I.M. daily. Increase dose up to 60 mg daily in one or two doses | None significant | Nausea, vomiting, diarrhea, cardiotoxicity (including degenerative myocarditis, pericarditis, and congestive heart failure), skin reactions, muscle weakness | Don't exceed recommended dose or extend therapy beyond 10 days. Enforce bed rest during and for several days after therapy.<br>    Drug may alter EKG tracings for 6 weeks. Take EKG before therapy, after fifth dose, after last dose, and 1 week after therapy.<br>    Don't administer drug intravenously. Although deep S.C. injection is preferred, I.M. injection is acceptable. To prevent necrosis and edema, rotate sites and apply warm soaks.<br>    Suspect emetine-induced reaction if diarrhea recurs after initial relief. |
| **gentamicin**<br>1.5 mg/kg I.V. or I.M. q 8 hours | *Bumetanide, ethacrynic acid, furosemide:* increased ototoxicity. Use together cautiously.<br>*I.V. penicillins:* separate gentamicin dose by at least 1 hour. Also, don't mix together in the same I.V. container.<br>*Nondepolarizing muscle relaxants:* increased neuromuscular blocking effects. Use together cautiously. | Nephrotoxicity (directly related to high blood levels), ototoxicity, skin rash | Weigh the patient, and obtain baseline renal function studies (output, specific gravity, urinalysis, blood urea nitrogen [BUN] and creatinine levels, creatinine clearance) before therapy begins. Monitor renal function during therapy; notify the doctor of signs of renal impairment. To minimize chemical irritation of renal tubules, keep the patient well hydrated during therapy.<br>    Evaluate the patient's hearing before and during therapy. Notify the doctor if patient complains of tinnitus, vertigo, or hearing loss.<br>    After completing I.V. infusion, flush the line with normal saline solution. |
| **iodoquinol**<br>**(diiodohydroxyquin)**<br>630 to 650 mg P.O. t.i.d. for 20 days | None significant | Optic neuritis, peripheral neuropathy, nausea, vomiting, skin reactions | Give drug after meals. Crush tablets and mix with applesauce or chocolate syrup.<br>    Tell patient to notify doctor if skin rash occurs.<br>    Instruct patient to have periodic ophthalmologic examinations during therapy. Wait 2 or 3 weeks before repeating therapy. |

## Anti-infectives (continued)

| Drug, dose, and route | Interactions | Side effects | Special considerations |
|---|---|---|---|
| **metronidazole**<br>500 to 750 mg P.O. t.i.d. for 5 to 10 days | *Alcohol:* disulfiram-like reaction (nausea, vomiting, headache, cramps, flushing) | Nausea, vomiting, anorexia, headache, metallic taste | Give drug with meals to minimize GI distress.<br>   Warn patient that drug may cause metallic taste and dark or red-brown urine. Also instruct him to avoid alcohol and alcohol-containing drugs for 48 hours after therapy.<br>   When drug is used to treat amebiasis, record number and character of stools. |
| **tetracycline**<br>250 to 500 mg P.O. q 6 hours | *Antacids (including NaHCO₃) and laxatives containing aluminum, calcium, or magnesium; food, milk, or other dairy products:* decreased antibiotic absorption. Give antibiotic 1 hour before or 2 hours after any of the above.<br>*Methoxyflurane:* may cause severe nephrotoxicity with tetracyclines. Monitor carefully. | Epigastric distress (nausea, vomiting, diarrhea); maculopapular and erythematous rashes; photosensitivity; urticaria; increased skin pigmentation | Tell patient that taking drug with milk or other dairy products, food, antacids, or iron products reduces its effectiveness. Instruct him to take each dose with a full glass of water on an empty stomach at least 1 hour before meals or 2 hours after and at least 1 hour before bedtime to prevent esophagitis.<br>   Advise patient to avoid direct sunlight and ultraviolet light; a sunscreen may help prevent photosensitivity. Inform patient that photosensitivity persists for some time after discontinuation of drug.<br>   Check drug expiration date. Outdated or deteriorated tetracycline may cause nephrotoxicity. |
| **tobramycin**<br>1.5 mg/kg I.V. or I.M. q 8 hours | *Bumetanide, ethacrynic acid, furosemide:* increased ototoxicity. Use together cautiously.<br>*I.V. penicillins:* Separate tobramycin dose by at least 1 hour. Also, don't mix together in same I.V. container.<br>*Nondepolarizing muscle relaxants:* increased neuromuscular blocking effects. Use together cautiously. | Nephrotoxicity (directly related to high blood levels), ototoxicity, skin rash | Weigh the patient, and obtain baseline renal function studies (output, specific gravity, urinalysis, BUN and creatinine levels, creatinine clearance) before therapy begins. Monitor renal function during therapy; notify doctor of signs of renal impairment.<br>   Evaluate the patient's hearing before and during therapy. Notify doctor if the patient complains of tinnitus, vertigo, or hearing loss. After I.V. infusion, flush line with normal saline solution. |

## Anti-inflammatories and immunosuppressants

| Drug, dose, and route | Interactions | Side effects | Special considerations |
|---|---|---|---|
| **azathioprine**<br>1 to 2 mg/kg P.O. daily | *Allopurinol:* impaired inactivation of azathioprine. Decrease azathioprine dose to one-quarter or one-third normal dose. | Bone marrow depression (including leukopenia, macrocytic anemia, pancytopenia, and thrombocytopenia) | Draw blood for hemoglobin, white blood cell (WBC), and platelet counts at least weekly or more frequently at start of therapy. Stop drug immediately if WBC count falls below 3,000/mm³ to prevent irreversible bone marrow depression.<br>   Because azathioprine is a potent immunosuppressant, instruct patient to report even mild infections (coryza, fever, sore throat, malaise). Also warn him that thinning of his hair is possible. |
| **corticotropin (ACTH)**<br>40 units S.C. or I.M. in four divided doses (aqueous); 40 units q 12 to 24 hours (gel or repository form) | None significant | Euphoria, insomnia, hypokalemia, dizziness, fluid retention, hyperglycemia | Give ACTH only as adjunctive therapy. Oral agents are preferred for long-term therapy.<br>   Note and record weight changes, fluid exchange, and resting blood pressure until minimal effective dose is achieved.<br>   Refrigerate reconstituted solution, and use within 24 hours.<br>   If administering gel, warm it to room temperature; draw into large needle (21G or 22G), and slowly give deep I.M. injection. Warn patient that injection is painful. |
| **hydrocortisone**<br>5 to 30 mg P.O. b.i.d., t.i.d., or q.i.d.<br><br>**prednisone**<br>2.5 to 15 mg P.O. b.i.d., t.i.d., or q.i.d. | *Amphotericin B, diuretics:* hypokalemia.<br>*Aspirin, indomethacin:* increased risk of GI distress and bleeding. Use together cautiously.<br>*Barbiturates, phenytoin, rifampin:* decreased corticosteroid effect. Corticosteroid dose may need to be increased. | Euphoria, insomnia, hypokalemia, hyperglycemia, peptic ulcer and GI irritation, fluid retention with possible hypertension and congestive heart failure | Warn patient on long-term therapy about cushingoid symptoms. Teach patient early signs of adrenal insufficiency (fatigue, muscle weakness, joint pain, fever, anorexia, nausea, dyspnea, dizziness, fainting). Monitor weight, blood pressure, and serum electrolytes. Patients with diabetes may need increased insulin; monitor urine glucose levels.<br>   Give once-daily doses in the morning for optimal effectiveness and less toxicity. Give P.O. dose with food when possible. Unless contraindicated, encourage salt-restricted diet rich in potassium and protein. Potassium supplement may be needed. |
| **sulfasalazine**<br>1.5 to 2 g P.O. daily in evenly divided doses q 6 hours | None significant | Nausea, vomiting, diarrhea, anorexia, generalized skin eruptions, photosensitivity | Instruct patient to take drug for as long as prescribed, even after he feels better.<br>   Warn him to avoid direct sunlight and ultraviolet light to prevent photosensitivity. Note that drug may color urine orange-yellow. To minimize GI side effects, administer after meals.<br>   Sulfasalazine is also available as an oral suspension and is chemically related to the sulfonamides. |

## Antilipemics

| Drug, dose, and route | Interactions | Side effects | Special considerations |
|---|---|---|---|
| **cholestyramine**<br>4 g before meals and at bedtime, not to exceed 32 g daily<br><br>**colestipol**<br>15 to 30 g P.O. daily in two to four doses | *Digitoxin, digoxin:* decreased digitalis effect from diminished gastrointestinal absorption<br>*Thyroid hormones:* decreased effects from diminished gastrointestinal absorption | Constipation, abdominal discomfort, nausea, skin rash | To prepare dose, sprinkle drug powder on surface of beverage or wet food. Let stand a few minutes; then stir. When mixing drug with carbonated beverage, stir slowly in large glass to prevent excessive foaming.<br>　Observe bowel habits; treat constipation as needed. Encourage a high-fiber diet and adequate fluids. If severe constipation develops, decrease dosage or discontinue drug, and provide a stool softener. |

## Digestants

| Drug, dose, and route | Interactions | Side effects | Special considerations |
|---|---|---|---|
| **medium-chain triglycerides**<br>15 ml P.O. t.i.d. or q.i.d. | None significant | Nausea, vomiting, diarrhea | To minimize GI side effects, give more frequent, smaller doses with meals or mixed with fruit juice or salad dressing.<br>　They are more easily absorbed than long-chain fats and do not require bile salts for emulsification. |
| **pancreatin**<br>325 mg to 1 g P.O. before or with meals<br><br>**pancrelipase**<br>1 to 3 capsules or tablets P.O. before or with meals | None significant | Nausea, diarrhea | Pancreatin therapy shouldn't delay or replace treatment of primary disorder.<br>　Use only after confirmed diagnosis of exocrine pancreatic insufficiency. Not effective in GI disorders unrelated to pancreatic enzyme deficiency.<br>　Adequate replacement decreases number of bowel movements and improves stool consistency. Don't crush or chew capsule as this may interfere with enteric coating. Adjust dosage to degree of maldigestion and malabsorption, amount of fat in diet, and enzyme activity of individual preparations. |

## Histamine$_2$ (H$_2$) receptor antagonists

| Drug, dose, and route | Interactions | Side effects | Special considerations |
|---|---|---|---|
| **cimetidine**<br>300 mg P.O. or I.V. t.i.d. with meals and h.s. for 4 to 6 weeks | *Antacids:* interfere with absorption of cimetidine. Separate cimetidine dose by at least 1 hour, if possible.<br>*Benzodiazepines, lidocaine, oral anticoagulants, metoprolol, phenytoin, propranolol, theophylline;* increased pharmacologic effects. Monitor for toxicity. | Blood dyscrasias, mental confusion, dizziness, mild diarrhea | When administering I.V. in 100 ml of diluent solution, avoid overly rapid infusion (risking circulatory overload). Some authorities recommend infusing the drug over at least 30 minutes.<br>　Elderly patients are more susceptible to cimetidine-induced mental confusion. Decrease dose in these patients and in those with hepatic or renal insufficiency.<br>　I.V. cimetidine is often used in critically ill patients to prevent GI bleeding. |
| **ranitidine**<br>150 mg P.O. b.i.d. for 4 to 6 weeks | *Antacids:* interfere with absorption of ranitidine. Separate ranitidine dose by at least 1 hour if possible. | Headache, dizziness | Use ranitidine if patient can't tolerate cimetidine or when cimetidine is ineffective. Ranitidine has fewer side effects and interactions and may be given without regard to meals. |

## Immune serums and vaccines

| Drug, dose, and route | Interactions | Side effects | Special considerations |
|---|---|---|---|
| **hepatitis B immune globulin (HBIG)**<br>0.06 ml/kg I.M. within 7 days after exposure; repeat in 28 days | *Live virus vaccines:* may interfere with immune response. Don't administer within 3 months of HBIG. | Local pain, tenderness at injection site | Give injections in buttocks or deltoid area.<br>　Use a new sterile syringe and needle for each HBIG dose.<br>　Draw back plunger of syringe to ensure that needle is not in blood vessel. Don't inject if blood or any unusual discoloration is present in syringe. |
| **hepatitis B vaccine**<br>Initial dose 1 ml I.M. followed by 1 ml I.M. 1 month later, then 1 ml I.M. 6 months after initial dose | None reported | Discomfort at injection site | Thoroughly agitate vial before injection to restore suspension. Use I.M. injection only.<br>　Store opened and unopened vials in refrigerator, but don't freeze.<br>　The recommended dosage regimen provides immunity for at least 5 years.<br>　Hepatitis B vaccine has *not* been associated with an increased incidence of AIDS (acquired immune deficiency syndrome). |
| **immune globulin (IG)**<br>0.02 ml/kg I.M. as soon as possible after exposure | *Live virus vaccines:* may interfere with immune response. Don't administer within 3 months of IG. | Local pain, tenderness at injection site | If dose exceeds 10 ml, divide and inject into different sites, preferably including buttocks. Avoid injecting more than 3 ml per site. Have emergency drugs ready to treat anaphylaxis.<br>　For patients with clotting abnormalities and small muscle mass, administer drug I.V., using 5% solution stabilized in 10% maltose (Gamimune). |

## Laxatives

| Drug, dose, and route | Interactions | Side effects | Special considerations |
|---|---|---|---|
| **bisacodyl**<br>10 to 15 mg P.O. or rectally in evening or before breakfast | None significant | Nausea, vomiting, abdominal cramps (with suppositories) | To avoid GI irritation, instruct patient to swallow tablet whole. Don't give drug with milk or antacids. Effective 6 to 10 hours after administration. Discourage excessive use.<br>Use tablet and suppository together to cleanse colon before and after surgery and before barium enema. |
| **docusate salts**<br>50 to 300 mg (docusate sodium) or 240 mg (docusate calcium or potassium) P.O. daily in the evening | None significant | Mild abdominal cramps, throat irritation | Use to prevent constipation but not to treat existing constipation. An emollient laxative or stool softener that doesn't stimulate intestinal peristalsis. Effective 12 to 72 hours after administration.<br>Laxative of choice in patients who should not strain during defecation, such as those recovering from myocardial infarction or rectal surgery; in disease of rectum and anus that makes passage of firm stool difficult; or postpartum constipation. |
| **magnesium salts**<br>15 g magnesium sulfate P.O. in glass of water; or 10 to 20 ml concentrated milk of magnesia P.O.; or 15 to 60 ml milk of magnesia P.O.; or 5 to 10 oz magnesium citrate at bedtime | None significant | Abdominal cramps, nausea | To make magnesium citrate more palatable, chill before using. A hyperosmolar, or "saline," laxative effective 30 minutes to 3 hours after administration.<br>Don't use drug longer than 1 week; frequent or prolonged use may cause dependence or "cathartic colon." Magnesium may accumulate in patients with renal insufficiency. |
| **psyllium**<br>1 to 2 rounded teaspoonfuls P.O. in full glass of liquid b.i.d. or t.i.d. | None significant | Abdominal cramps | To mask grittiness, mix with at least 8 oz (240 ml) of cold, pleasant-tasting liquid. Stir only a few seconds, then have patient drink mixture immediately or it will congeal. Offer an additional glass of liquid.<br>A nontoxic, bulk-forming laxative effective 12 to 72 hours after administration. Warn patient that taking drug before meals may reduce appetite.<br>Since all forms of Metamucil brand contain sugar, use different brands of psyllium for diabetic patients. |

## Miscellaneous gastrointestinal drugs

| Drug, dose, and route | Interactions | Side effects | Special considerations |
|---|---|---|---|
| **ferrous sulfate**<br>*For iron deficiency:*<br>750 mg to 1.5 g P.O. in divided doses t.i.d. | *Antacids, cholestyramine resin, pancreatic extracts, vitamin E:* decreased iron absorption. Separate doses, if possible.<br>*Chloramphenicol:* watch for delayed response to iron therapy. | Nausea, vomiting, constipation | Give liquid iron preparation with glass straw to avoid staining teeth.<br>Record color and amount of stool. Oral iron may blacken stools and cause constipation. Teach patient dietary measures for preventing constipation.<br>Monitor hemoglobin and reticulocyte counts during therapy. |
| **phytonadione (vitamin K)**<br>*For hypoprothrombinemia:*<br>2 to 25 mg P.O., S.C., I.V., or I.M., depending on severity; dose may be repeated | *Cholestyramine resin, mineral oil:* inhibited GI absorption of oral vitamin K. Use together cautiously. | Pain and swelling at injection site, transient hypotension after I.V. administration | Monitor partial thromboplastin time to determine effective dose.<br>Protect parenteral product from light by wrapping infusion container in aluminum foil.<br>Administer I.V. by slow infusion (over 2 to 3 hours). Mix in normal saline solution, $D_5W$, or dextrose 5% in normal saline solution. Observe for signs of flushing, weakness, tachycardia, and hypotension. |
| **spironolactone**<br>*For diuresis:*<br>25 to 100 mg P.O. daily in divided doses | *Potassium preparations:* may result in hyperkalemia. Use together cautiously. | Hyperkalemia, gynecomastia in males, menstrual disturbances | Warn patient to avoid excessive ingestion of potassium-rich foods or potassium-containing salt substitutes. Give drug with meals. Elderly patients are especially susceptible to excessive diuresis. |
| **sucralfate**<br>*For duodenal ulcer:*<br>1 g P.O. b.i.d. 1 hour before meals and h.s. | *Antacids:* may decrease binding of sucralfate to gastroduodenal mucosa, impairing effectiveness. Separate sucralfate dose by at least 30 minutes. | Constipation | Instruct patient to take drug on an empty stomach 1 hour before each meal and at bedtime.<br>Pain and ulcer symptoms may subside within first few weeks of therapy. For proper healing, instruct patient to complete prescribed regimen.<br>Monitor for severe, persistent constipation. |
| **vasopressin**<br>*For GI hemorrhage:*<br>20 units diluted with 20 to 100 ml 0.9% NaCl or $D_5W$ and infused I.V. over 5 to 30 minutes; or intraarterially at 0.2 to 0.4 unit/min | None significant | Angina (especially in patients with vascular disease), pallor, abdominal cramps | Repeated doses may be given every 2 to 4 hours but may decrease drug effectiveness.<br>Use an infusion pump, especially when administering via intraarterial infusion. |

# Selected References and Acknowledgments

## Selected References

Alavi, Abass, and Arger, Peter. *Abdomen*. Multiple Imaging Procedures Series. New York: Grune & Stratton, 1980.

♦

Anthony, Catherine P., and Thibodeau, Gary A. *Textbook of Anatomy and Physiology*, 11th ed. St. Louis: C.V. Mosby Co., 1983.

♦

Bachrach, William, et al. "Grand Rounds in Critical Care: Problems in Swallowing and Esophageal Carcinoma," *Heart & Lung* 10(3):525-31, May/June 1981.

♦

Broadwell, Debra C., and Jackson, Bettie S. *Principles of Ostomy Care*. St. Louis: C.V. Mosby Co., 1982.

♦

Brunner, Lillian S., and Suddarth, Doris S. *Textbook of Medical-Surgical Nursing*, 4th ed. Philadelphia: J.B. Lippincott Co., 1980.

♦

Brunner, Lillian S., and Suddarth, Doris. *The Lippincott Manual of Nursing Practice*, 3rd ed. Philadelphia: J.B. Lippincott Co., 1982.

♦

Cassmeyer, Virginia L., and Greig, Judith L. "Problems of the Liver and Related Structures," *Medical-Surgical Nursing: Concepts and Clinical Practice*, 2nd ed. Edited by Phipps, Wilma J., et al. St. Louis: C.V. Mosby Co., 1983.

♦

Chernoff, R. "Nutritional Support: Formulas and Delivery of Enteral Feeding. I: Enteral formulas; II: Delivery systems," *Journal of the American Dietetic Association* 79(4):426-29, 430-32, October 1981.

♦

Cohen, Sidney. *Clinical Gastroenterology: A Problem-Oriented Approach*. Biomedical Engineering and Health Systems Series. New York: John Wiley & Sons, 1982.

♦

Fields, Willa L., and McGinn-Campbell, Karen M. *Introduction to Health Assessment*. Reston, Va.: Reston Publishing Co., 1983.

♦

Given, Barbara A., and Simmons, Sandra J. *Gastroenterology in Clinical Nursing*, 3rd ed. St. Louis: C.V. Mosby Co., 1979.

♦

Goodhart, Robert S., and Shils, Maurice E. *Modern Nutrition in Health and Disease*, 6th ed. Philadelphia: Lea & Febiger, 1980.

Greenberger, Norton J., and McPhee, Mark S. "Diseases of the Gallbladder and Bile Ducts," in *Harrison's Principles of Internal Medicine*, vol. 2, 10th ed. New York: McGraw-Hill Book Co., 1983.

♦

Greenberger, Norton J. *Gastrointestinal Disorders: A Pathophysiological Approach*. Chicago: Year Book Medical Pubs., 1980.

♦

Groer, Maureen W., and Shekleton, Maureen E. *Basic Pathophysiology: A Conceptual Approach*, 2nd ed. St. Louis: C.V. Mosby Co., 1983.

♦

Guthrie, Helen. *Introductory Nutrition*, 5th ed. St. Louis: C.V. Mosby Co., 1983.

♦

Guyton, Arthur C. *Human Physiology and Mechanisms of Disease*, 3rd ed. Philadelphia: W.B. Saunders Co., 1982.

♦

Hurwitz, Alfred L., et al. *Disorders of Esophageal Motility*. Philadelphia: W.B. Saunders Co., 1979.

♦

Hui, Yiu H. *Human Nutrition and Diet Therapy*. Monterey, Calif.: Brooks/Cole Publishing Co., 1983.

♦

Kaye, Donald, and Rose, Louis F. *Fundamentals of Internal Medicine*. St. Louis: C.V. Mosby Co., 1983.

♦

Kirsner, J.B., and Shorter, R.G. "Recent Developments in 'Nonspecific' Inflammatory Bowel Disease," Parts 1, 2. *The New England Journal of Medicine* 306 (April 1; April 8, 1982):775-85, 837-48.

♦

Krause, Marie V., and Mahan, Kathleen L. *Food, Nutrition, and Diet Therapy*, 6th ed. Philadelphia: W.B. Saunders Co., 1979.

♦

Kurtz, Robert C., ed. *Nutrition in Gastrointestinal Disease*, vol. 1. Contemporary Issues in Clinical Nutrition Series. New York: Churchill Livingstone, 1981.

♦

Lewis, S., and Collier, I. *Medical-Surgical Nursing: Assessment and Management of Clinical Problems*. New York: McGraw-Hill Book Co., 1983.

♦

Pierce, L. "Symposium on Diseases of the Liver. Anatomy and Physiology of the Liver; in Relation to Clinical Assessment," *Nursing Clinics of North America* 12:259-73, June 1977.

Rice, Hazel V. *Gastrointestinal Nursing*. Nursing Outline Series. New Hyde Park, N.Y.: Medical Examination Publishing Co., 1978.

♦

Romanes, G.J., ed. *Cunningham's Textbook of Anatomy*, 12th ed. New York: Oxford University Press, 1981.

♦

Sarfeh, I.J., et al. "Results of Surgical Management of Hemorrhagic Gastritis in Patients with Gastroesophageal Varices," *Surgery, Gynecology and Obstetrics* 155(2):167-70, August 1982.

♦

Sleisenger, Marvin H., and Fordtran, John S. *Gastrointestinal Disease: Pathophysiology, Diagnosis, Management*, 3rd ed. Philadelphia: W.B. Saunders Co., 1983.

♦

Spence, Alexander P., and Mason, Elliott B. *Human Anatomy and Physiology*, 2nd ed. Menlo Park, Calif.: Benjamin/Cummings Pub. Co., 1983.

♦

Spiro, Howard M. *Clinical Gastroenterology*, 3rd ed. New York: Macmillan Publishing Co., 1983.

♦

Thorpe, C.J., and Caprini, J.A. "Gallbladder Disease: Current Trends and Treatments," *American Journal of Nursing* 80:2181-85, December 1980.

♦

Weinsier, R.L., et al. "Hospital Malnutrition: A Prospective Evaluation of General Medical Patients During the Course of Hospitalization," *American Journal of Clinical Nutrition* 32(2):418-26, February 1979.

♦

Sakai, Yoshihiro. *Practical Fiberoptic Colonoscopy*. New York: Igaku-Shoin Medical Pubs., 1981.

## Acknowledgments

♦ p. 44 Bottom photo courtesy of Igor Laufer, MD, Department of Radiology, Hospital of the University of Pennsylvania, Philadelphia.

♦ p. 63 Photo courtesy of Lloyd R. Garren, MD, Wilmington Medical Center, and Mary L. Garren, MD, PA, Union Hospital, Elkton, Md.

♦ p. 66 Chart courtesy of The Metropolitan Life Insurance Company, New York.

♦ p. 80 Photo courtesy of John Yardley, MD, The Johns Hopkins Hospital, Baltimore.

# INDEX

i = illustration; t = table

i = illustration; t = table

i = illustration; t = table

i = illustration; t = table

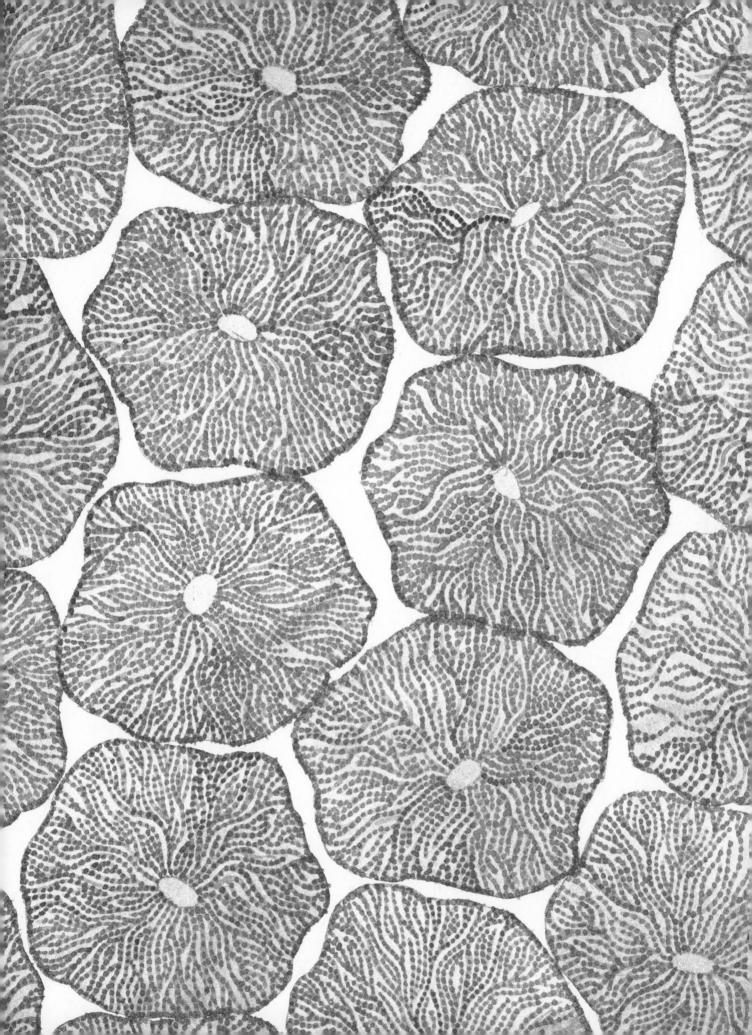